They're Mine and I'm Keeping Them

or

How Freezing My Breast,

Saved My Breast

by

Laura Ross-Paul
Alexander Paul
Dr. Peter Littrup

Contents

Publisher's Note

The information and materials contained in this book are for informational purposes only. It should not be relied upon as medical advice. The purpose of this book is to provide information about cryoablation. It is not intended to be a substitute for professional medical advice, diagnosis or treatment. Always seek the advice of your physician or other qualified health care provider with any questions you may have regarding a medical condition or treatment and before undertaking a new healthcare regimen. Never disregard professional medical advice or delay in seeking it because of something you have read in this book.

No warranties are given in relation to any medical information or references given in this book. No liability will accrue to the authors or publishers in the event that a reader suffers a loss in any way connected to use of information from this book.

Introduction

Breast cancer! The diagnosis all women fear and hope to avoid. In 2003, tests revealed Laura Ross-Paul had three tumors spread around her breast in a way that a lumpectomy was not an option. Doctors advised a mastectomy.

Laura resisted a mastectomy and wanted to explore alternatives that would allow her to keep her breast. I was fortunate to find Dr. Littrup at Karmanos Cancer Center in Detroit and he consented to a cryoablation treatment of Laura. As a result, she became the first woman in America to avoid a mastectomy by having her tumors frozen using a treatment called cryoablation.

Not only did Laura's cryoablation allow her to keep her breast, it also might have helped to prevent a recurrence of her cancer, because cryoablation often results in an "immune effect."

Cancer survives in the body by camouflaging itself from the immune system. After a tumor is frozen, the body absorbs the dead tissue. The protein structure of the tumor remains intact after freezing, so the immune system can "see" the cancer and recognize that it is a "foreign body." When it does, this triggers a complex immune process that often builds antibodies to the cancer. These antibodies then kill other tumors throughout the body. This is the "immune effect."

Unfortunately, the immune effect does not always occur after cryoablation. Researchers believe this is because some patients lack cytokines, a necessary protein element of the immune effect. A challenge for researchers in America now is to explore the effectiveness of a "cytokine boost vaccination," or some other method, which might be combined with cryoablation to universally induce the immune effect and thus prevent a cancer recurrence.

Research in the United States has moved slowly regarding the immune effect triggered by cryoablation. In fact, cryoablation is still rarely used as of early 2013 for the treatment of breast cancer in America, despite the fact that it could save women from a mastectomy.

This is not the case internationally and especially in China. In late 2012, Laura accompanied a friend, Fe Zahorodniuk of Alberta, Canada, to FUDA hospital in Guangzhou, China. Fe had previously had a lumpectomy for breast cancer in Canada. After that treatment, she was diagnosed with a recurrence in 2012. She was facing a double mastectomy and traditional chemotherapy. Fe, like Laura, did not want to lose her breast and contacted Laura through our website, KeepingThem. com.

After several months of cryoablation treatment combined with newly developed immune system therapies at FUDA hospital, advanced testing proved Fe to be cancer free—and she saved her breasts.

Part One of *They're Mine and I'm Keeping Them* tells the story of Laura's healing journey. It was not a simple journey; it was a difficult odyssey.

Part Two offers advice regarding obtaining breast cancer cryoablation and advice on other matters particular to follow-up treatment.

Part Three details the treatments received by Fe and the travels of Alex and Laura to receive themselves the CIC therapy offered at FUDA Hospital in Guangzhou, China.

Breast cancer cryoablation is still considered an experimental treatment by the medical community and insurance companies in America, which greatly impairs its availability. Laura, Dr. Littrup and I, hope that this book helps speed the arrival of the day when the therapies offered in China are available in the United States and covered by insurance so that other women can cure their cancer and save their breasts. Perhaps someday, American women diagnosed with breast cancer and advised to have a mastectomy might be able to say, as Laura did years ago, "They're mine and I'm keeping them."

Author's Note

Laura, Dr. Littrup and I (Alex Paul) combined our efforts in this book with the goal of increasing awareness in the world about the opportunity cryoablation presents for breast cancer patients worldwide.

Laura provided me with her journal of her cancer treatment in 2003 and after. I admit to being stumped at first as to how to tell her story and not let it devolve into a lengthy technical paper on the virtues of cryoablation. I want to give a strong thank you to Elizabeth Lyon, my editor, who went over the very earliest manuscript with me. She suggested that I draw on my fiction writing because from what she knew of Laura's story, it was a perfect example of Joseph Campbell's hero's journey. Once I looked at the story in this manner, all the elements of the story fell into place for me. I then edited Laura's journal for content and clarity so that it would match the story flow of the hero's journey and this became the "spine" of the book.

In the case of Dr. Littrup's contribution, he was at first reluctant to get involved due to the time restrictions given his operating and treatment schedule added to his research work and inventions. But Laura and I were convinced that the book would be richer with his contribution and, of course, have more credibility.

I was able to convince Dr. Littrup that his time involvement would only consist of some taped interviews, which I could then use to ghostwrite his sections of the book. With that as the goal, he allowed me to travel to Detroit where we spent a long weekend in August going over the fascinating details of his life. I became very excited because the story of his life is riveting; all the way from the family history of helping Jews escape the Nazis during WWII to his personal medical miracle of survival.

During the interviews I drew on my fiction background and asked him all the questions I used to develop my fictional characters: what was your nickname in high school (the answer was a delightful and interesting surprise), what is your favorite book, etc. This filled out his persona beyond just that of his medical writing and led me to discover his amazing personal life, which I feel adds richness to the book as well.

To my delight, Dr. Littrup grew more interested in the project after I sent him his early chapters and he added even more details so that, in the end, his chapters are a blend of my ghostwriting and his own contributions, which I simply edited to blend in. Dr. Littrup is one of the most amazing men I've had the good fortune to meet in my life and I sincerely appreciate this opportunity to work with him and learn about his life.

Once armed with Laura's journal and Dr. Littrup's chapters, I took on the role of the book's narrator to weave the story together as well as add my own perspective of being a husband to a wife going through breast cancer. What an amazing and happy thing it is to be finishing up this book with Laura now an 11-year cancer survivor! Her courage and faith are an endless inspiration to me.

To keep the various authors identified, Laura's sections are headed by the label "Laura" in bolded text while "Alex" appears in bolded text headers when we switch back and forth. As well, my writing appears in regular text throughout the book while the combined efforts of Dr. Littrup and myself are in regular text but set out in separate chapters to show that the writing is from Dr. Littrup's point of view.

I also want to congratulate Laura for the passages in Section 3 of the book where she describes her first trip to China. This writing was done with very little editing by myself and got the attention of the people at FUDA who are now translating that section of the book into Chinese in order to provide information about their work at FUDA.

I sincerely hope that the long hours I spent writing this book will help speed the arrival of the day when the therapies offered in China are covered by insurance and are readily available in the United States. That was my goal long ago when I observed the line of women registering for a mastectomy on the morning that Laura saved her breast by cryoablation. I have spent a large part of my life now writing this to make their outcomes less of a loss and much more of a triumph over cancer. If we do in America what they have already done at FUDA Hospital in Guangzhou, China, that will be the case.

I have a dream that someday other women besides Laura will be able to treat their cancer without having to lose their breasts. Someday, American women diag-nosed with breast cancer and advised to have a mastectomy might be able to say, as Laura did years ago, "They're mine and I'm keeping them!"

Thank you reader for this opportunity to write and help you learn about this important subject.

Finally, Laura Ross-Paul is a well-known American artist. It is, therefore, only natural that we used her beautiful imagery on the book's cover as well as including some of her paintings in the book. This is especially true, because she painted these images while dealing with her cancer treatment. These paintings tell the story of Laura processing her cancer experience through her personal visual language.

Curator and reviewer comments regarding the images are included to give the reader insight into the work. If you would like to see more of Laura's amazing artwork, go to FroelickGallery.com or LauraRoss-Paul. com.

Foreword by Dr. Littrup

The search for miracles is a very personal journey, while the fulfillment of a dream is in the eye of the beholder. May we all dare to dream so that we preserve the chance that it can come true.

It is important in a work like this to distinguish between the scientific and factual content and the emotional and spiritual content. As a doctor exposed each day to patients newly diagnosed with cancer, I find that an almost universal response of these patients is to go through the emotional stages of denial, anger, bargaining, depression, and finally acceptance. For each patient, treatment choices should lead to an eventual peace of mind by delicately navigating the balance between quality and quantity of life. As physicians, I believe we are there to provide them with honest, compassionate options that empower them to guide their own journey.

Laura and her husband Alex were no exception to this phenomenon, and their efforts to find a miraculous cure to Laura's breast cancer are quite typical. Fervent belief in miraculous cures may help some patients through their initial stages of denial, anger, and bargaining, while staving off the relentless onslaught of depression from the word "cancer." Some may call this "magical thinking," yet, who am I to deny anyone the hope that a miracle might indeed provide them a chance to beat the odds?

In my own life, I survived a torn aorta through the intervention of a good friend who was a physician, and who recognized my symptoms and rushed me to the hospital. I was perhaps less than a minute from dying when just the right surgeons began just the right surgery. If I had been anywhere else at any other time, I am sure I would have died. Was that a miracle? Perhaps my surgical intervention was more straightforward than the ill-defined miracle healing that Laura hoped for as she describes in this book. However, I am certain a miracle occurred for me, since my second chance at life had worse odds than most cancer patients.

It is in that spirit that I have joined them in writing this book. I have chosen not to judge or condemn any of their efforts at spiritual healing. Instead, I am glad that at the end of their quest for a miraculous healing, they came to Karmanos Cancer Institute and we provided Laura with a fully informed decision to pursue a newer application of a long-established cancer treatment in the form of cryoablation. There are probably many conservative pundits in the medical community who would say that breast cancer cryoablation is an unproven treatment that is equivalent to the false hopes given by psychic surgeons for a purely spiritual healing. I draw a careful but firm line between the sublime and the ridiculous. Simply because we don't have long-term breast cryoablation outcomes using rapidly advancing cryotechnology does *not* allow those skeptics the right to neglect or dismiss years of established research with cryobiology and the crucial temperature profiles needed to kill *any* tissue.

Such ill-conceived criticisms against the potential of breast cryoablation are highly suspect of self-serving attempts to preserve the status quo of breast cancer treatments. Similar to prostate cryoablation only gaining full acceptance when urologists were able to embrace it as "their" procedure, breast cryoablation may suffer similar delays in acceptance. However, medical politics are *not* the fault of breast cancer patients and they should *not* be held captive to paternalistic viewpoints that would ban cryoablation until one medical specialty could claim cryoablation as their own. Unfortunately, until broad-based cryoablation training programs are available that emphasize experienced physicians performing cryoablation, patients will most likely have to pay for it themselves. Under these delicate circumstances, we must all seek honest, cost-effective solutions to overcome a transition period that may plague many areas of image-guided therapy.

The greatest area of concern I have for this book relates to patients who can't afford a plane ticket, let alone a long car ride and hotel in another city, to get what they believe is the best health care for them. This raises much larger questions about equal access to affordable, state-of-the-art health care, which is beyond the scope of any book on breast cancer treatment options. However, I want to make it clear that my desire to develop a cost-effective procedure and cryotechnology were also a byproduct of watching the exorbitant billing ordeal the Pauls experienced in seeking cryoablation. Those who may dismiss this book as a clever marketing ploy are doing a disservice to medical progress for a viable cancer treatment option.

I certainly don't espouse cryoablation for all breast cancer patients since this is a private decision that should be tailored toward each patient's peace of mind. Likewise, I don't want any patient to feel they made the wrong choice if they have already been treated, or are about to engage in treatment they have carefully considered and accepted. Hopefully, any positive attention we generate from this book will emphasize affordable cryoablation options for all breast cancer patients.

I sincerely believe this book presents, for the first time, a genuine opportunity to help change the focus of breast cancer treatments toward more earnest attempts at complete breast conservation. In combination with other therapies, cryoablation may thus become a solid piece of the puzzle that ultimately offers a durable, cosmetically pleasing cure for breast cancer in the future. I am grateful to all who have dared to help me pursue this dream.

Part One: A Healing Journey

Chapter 1: A Warning from the Mammogram

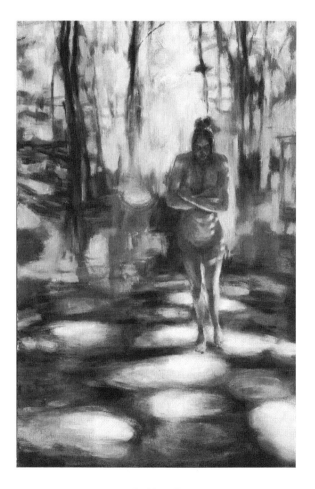

"Filter"

21

The psyche, the soul, the essences of the individual and how that individual fights for, negotiates or embraces the precariousness of existence has long been the subject of painter Ross-Paul's art . . . the protagonist in these new paintings are contemplative rather than active; intensely quiet rather than intensely emotional.

"They are, it appears, in a state of suspended animation. They are thinking. They are also naked."

—Teri Hopkins, curator for the Marylhurst Art Gym, writing for the catalog for the 2006 exhibit, "Naked" Froelick Gallery, Portland, Oregon

Laura

2/ 14/ 2003, Valentine's Day

A funny day to be having a mammogram, but the first date I could get after my first mammogram in January showed some unusual tissue and they called me back. So today, on the day of love and hearts, the young, energetic doctor gave me the news after the procedure. This second mammogram has confirmed there are two irregularities close together on the left side of my left breast.

His advice was rapid-fire, concluding with his opinion that a surgical biopsy would be the best course. This could cause a large hole. It would be the safest way to find out if it is cancer. However, what if it's not? He seemed so sure; it was like handing me a death sentence within minutes of my mammogram.

It's funny how you live your life the best you can, thinking headway is still possible as long as your health exists. I've been so proactive about my health: exercise, diet, spiritual work to help with stress. All the while I thought I was buying myself time, and maybe I am.

My first thought as I was driving home was, it has been good so far. I feel I've made it further along than my mom got to go, dying as she did at forty-four from breast cancer. My second thought was that I didn't want to share Alex or the kids with another woman that he would marry if I die! No, no, no. It's an idea I can't easily give into.

The lines in my palm have been warning me that some big life changes might be coming up—I guess I thought it would be my heart, perhaps a heart attack, happening rapidly and decisively. As it was, a stranger was telling me within three minutes of my mammogram that I should get a big chunk cut out of my breast!

There is an axe in the ceiling, hanging over your head your whole life. Then one day, it drops.

At least reading my palm tells me that success comes about the time my life starts falling apart!

Sunset. It's so beautiful here. I've read that as you grow older, it only gets better, prettier, and less hard, less challenging. Or maybe more challenging. Nevertheless, many of my personal challenges are past me. I hope this one turns out to be insignificant.

What will I do if it turns out to be bad? That my time is limited? What will I do? Paint portraits of the family—some with me if they want. Or create the watercolors for the acupuncture charts I've thought about doing for years; do them if I still can to pay back the alternative health community?

I used to worry, can I get ten more years? This was all I wanted during my thirties when I had another health scare. Then I reckoned I needed ten more years to accomplish a body of artistic work big enough and strong enough to leave a mark, a mark with my name on it. I have that now. I also have three great kids who would miss me but don't need me anymore. Only in the way you always need your mom. I have to fight! I hated losing my mom to breast cancer.

* * *

Alex

The call from Laura came as I was visiting my mother, Emily Paul, at her apartment in the retirement home I had built ten years earlier.

"I just got out of my second mammogram," Laura said. "There's a suspicious area in my left breast. The doctor thinks it's cancer and he wants me to see a surgeon and get a biopsy!"

"You're kidding!" The words refused to sink into my brain. Laura's mom had died of breast cancer at age forty-four. Laura had spent ten years on and off breast-feeding our three children, which we always thought was the ultimate insurance policy against breast cancer. Yet here she was, harboring "something suspicious" in her left breast.

We agreed it was probably nothing and the biopsy would show that it was benign. Therefore, we decided not to tell the kids, our friends, or anyone at all, until we had more information. Telling anyone felt like we would somehow make it real, that our friends would regard us differently. Somehow, there would be a stigma or a shame.

I had to tell my mom, however, because she could see how upset I was when I hung up.

"Laura might have breast cancer." The words did not come out easily. My father had died of prostate cancer in 1996. Now, only seven years later, cancer had returned to our family.

At the time, my mother was a tall, handsome, English woman in her eighties. She had survived a generous portion of misfortune during her life as many did who lived through World War II. Her fifteen-year-old brother had died of a now easily treated allergic reaction when she was just seven.

Even worse, the Japanese invaded Hong Kong on December 8th, 1941 at almost the same moment they attacked Pearl Harbor on December 7th on the other side of the International Date Line.

My parents escaped Hong Kong before the attack on December 3rd, on the last ship to leave before the war started, leaving behind my mother's family of two teenage sisters and her parents. The Japanese conquered Hong Kong on Christmas Day, 1941. It was called Black Christmas due to the horrors of rape, murder and torture committed by the Japanese on the Chinese in the city.

The English prisoners were treated more favorably, though not according to international law. They were put into concentration camps with meager rations and the men had to do forced labor.

My grandmother had the foresight to sew gold coins and jewels into their clothing. They used it to buy extra food from the guards and managed to avoid starving to death in the camp.

My parents' flight from Hong Kong ended in Canada where my father joined the Canadian army and went on to fight in Italy and then Holland during the D-Day invasion. He rarely spoke of his combat experience. The war came out in odd ways, though. I wanted to learn to hunt deer as a boy because we lived in Mill City, a small logging town in the Cascade Range. He refused to take me, saying that he never wanted to kill another living creature if he didn't have to.

My mother served as a lieutenant in the Canadian WAC during the war. My father survived and returned home. However my grandfather had eaten little food in order to have enough for his daughters and he died aboard ship on their way home to England. My grandmother came to Canada to be with my parents. The only memory I have of her is visiting her at her death bed and holding a frail, brown spotted hand that limply dangled over the edge of the bed for her four-year-old grandson to hold.

My mother passed away in 2008 and, going through her photo albums, I found a small picture, a black and white shot of a huge, white, ocean liner leaving Hong Kong. It was taken from the dock by my grandfather and he had written on the back, *Don and Edie, Dec. 3, 1941, steaming from HK.*

I cried over that picture because I realized when my mother and grandfather had parted, they both assumed they would see each other again. In fact, in those belongings I found a monthly pass for December on the Star Ferry, bought by my grandfather. He obviously had no idea the invasion was so imminent.

This was a stark reminder of how fragile our lives are, and a reminder that we should cherish the time we have with our loved ones.

Confronted with Laura's cancer, my mother offered advice.

"Life can bring you challenges, but it does no good to panic. Just meet it head on and, with God's grace, you'll survive."

I headed home to have a Valentine's Day "Date Dinner" with my lovely wife. Her sorority used to invite their boyfriends to an elaborate dinner, a custom which she maintained in marriage.

Laura and I met in the fall of 1969 and, by January of 1970, we were married. So our first "Valentine's Date Dinner" at her sorority was actually as husband and wife at the ages of twenty and twenty-two! I remember feeling slightly old and married at the time. How silly we are to judge ourselves.

Our kids have difficulty believing we got married at such a young age now that they are all older. I was a senior in engineering and held a student government position as senator of the engineering school at Oregon State University.

Laura was a cute, athletic, popular, blonde sorority girl with hidden connections to an anti-war, underground newspaper, *The Scab Sheet*. As cover artist, she sold many of their papers with her provocative and powerful front page, political cartoons.

Our common interest in ending the Vietnam War gave us an immediate platform for long discussions about life and politics. Those earnest and idealistic late night talks quickly led to love.

Laura at fifty-four was as bright and vivacious as she was in college when I first eyed her: medium height, slim, blonde hair, blue eyes, and a mole on her left cheek that was a mark of beauty to me. An athlete, she had climbed 11,000-foot Mt. Hood at the age of fifteen. She was an outdoor person, skier, Campfire Girl, and even a camp bugler.

What more could an engineer—who was also a skier, surfer, hunter and angler—have looked for in a wife? The way I imagined our lives when we were first married was that Laura would ski with me all winter, followed by camping and fishing throughout the Oregon spring. We would spend our summers camping and surfing, which would naturally lead to camping and hunting in the fall. Around Thanksgiving and the end of hunting season, we'd be at the beginning of ski season again!

All the big items—work, children, house—were just small details in the grand scheme of enjoying Oregon's outdoors! It turned out that she was game for the outdoors but, like my father, averse to killing. So we camped, skied and surfed our way through life. I thought at the time: what more than love of the outdoors could be important in finding a wife? Well, intelligence, a passion for life, careers, and raising a family were all goals we agreed on. No wonder we married within four months of our first date!

Our thirteen-year-old daughter Emma got home from school and was excited to share "date dinner night" with us because she had discovered lots of boys were interested in her. To prove it, she dumped half a backpack's worth of valentines on the dining room table! This pleasantly interrupted our hushed conversation about cancer, but leaving that morbid topic was more than welcome.

Her dark brown eyes sparkled and her ponytail bobbed around during dinner as she related all the gossip about the romantic lives of her friends. Emma had one special boy, a tall, eighth-grade basketball player, from another school no less! She declared she would move forward with caution. Eighth-grade romance! Passion and disaster greater than any soap opera. And a welcome breath of life intruding on Laura's sad news.

During dishes and homework time, Laura told me she had scheduled the biopsy. Trying to prepare for bad news, our conversation turned to her wish for nontraditional healing.

In the early 1980s my father had experienced a successful treatment of his prostate cancer by a Philippine "psychic surgeon." Despite my initial skepticism, a doctor later confirmed after an exam that the tumor had vanished since the last doctor's visit only two weeks earlier! My father lived a healthy life for another sixteen years.

This wasn't our only experience with the availability of miracle cures. In 1992, Laura's doctors had found "something suspicious" in the same area now suffering from breast cancer. We visited a woman faith healer who lived on a ranch in the desert outside Reno, Nevada. A treatment like my father's had the same result; no cancer was found by the doctors.

We thought of going back to this miracle healer of the desert but discovered she had died. We learned that her son, Carlos, was carrying on her work and we decided over dishes to locate Carlos and visit him.

The thought that Laura might have cancer kept coming back into my mind later that evening. I found myself forgetting she might have cancer and then out of the blue, I would remember.

A sense of panic would rush over me every time, requiring me to force myself to be calm as my mother had advised. I soon realized panic would just wear me down if I kept giving into it.

But later, out of the blue, my brain would shout, *Laura might have cancer,* and start the whole process over again. I couldn't imagine what she might be going through. It was making me panic and I didn't even have cancer! I sure was failing to take my mother's advice!

I pretended to watch TV after dishes. My life felt like a speeding train. I was the train's engineer. My train had run straight on its happy tracks for years after college, resulting in Laura's wonderful art career, a successful business for me, the raising of three healthy children, and now, following my success in business, I was beginning to gain success in my writing career, a career Laura had encouraged me to pursue.

I had written a novel, *Suicide Wall,* a story about Vietnam veterans and suicide, and it was the subject of numerous radio talk shows and was selling on Amazon.com. I was turning to a second project at the onset of Laura's cancer. This time I was writing a young adult adventure novel set in prehistory.

However, "something suspicious," felt like our train of life was heading down the wrong tracks thanks to some evil gremlins who had secretly pulled a switch a while ago and turned the train toward a new, sad, destination.

Minus Laura's cancer, our "ride in the train of life" should have continued through a happy, broad valley of green meadows, smiling people, and red barns nestled among tall oak trees until we were both very old and surrounded by great-grandchildren.

Now cancer gremlins seemed intent on running our "life tracks" up a narrow ravine cutting into dark mountains with thunderclouds, rain and lightning visible from far away! This wasn't the life I'd planned!

Determined to save Laura and keep our happiness on track, I turned to the Internet that night after Laura went to bed to learn more about breast cancer.

It strikes one out of eight women. Depending on the severity, or stage of the cancer before treatment, the chances of surviving five years from detection and treatment are nearly 98 percent with early discovery, but only 16 percent if discovered after it has spread to other parts of the body.

Having cancer is like being forced to play Russian roulette. You try everything you can think of to avoid getting involved: no smoking, exercise, diet. But once you have it, there's a gun at your head and it might go off no matter what you do! You're forced to play and your only friend is the odds, but they are no comfort. Even if there's only one of six chambers with a bullet in it, knowing the pistol holds one bullet is not reassuring, even though the odds are it won't fire, because if it does fire, it's game over.

Depression set in as I learned breast cancer has no guaranteed cure. It's not like the flu that you deal with and it goes away. No, with breast cancer, you pick your treatment and hope.

A miracle healing by Carlos was becoming a much more appealing option. It would be so nice for the cancer to simply vanish and we return to our old life before cancer.

I went to bed late but then woke at 4:30 a.m. The first thought I had was Laura has cancer! The adrenaline surge propelled me to my computer. Fear drove my fingers. Somewhere there had to be a cure. As long as I was trying to find a cure, I was somehow saving her life.

In the back of my mind I kept wondering, how could Laura have cancer? She was a skier, a jogger, and at fifty-four, she had many years left to pursue her successful career as a celebrated Oregon artist. She also had me and three kids that didn't want her to pass away.

With everything to live for it seemed impossible she could die so young. I wanted faith healing! Yet a chilling bumper sticker I had seen once crossed my mind. It had read, *Even non-smokers die eventually.*

* * *

Laura

2/15/2003, Saturday

Interesting news. I called my older sister today and she's had three operations to remove lumps. She has fibrocystic disease of the breasts, which causes the breast to make cysts. So far, they have all been benign. She says bad mammogram results don't even worry her anymore. She says a simple day-surgery procedure removes the cysts. It really hurts afterward, and you need at least a day to recover. I'm not so worried now.

***

Alex

I rejoiced learning that the "something suspicious" might be a cyst like Laura's sister. But we didn't want to wait to plan a visit to a faith healer until after the biopsy, because there's a time pressure to having cancer and every day you don't treat it, you risk it breaking out into the body and making your survival odds lower. So I focused on visiting the faith healer, just in case.

I had reservations about faith healing. In fact, the very concept of miracle healings makes me angry in a way. Here's why. If they work sometimes, but not others, it just seems like God, the source of all miracles is unfair.

Everyone wants a healing, so is it a matter of faith? If you don't have enough faith it doesn't work? But how do you "build faith"? Or is it just random luck? Surely, a miracle healing could not be a matter of luck. Whatever the mechanism, it seems unfair if it doesn't work every time.

However, I put those skeptical feelings aside and arranged Laura's visit. Miraculously, which seemed a good omen, Carlos had scheduled a West Coast visit months ago and would be out here in days! And he had openings.

I quickly booked flights, a car and a motel in Napa where he would be working.

One problem: Laura's biopsy was the afternoon we were to fly down. I so wished Laura could visit Carlos first, then have the biopsy. It would build our faith if the doctor could find nothing, a scientific confirmation of a healing.

And the reverse was true. By having the biopsy before the faith healing, well, it seemed like asking for failure. However, Laura decided she wanted to keep her biopsy appointment, reasoning it was better to know if she had a malignant tumor before visiting Carlos. Then if he said he had removed it, we'd definitely have proof a miracle healing occurred, especially if it's absence was confirmed by a second biopsy.

I didn't object. It was Laura's illness, not mine. Her peace of mind was uppermost.

On biopsy day, the same day we were flying to see Carlos the healer, I joined Laura for the appointment. I have always liked the people and the excellent care we have received from our HMO's local hospital. But today, it struck me I always expected a cure when I visited. This time a cure might prove elusive leading to Laura's early death.

Now the hospital of hope had become part of my new life where thoughts of breast cancer randomly entered my brain. It was like kids throwing fire crackers on July 5th. It stirs your adrenaline but annoys you.

I just wanted us to run away. But no matter where we ran, the cancer would still be inside Laura. I didn't want to be in the hospital at all, even though I had to be supportive.

I couldn't help but feel this hospital should have nothing to do with us. We're young and active; why only a few weeks ago we had gone skiing! Skiers only need hospitals when they break a leg. Cancer didn't seem like part of our reality, and yet here we were.

Laura checked in. A patient came out of the exam room and, spying a friend in the lobby, sat by her and chatted. It was impossible not to hear their conversation about her next operation, a "rebuild."

She'd had a mastectomy. Now it was time for the rebuild. After the rebuild would come the nipple tattoos. The only rebuilds I've known involve someone putting a big block Chevy into their '65 Malibu. This woman was as enthusiastic about her pending rebuild as my hot-rodding friends.

I could see this upset Laura. Cancer had thrust Laura into thinking she might need a rebuild. After a long wait, distressing because our flight was imminent, a nurse showed us into the exam room, asked Laura questions, then said the surgeon would arrive in half an hour.

"We have a six o'clock flight. Can we make it if I keep this appointment?" Laura asked.

I prayed the nurse would say no and force a reschedule. Then Carlos could remove the lump, the biopsy would find nothing and we wouldn't need to ponder a rebuild.

"She'll be in soon," the nurse replied. "You'll make it." The half hour came and went, and by three-thirty we were ready to leave since check-in for the flight cut off at five.

In walked the surgeon. A large woman, she filled the room with her energy, presence, and authority. She entered the room the way I imagined a knight entering a castle would a thousand years ago. Unheard heralds brayed their trumpets. We stiffened to attention, the drowsiness of waiting cut off by the adrenaline of our fear. The surgeon, the killer of cancer! For her to exist, cancer had to be a reality, a deadly disease.

I felt dwarfed, hopeless and stupid to hope Laura was healthy or that a faith healer I didn't have much faith in could miraculously remove the tumor this surgeon would surely find.

Laura's surgeon was pleasant but serious. She should be serious; she battled daily with one of the Four

Horsemen of the Apocalypse. She quickly placed her hands on Laura's breast and poked around as Laura winced in pain. The surgeon found the lump and gave it a hard squeeze.

"Okay, here it is, you can tell it's there," she said. "I'll get it prepped."

She swabbed a portion of Laura's breast with red liquid antiseptic, put on latex gloves, then reached for an instrument, a long needle.

The needle, the lance, the knight's weapon, came in a sterile plastic bag. It rested on a clean white cloth draped over a stainless steel table. It seemed full of intent and ceremony, a sterile sacrament on communion day.

The surgeon gave Laura a local anesthetic shot and I looked away. I could not stand watching my wife suffer. After tearing the plastic to expose the sharp needle, the surgeon spoke.

"Okay, I'm ready."

"All right," Laura replied softly.

The surgeon blocked my view and jabbed with her arm. A snip, the sound of vegetables cut on a granite countertop, filled the room. She whisked the lance/needle into its bag. A bandage, a promise of analysis, and a good-bye left us alone only minutes later. We were silently walking across the top, open floor of the parking structure on the way to our car and flight.

The last rays of sunset sky had the drama of a symphony. Southwest wind pushed broken clouds above over our hunched, hurried figures. The last rays of light angling through cloud tops only promised a long, dark, cold night, which crowded out hope. We drove in defeated silence.

"Do you think Carlos is going to work?" Laura finally asked near the airport. The cross-town ride had passed with no conversation.

"Yes, I do," I lied. Despite my father's miracle, I felt little hope. Laura's cancer seemed bigger, more certain, more real.

"But what do we do if the tissue report shows I have a malignant tumor, and Carlos removes something and says I'm healed?" Laura asked. Her question jarred me from thoughts of my father's cancer. He was dead and irretrievable. I could still save my wife.

"You'll just have to get a second biopsy," I reassured her while masking my apprehension.

The flight was delayed and we didn't even leave the San Francisco airport car rental until after nine. I had asked for the "Hertz Never Lost" GPS unit. Crossing the Bay Bridge, it told me to make a turn, not the right one. We emerged in a rough neighborhood, somewhere in Oakland. I pulled over and tried to figure out how the "Never Lost?" unit worked, when a car rushed up to us and stopped with a screech.

Though startled, I rolled down the window when I saw it was a police officer in an undercover car.

"Are you folks lost?"

"Totally!" A guardian angel could not have flown to our side faster or given better directions. He didn't try to direct us, he led us back to the freeway! I am a big fan of policemen; my father was one in Canada before entering the war. They're really good guys.

We dragged into "The Chateau Inn" after eleven.

The Chateau Inn—read motel—felt like a ski area in summer. A huge, empty parking lot shouts, "You're not here at the right time!" Instead of skiing, we had missed the wine tasting season. Then, the night clerk confided, tourists overflowed the valley. Given the midweek in off-season mid-February we had our pick of spacious rooms at a low price. The feeling of joy at getting a bargain soon dissolved in the realization that we didn't want to be here! We collapsed in bed to Jay Leno and hopes of Carlos in the morning.

Napa is an odd blend of upscale wine and low-rent rural. The morning sun revealed we were not far from the healing house. The stairs of the old, hippie house creaked. An ex-hippie woman our age gave us a warm welcome into her combination home, candle and spiritual shop and healing center. Shelves in her living room and displays in her kitchen offered everything from books on massage to books on healing, to teas and soap and gems.

I have learned not to judge people by their circumstances. If healers were "proper," they would have huge clinics, insurance billing and busy schedules. They would not wear stethoscopes. No need. Carlos's mother used to "scan" our bodies by holding a towel in front of us. How she could "see" through the towel, or through our bodies, I have no idea. Results were all that mattered.

Laura spent an hour alone with Carlos. He doesn't allow cameras or guests in a healing room. I slumbered in a rocking chair, the morning sun creeping slowly towards me across a black cat sleeping on a throw rug. Lilting soft music and incense smoke washed the room. I felt like I was in a museum in 1968.

Laura came out and Carlos asked me in. He had found a growth, though it was not a tumor. He had managed to remove part of it, but Laura needed to come see him tomorrow to get the rest out. He assured me she was cancer free. This statement relieved yet worried me.

While the scene reminded me of my father's miracle healing years earlier, I still felt anxious. The engineer in me said only a new mammogram and biopsy would prove Laura cancer free.

Later that day we sat around the pool and Laura worked on her journal. It was sunny but cool, so we didn't swim, just sunned. Despite the chance to ski and snowboard in the mountains, Oregonians endure their winter rains more than enjoy them. We emerge each spring with heads turned down out of the habit of avoiding rain for so long.

When the sun comes out in Oregon it's a surprise, an afterthought of nature we have to grow familiar with again, like an old friend returning home after a long absence.

The white concrete at our backs reflected the sun and the warmth felt good. The walls reminded me of Greek villages I had visited one winter. I resolved then that once Laura was free of cancer, whether by miracle or medicine, we would celebrate in Greece or somewhere Mediterranean.

Laura

2/20/2003

Napa Valley, California

Sitting by the pool at the Chateau Inn. This morning the spiritual healer, Carlos, worked on me.

Yesterday, before we left Portland to come see Carlos, we went to see the surgeon Dr. Fancher recommended for my biopsy. Dr. Fancher, my regular doctor, is convinced I have breast cancer based on the radiologist's description of my second mammogram. I wonder if my mom's cancer history has influenced their thinking.

I related my sister's fibroid cyst condition to Dr. Fancher on the phone, but he seemed doubtful this is what I have. He recommended I have the tumors surgically removed. The surgeon surprised me yesterday when she said she could feel them (I could not), and since she could feel them, she decided to biopsy them on the spot. It was over in three clicks of a long needle.

"Dazzle," my nickname for my camp and high school buddy, went down this breast cancer road during Christmas, only a month earlier. She told me the steps of her treatment. It began with an irregular mammogram showing displacement of calcifications. Her second step was an office biopsy, which indicated a malignant tumor. An operation, a lumpectomy, followed, where they took out her tumors and some lymph nodes. Yikes! I'm now at step number two, the office biopsy. The idea of an office biopsy relieved me in a way. I thought I would need a biopsy using surgery.

Not needing a surgical biopsy gave me hope, as it was the least invasive way to find out if I have a malignancy. So afterwards, we were on to Napa and Carlos, and now here I am journaling at the Chateau!

Last night, the three-quarter-full moon rose over the bay as we crossed the Bay Bridge. The silhouette of lacy dark trees against the moon and the moonlight reflecting off the water were so beautiful, especially when countered by the filthy interior of the Bay Bridge.

The all-consuming flashes of beauty throughout the trip kept surprising me. As we drove to the Portland airport earlier, I glimpsed a huge plane landing with its landing lights on. Dramatic rain clouds coming in from the Pacific and the silver blue of the just-rained-upon city in the background silhouetted the plane, with the elongated triangle of shimmering landing strip in front.

Alex was accommodating and did not object to our going to the seventh floor. I snapped photos from the roof of the parking structure while he stood with our luggage in the last of a rain shower. He arranged this whole trip and has been such a dear to be with. He makes me laugh so much, tells me interesting news, and gives me hope in general. This state of fear and anxiety has a firm grip on me and I appreciate the breaks he gives me.

Carlos says I don't have cancer. We'll see on Friday when I get back. I'll find out the result of the biopsy. Carlos says to ask for a second opinion if they do find a tumor after the first biopsy, and not to let them operate on me until I have that second opinion.

Chapter 2: Dr. Littrup—The Making of a Pioneer, a Heretic, or a Difference?

Dr. Littrup

As a child, I always felt bound for a strange destiny. I had a weird feeling about my life as I grew up, but I didn't know why. When I turned eleven, my mother told me that she had considered abortion when she found out she was pregnant with me.

The idea of never arriving on this planet shocked me and has haunted me ever since. For years, I wondered if my birth meant I had something important to do while I was here. As a child, I heard stories of my mother and grandfather and their participation in the Danish underground. I think those stories added to my sense that people can have an important destiny.

I grew up around Detroit, but my parents were from Denmark. They met and married after the Second World War. My father was a mechanical engineer during the war, while my mother worked for the railroad and helped the Danish underground smuggle Jews to safety in Sweden.

My mother was the daughter of a ship's captain, Peter Rasmussen Petersen. After World War II,

The King of Denmark knighted him for his heroic career in the merchant marines. However, his official autobiography said that the knighting was a result of him saving lives when ships were in distress, all prior to World War II. The official autobiography from the state never revealed any other reason for his knighting.

I learned years later that the official state biography withheld stories about his participation in the underground during WWII because there was a fear of Nazi retribution even after the war. The long arm of the Gestapo still held power, real or imagined, long after the defeat of Germany.

Now that my grandfather and my mother have both passed away, I can safely, and proudly, relate what I believe to be the most important reason my grandfather was knighted; he and my mother helped dozens, if not hundreds, of Danish Jews escape certain death in the Nazi concentration camps.

My mother worked for DSB, the Danish national railway. Her job allowed her to phone ahead and notify my grandfather of the imminent arrival of German armored trains.

My grandfather captained a train ferry, which carried these armored trains from Helsingor, Denmark to Halsingborg, Sweden through the narrow Oresund Strait. From Halsingborg, the trains would continue to Russia or Norway with their loads of armaments destined for the German war effort.

The rail car's heavy armor meant there were few guards on the train since they were immune to light arms attack by the Danish underground. With few guards, the trains became an ideal method for smuggling Jews to freedom.

Jews escaping to the north from Copenhagen lashed themselves to the underside of the armored trains and arrived at Helsingor nearly frozen. Members of the underground would cut them free. My grandfather and others then sheltered them until they had recovered.

When no guards were looking while the crews prepared the railcars for boarding his ship, my grandfather would signal the escaping Jews to sneak back underneath the trains. There they hid themselves above the axles during the short passage across the strait.

Once the railcars rolled off the ship after docking in neutral Sweden, the guards no longer paid attention to the train since it was safe from attack in Sweden. The Jews would roll out from under the train after the guards left and walk to freedom.

Thousands of Danish citizens collaborated in this effort. Hundreds of tiny boats, from fishing boats to rowboats, also ferried small groups of Jews across the Oresund at night. Before she died, my mother recalled having to drug infants and toddlers with chloral hydrate to keep them quiet for several hours of transport. The risk of such primitive anesthesia outweighed the certain death if a child made the slightest sound. Estimates suggest that 99 percent of all Danish Jews escaped their fate in the Nazi concentration camps by fleeing to Sweden.

My father, Gunnar Littrup, was an engineer on a small ship in the Danish Navy until the military was sent home after their rapid capitulation to the German invasion. He met and married my mother just after the end of World War II. My parents soon had my older sister, but they divorced when she was only two. My father left Denmark soon after the divorce and joined his older brothers who had previously emigrated to America.

My father used to joke that he left little Denmark because it was not big enough for him and his father-in-law. I met my grandfather before he died, but I was only two years old. By all accounts, he was a charismatic man who had lived an astounding life during the transition from sail to steamships. After learning more about my grandfather, I was able to understand my father's feeling that grandfather was indeed, larger than life.

Seven years after their divorce, my father returned to Denmark to visit my sister. During this visit, my parents discovered that neither had remarried, so they decided to marry for a second time, and my mother came to America with her new, for the second time, husband.

Despite my mother's first reservations about delivering me into the world and her resulting thoughts of abortion, once they decided to have me, my parents committed to raising me despite their sometimes, dissimilar spirits. I always felt blessed by their love and nurturing. They always made time to help or guide my energies and enthusiasm.

Tales of my mother's willingness to risk all to make a difference in the world had a big influence on me. Her courage made me willing to take risks, to venture into new territory, to question existing beliefs. Her example made me determined to make a difference in medicine.

From my father came my analytical bent for clever engineering solutions if a problem so required. Moreover, as a practical engineer, the KISS principle—Keep It Simple Stupid—guided my father with a firm hand and it influenced me as well!

I took an unusual road to a medical career. I was born in 1959 in Flint, Michigan. Flint is not a breeding ground of scholars, Michael Moore aside. Flint is a blue-collar city 50 miles north of Detroit.

My father had been an engineer running a chocolate factory in Denmark prior to coming to America and joining his brothers in Flint. His English had not been good enough to gain employment as an engineer with General Motors. However, he relied on the fact that he had a journeyman's card as a tool-and-die maker and landed a good paying job with GM at their factory in Flint. My mother and sister joined him there when they remarried, and then I came along.

When I was in the fourth grade, my father received a promotion from the tool and die shop to the white collar engineering department at GM's Tech Center in Sterling Heights, Michigan. My father had only asked for a transfer within the same factory that would pay 10 cents more an hour. Instead, since his English had improved, and they needed engineers, they bumped him up to the Tech Center. I remember the family going out to buy white shirts, since the only ones my father owned literally had blue collars.

Dad was proud of his promotion, and he often told me, "Peter, you only need to know three things to make it in America: work hard, be honest but most of all, use your talent!"

My father taught me another very important lesson after we moved into Sterling Heights. It was a "white-flight" neighborhood full of people who had moved north from Detroit after the 1967 riots. Racism was in the air, and in short order my new friends had taught me the "N"-word.

I used that word one evening, not even knowing at age nine that it was a derogatory comment. Dad replied,

"Peter, did you know your father was a nigger when he came to this country?"

They say as a kid you don't have the ability to form abstract thoughts until about age eleven, and I remember thinking as a nine-year-old, "Whoa, my dad used to be black!" I wondered for a second how that could be, and also wondered if I might turn black soon and then return to white later, like those Lipizanner stallion horses I had just seen in the circus. Perhaps this was some trait unique to people from Denmark? I had no idea, and I wondered if this was another one of those things my parents hadn't told me about being Danish in America.

My father soon educated me by going on to say, "A nigger is someone who isn't given the respect or opportunity to use their God-given talents. You will be fortunate if you choose to use your talents, so remember we are all God's children!" This from a relatively quiet engineer.

Ignorance and racism are mutual friends that my parents taught me to avoid with a passion. My father stunned me with this short comment about my own ignorance. It changed my life. He taught me to see people without racial bias, only cultural differences.

During the seventh grade in Sterling Heights, I decided to become a doctor while dissecting frogs in science class. Up to that time, I had wanted to become an engineer like my father because I loved complex machinery. However, when I opened that frog, the thought gripped me that here was one complex piece of equipment! From that point on, I only wanted to be a doctor.

When I entered Warren High School, which was on the border of Sterling Heights, it didn't take long for my classmates to give me the nickname, "Pete the Feet."

I was only 5'4" tall, but had size 13 feet. I guess I was like a puppy with big paws that had yet to grow, which I eventually did. However, in my early high school years, those big feet proved to be an advantage while swimming.

I swam with an AAU (Amateur Athletic Union) club in grade school, and had given it up in the seventh grade for karate. The summer between my sophomore and junior year in high school, I decided to go back to swimming for the AAU club. On the high school swim team during my sophomore year, I had been a slow "Lane 6" backstroke swimmer. However, the AAU club had transformed itself from a community club to one that trained kids, not for state meets, but for Nationals.

They told me I was too slow to train with guys my age, so the only place they could fit me in was in the lane for the eleven-year-old girls! Nothing motivates a fifteen-year-old boy more than telling him he needs to train with his equals, and then showing him that those equals are eleven-year-old girls.

That fall, before I began competing in swimming, I went small game hunting. It was my first time hunting and I had bought some cheap shells on my summer lifeguard's budget. My shotgun jammed as I loaded it before we headed out into the field to hunt, so I held the gun with the barrel under my arm while my friend tried to remove the shell. The gun went off with the muzzle right by my chest. I looked down and so much blood covered my coat that I thought for a second I was dying. Fortunately, the only damage was from the muzzle blast, the shot just grazed me on a perfect tangent. Nevertheless, the blast burned off a wide spot of skin.

I showed up for my first swim meet with a big plastic patch on my side and feeling like a freak. No one knew how I would do, because I'd been training with little girls all summer. I won the race, and even better, beat the high school record in the 500-yard freestyle by seven seconds!

That little piece of success changed my outlook on life. It confirmed my father's advice: if you worked hard in America, you could succeed. It made me realize that if I put enough concentrated effort into something, I could succeed.

Only 20 percent of graduating seniors from my high school went on to college of any sort. And back then, there were good paying jobs to be had in the Detroit auto industry. I felt like a rebel wanting to become a doctor. Many of my friends went to work in the auto industry right out of high school, and soon they had cars, boats and houses.

I had to put myself through college, working in a tool-and-die shop every summer and lifeguarding on weekends during the school year. In the tool-and-die shop, I drilled holes in steel plates, swept floors, and filed rough edges off metal parts. This was boring work, but I found great enjoyment in it because the shop fore-man showed me how to operate nearly every piece of equipment in the shop, from complex drill presses to Bridgeports and lathes. He complimented me on my abil-ity to be a quick study in learning mechanical skills, and it filled my belly with a longing to translate these skills into medicine someday.

That job also taught me the value of cleverness. Cleverness was being able to solve problems with noth-ing besides the resources available. I learned that clever solutions sometimes turned out even better than any planned scheme because you developed an innovative, hands-on approach.

I entered pre-med at the University of Michigan in Ann Arbor. Three and a half years later, in December 1980, I graduated with a double major: honors physiology and biological anthropology.

A wonderful research mentor and physiology professor at the med school, Dr. Richard Malvin, sponsored my honors thesis. His final advice as I left for medical school was, "Just do good science!"

I entered medical school at the University of Michigan in 1981 and received my degree in medicine in 1985. Finally, I was a doctor but not yet a radiologist. I had decided during medical school to become a radiologist after publishing some of the first articles on the new field of Magnetic Resonance Imaging, MRI. The idea of seeing into the body electronically fascinated me.

Other things fascinated me in my life, such as one Martha Appledorn, whom I met during my third year of medical school. We married on November 23, 1985 in Birmingham, Michigan, just after I started an internship in Ann Arbor at St. Joseph's Mercy Hospital.

The road to becoming a practicing radiologist is paved with the building blocks of a long apprenticeship. The first step in this training is to practice medicine as an intern at a hospital under the watchful eyes of various older doctors.

In my case, one of these older doctors was Fred Lee, Sr. I learned at our first meeting that he had prostate cancer and had only twelve to twenty-four months to live. He had such a profound passion for life, despite his apparent terminal diagnosis, that I chose to spend a month's rotation during my internship helping him with his new life's work—the screening and treatment of prostate cancer.

During that time, I watched Fred give his body and soul to fighting prostate cancer. He used an unusual combination of I^{125} seed implants (radioactive iodine pellets) followed by hyperthermia (heat) and combined with an external beam radiation boost to kill his tumor. Fred then followed up with chemo-hormonal therapy called Emcyt to kill the cancer that had spread to his lymph nodes.

Perhaps because of his willingness to choose such an intensive, yet avant-garde approach, he is still alive twenty years later, with no evidence of disease. His victory over cancer was an incredible inspiration to me.

Here was a man who had used medicine, though in an unorthodox way, to save his own life. To me he was the personal embodiment of the Hippocratic Oath: to "Doctor, do no harm—and heal yourself while you're at it!"

Then it came time for me to leave Fred and become a radiology resident, residency being the next stage of a doctor's career after serving an internship. However, I wanted to stay on with Fred and help him with his quest. The one-month rotation I had served with Fred in 1985 had inspired me. This was a difficult decision, but my wife supported it, saying, "I don't want you to look back and regret a passed opportunity to work with Fred. Just make sure you still have a radiology residency waiting for you in Boston."

Harvard's prestigious New England Deaconess Hospital in Boston agreed to defer my residency, so I stayed on with Fred in Ann Arbor for a year of intensive research that we called a "Fellowship" before I even started my residency.

My year of research with Fred spanned the years 1986 and 1987 and it was very exciting. Fred's initial focus was to develop a more efficient, lower-cost approach for detecting prostate cancer by using ultrasound. We could see cancerous spots with ultrasound, but we had to confirm their location to prove that ultrasound was working.

Fred and I developed a now commonly used needle biopsy technique for prostate diagnosis. This new biopsy technique could occur in an outpatient setting, meaning outside a hospital, since it required no anesthetic. I traveled to a conference in Denmark of all places, and brought back a Swedish, automated biopsy needle, called the Radiplast.

This device revolutionized prostate biopsy because it made the process of sampling prostate tissue more consistently precise and less difficult to perform. When Fred lectured on it, he frequently called the little clicking sound the Radiplast gun made when it took a tissue sample for biopsy, the "shot heard around the world." This machine proved so successful that it was eventually licensed and distributed by the large medical company, C.R. Bard, giving it the name the Bard gun, which it is known by to this day.

During this fellowship with Fred, I was learning more about myself. I enjoyed bringing machinery into use to help the "human machine." I think this was a throwback to my lineage as an automotive engineer's son with tool-and-die shop experience.

Fred and I started a multicenter trial during that year. In our trial we compared the efficacy of ultrasound,

PSA (a blood protein test that can indicate prostate cancer), and the traditional digital rectal exam. This was the American Cancer Society National Prostate Cancer Detection Project (ACS NPCDP). It was during this trial that I met Dr. Gerald Murphy, the Chairman of the trial and Chief Medical Officer of the ACS, who was a fireball of inspiration and intellectual mentorship.

The ACS NPCDP that Gerald Murphy, Fred Lee, and I started was the first head-to-head-to-head comparison of different methods of detecting prostate cancer: PSA (prostate specific antigen), DRE (digital rectal exam), and TRUS (Transrectal Ultrasound: literally, a hunt for tumors using an ultrasound).

This comparison showed that PSA and TRUS were twice as effective as DRE in detecting the presence of prostate cancer. The results of our trial ignited the now standard use of the 1-2 punch of PSA and TRUS combined with a simple biopsy.

In the middle of this work, I continued doing other research with Fred. I realized an aspect of research that I did not enjoy involved using dogs as research patients. I am a dog lover, yet the scientific world demands that a pure researcher show little emotion about animals. The rule is that work done on these animals saves human lives. While this is undoubtedly true, I had a difficult time tolerating the work I did in experiments on dogs where we used lasers and microwaves to operate on the healthy prostates of dogs.

It upset me that I couldn't reveal my empathy for dogs in this scientific forum. I could tell they weren't happy campers even though dogs couldn't "tell me where it hurt" or fill out a pain questionnaire. Animal research with dogs gave me the heebie-jeebies in addition to a severe dose of guilt. I had to abide by my training, however, which taught me to varnish over any emotion with the hard lacquer of premeditated science.

The information and science we developed in this research translated into the first attempts done anywhere to destroy human prostate tumors using a laser, so the work with dogs definitely had scientific purpose. Still, I was relieved when my research work involving dogs ended.

The work Fred and I did using ultrasound guidance expanded into using ultrasound during the insertion of radioactive Iodine pellets, I^{125}, into the prostate. All this work, and the work we also did performing laser ablation of prostate tumors, would bear fruit later in my residency at Harvard's Deaconess.

Fred Lee's paternal friendship, as well as his surprising and wonderful cancer remission during that year, made an exciting year of research into a truly extraordinary experience for me. When the year of my research fellowship with Fred Lee ended in 1987, Martha and I moved on to Boston and the four-year radiology residency Deaconess had kindly held open for me.

Soon after arriving at Deaconess, I found the Chairman of Radiology, Dr. Mel Clouse, to be enthusiastic and very encouraging of my research. He placed me under the tutelage of Dr. Bob Kane, a superb ultrasound director, who also monitored my traditional tasks as a radiology resident at Deaconess. At the same time, I became supervisor of a laser laboratory at another Harvard institution, the Peter Bent Brigham Hospital.

In addition to all these duties, the American Cancer Society appointed me as the principal investigator for their NPCDP trial in Boston during my first year at

Deaconess. This was the trial that Fred and I had started the previous year. As principal investigator for the trial in Boston, I began performing prostate ultrasounds with Professor Kane.

Professor Kane was an experienced radiologist and ultrasound maven, but had not yet used ultrasound for detecting prostate cancer. The day I started working with him at "the Deek" (Deaconess), he pronounced jokingly, "If I have to learn *any* ultrasound from a first-year resident, then I'll make sure you know *every* other facet of ultrasound!"

I simply stuck out my hand and said, "You have a deal, sir."

My residency lasted four years. The first two years were spent at Deaconess, with a third year at Massachusetts General Hospital. During my Deaconess residency, I wrote several papers on the prostate cancer detection work I had done earlier with Fred Lee and had continued during my time as principal investigator in the Boston ACS-NPCDP clinical trial. In 1988, our team of "Lee, Littrup" published three papers in medical journals—a rare accomplishment for a resident.

This publishing success during the years away from Fred Lee made me realize how important he had been in my life. Beyond our prolific publishing, he had impressed me with the five great kids he had raised with his wife Ethel. To honor Fred's influence in my life, my wife and I decided to name our firstborn son Gerrit Lee Littrup.

I received one of the first two-year research fellowships from the Radiology Society of North America during my last year of residency at Deaconess. With the residency completed, I returned to Ann Arbor, Michigan to spend the last year of my fellowship doing research with

Fred Lee at St. Joseph Mercy hospital in Ann Arbor. And in an odd coincidence, our second son, Gunnar Vagn Littrup, arrived on Fred's birthday!

During this fellowship, I developed the first laser balloon treatment for reducing an enlarged prostate. Ultrasound guidance allowed this operation to occur and MRI provided great follow-up. This work was just beginning as I finished the ACS-NPCDP prostate cancer screening research.

My publishing success continued with my return to working with Fred. This led to another opportunity to study the economics of cancer screening. During one of the regular meetings of the ACS-NPCDP, I casually asked Dr. Murphy, the renowned chairman of the committee, whether cost-savings would result from efficient prostate cancer screening.

"You know, by finding cancers earlier, we should be treating them more cost-effectively," I suggested.

Dr. Murphy simply smiled and replied that Allen Goodman, a health economist at Wayne State University, had written a textbook on health economics. Dr. Murphy then added that he expected a draft of a collaborative paper between Allen Goodman and me by the next quarterly meeting of the committee.

Dr. Goodman and I met and decided to accept Dr. Murphy's challenge. Within a year, Dr. Murphy joined our effort and together we published a paper entitled, "The Benefit and Cost of Prostate Cancer Early Detection" in *A Cancer Journal for Clinicians*.

Some doctors challenged the results of our study, despite the scientific rigor we displayed. Many urologists resisted adoption of transrectal ultrasound since they considered the digital rectal exam, DRE, to be the gold standard of prostate tumor detection. At that time, in the early 1990s, many urologists also considered the PSA (Prostate Specific Antigen) blood test to be "experimental" and unproved, and so they rejected this test as well.

However, Dr. Murphy overcame these objections when he recommended the American Cancer Society adopt these new diagnostic techniques in a landmark meeting in October 1991 at Sea Island, GA.

I didn't recognize the impact my paper would have when I wrote it. However, during one of our last meetings, Dr. Murphy countered a self-deprecating remark I made about my "boring" benefit-cost paper.

"Peter, you have no idea how much difference you've already made in treating this disease!"

No matter what other compliment I may receive in my medical career, I'll always treasure that remark from a cancer "giant" like Dr. Murphy. In 1991, Prostate Cancer Awareness Month launched this new screening tool as a community-based detection effort across America. Dr. David Crawford chaired this effort.

The American Urologic Association quickly did a 180-degree reversal on their "experimental" stance and advised that all urology residency programs should teach TRUS with biopsy as a follow-up to PSA testing. Even with this, the Europeans, Canadians, and the American Academy of Family Practice objected to these new screening techniques. They claimed the advanced screening led to too many unnecessary surgeries. Since surgery had a one to two percent mortality rate in and of itself, subjecting people to potentially unnecessary surgery was more lethal than letting their cancer go undetected.

This comment had a profound effect on me, because prostate cancer needed an approach on several levels. First, we had to get better at detecting it, which my research had proved was not only possible but cost-effective. Second, we had to get better at treating the patient so one to two percent of the patients treated didn't die because of our treatment.

The mortality rate of the surgery was not a reason to "not detect cancer better!" It was a reason to improve treatment. The desire to improve treatment stayed in the back of my mind as I continued my medical career.

Looking back on this controversy, I have to say that so far in my career, I am most proud of being a part of the early detection "boom" in prostate cancer. This increased emphasis on early detection resulted in a reported increase in prostate cancer incidence, peaking around 1992. There wasn't an actual higher rate of cancer in those years during the implementation of PSA early detection. Instead, the number of cases of prostate cancer increased because they had previously gone unnoticed without PSA testing.

This increased detection "boom" translated into lower prostate cancer mortality on a per capita basis by 2005. I continued my research interests, but now focused my desires to help improve cancer treatment, rather than just "opening Pandora's box" with screening and not providing a good solution.

Once I began work back at St. Joe's in July of 1985, I also began running prostate cancer detection/screening programs in African-American churches around Ann Arbor, as well as continuing the ablation research. Frankly, I did my screening in the African-American community because of the statistics we had discovered in the

ACS-NPCDP. This would not have been possible without the help of a wonderful young assistant, John Newby, who was trying to get into medical school but also wanted to help his community. His willingness to embrace a white physician and help transcend the distrust that much of the African American community holds for the medical establishment warmed my heart. It stirred a ghostly feeling of my heritage. Seeing no color in your fellow man for the sake of humanity and better medicine felt like a small taste of the pride the Danes must have sensed when helping their Jewish countrymen overcome the deadly bitterness of any racism.

My experience in Boston had also shown me the genuine need for medical outreach to this community. The ACS had long known that African-American men had twice the incidence of prostate cancer as the US general male population and nearly three times the death rate. While our ACS NPCDP centers had been in metropolitan areas with large African-American populations, they only represented seven percent of our trial patients. In other words, they were not voluntarily coming in for testing like the non-African-American population.

In fact, the high prevalence of prostate cancer in African-Americans was the third most important factor in my benefit-cost analysis with Dr. Goodman, so screening should be even more cost-effective in high-risk groups.

It also made me realize that after test specificity, that is, lowering the false positives, we also needed to focus on the second most important factor in controlling screening costs—finding a better early treatment method. I began to imagine what might work.

Therefore, the fellowship I received from the Radiology Society of North America (RSNA) in 1991-2, allowed me to build on the work I had done in 1986 with interstitial laser treatments guided by TRUS. The hope for this research was that microwave or laser tissue ablation through a balloon catheter would prove successful in killing tissue around the urethra to allow men to urinate better. Even though drugs were eventually developed to treat most *benign* symptoms of prostate disease, development of image-guided treatments gave me wonderful experience to expand future treatment options for *cancer*. This led to my ACS Junior Faculty Award that tried to explore the possibility for laser ablation of local prostate cancer.

The prostate is a small organ buried in a sensitive and delicate part of the body. My desire to do as little surgical harm as possible to the patient drove my interest in using small probes. At the same time, I had to make sure the probe killed the tumor.

I diligently performed my laser research on the effects of heat ablation while knowing that freezing was also potentially effective in treating prostate cancer. I wanted to help develop a new way of dealing with prostate cancer, yet I had no bias against any particular method as long as it helped the patient.

Earlier, when I was at Deaconess, I had studied cryoablation and the work of Dr. Gary Onik, a pioneer in the field. He had been at Deaconess and had left a year before I arrived. But during my residency with Dr. Kane, we had continued Gary's work with cryoablation of liver tumors. I became fascinated by the potential—and the problems—of cryoablation.

I initially avoided cryoablation during my Deaconess residency because the primary application used relatively archaic equipment. The cryoprobes were thicker than a pencil (that is 8 mm, 0.33 in), which routinely caused bleeding after removal from the patient.

These cryoprobes were thick because while a small, inner tube carried *liquid* nitrogen into the body down to the tip of the probe, a larger outer tube had to carry the *gaseous* nitrogen back out of the probe. The large outer tube encased the inner tube, like the lead in a pencil. At the tip of the probe, the liquid nitrogen expands into a gas. This "evaporation" causes most of the freezing power at the tip of the probe.

Liquid nitrogen expands 200 times when it turns into a gas. With this expansion rate, the large outer tube still did not allow for enough expansion of the gas. As a result, the gas invariably caused vapor lock in probes with a smaller diameter than 3 mm. Vapor lock occurs when no more liquid can travel down the probe because the large amount of gas produced at the tip cannot get out fast enough.

This all resulted in an awkward procedure because the large probe made it impossible to safely put it through the skin. In fact, a surgeon had to patch the 8 mm holes after the removal of the cryoprobes from the liver. If the probe had been smaller, like the size of a needle, the body could have healed itself with minimal bleeding.

However, in September 1991, I received a fateful call from Gary Onik, who had moved on from Deaconess to Pittsburgh's Allegheny General. Previously, I had told him that I thought the future of cryosurgery lay in small probes, or needles, and that if he did manage to get them smaller, to give me a call.

Even though I was able to "see" some of the earliest laser ablations by ultrasound, the visibility could not compare to the larger size and clarity of developing ice that Gary Onik had recorded in all his cryoablation research. In this work, he originally froze human liver tumors using intraoperative ultrasound to guide the whole process.

During the call, Gary related the exciting breakthroughs he had achieved for use in the prostate. He called to tell me the new cryoablation equipment he helped develop with other cryo gurus (Drs. Boris Rubinsky and John Baust) could now deliver liquid nitrogen down cryoprobes thinner than a straw (i.e., 3 mm).

In the fall of 1991, I went out to visit Gary at Allegheny Hospital in Pittsburgh to watch one of the first human prostate cryoablation procedures. Even though I was finishing the second year of my RSNA research fellowship and had just submitted for an American Cancer Society Jr. Faculty Research Award for continued work with interstitial prostate laser therapy, the promise of cryoablation with smaller probes produced one of those "Aha!" moments.

This moment occurred after I saw Dr. Onik perform prostate cryoablation with the smaller probes. I had followed his patient into the recovery area to see him wake up from anesthesia. The patient exhibited symptoms of pain, which appeared similar to the pain I had witnessed in dogs following heat-based prostate ablations.

So I asked the patient where his pain was and, to my astonishment, he pointed to his throat! Instead of any pain related to the pelvis/prostate, only his throat bothered him from the anesthesia endotracheal tube.

This astounded me. A light bulb went off when I saw the low postoperative pain resulting from cryoablation. Freezing the entire prostate appeared to produce much less pain in humans than heating only a portion of the prostate by small laser fibers in dogs.

During that short visit with Gary, I changed a few facets of his procedure. I suggested that he should freeze the front of the prostate first and carefully monitor the freeze in the front while we could still see inside before we turned the cryoprobes on in the back of the prostate. Previously he had been working in the reverse order. However, because ice is such a good sound absorber, and ultrasound looks at the freeze from the back of the prostate, the frozen tissue at the back caused such a shadow that it obscured seeing any freezing at the front of the prostate. By reversing the freezing order, Gary was able to increase his control of the entire prostate destruction. He declared that I had to become one of their first cryomachine users.

Soon after I returned to St. Joseph's Memorial Hospital in Ann Arbor, Fred Lee and I began to offer the first cryoablation treatments of the prostate in Michigan, and never looked back.

Gary's new equipment, made by Cryomedical Sciences, Inc., allowed the first breakthrough of clinical cryoablation by producing slim, yet powerful, 3-mm probes that allowed percutaneous, or "through the skin," treatment of the prostate. The field of cryoablation had just opened the door for applications in urology.

However, urologists wanted nothing to do with cryoablation for prostate cancer, despite this important progress in prostate cancer treatment. Instead, urologists rejected it, displaying an "NIH" i.e., "Not Invented Here" attitude.

Prostate cryoablation was treating a disease on the urologist's turf. Radiologists had pioneered the procedure since they were comfortable guiding a treatment by ultrasound. Traditional urologic surgeons who observed the radiologist's work directly initially rejected cryoablation because it was NIH, not invented here.

A couple of straight-shooting, just plain good guys, who also happened to be superb urologists (Drs. J. Edson Pontes and Jim Monte), sensed my frustration with the initial rejection of cryoablation by urologic surgeons. They suggested that if I wanted to see cryoablation adopted for prostate cancer treatment, I needed to prove I could see the ice ball on ultrasound and kill cancerous tissue as accurately as Fred and I claimed. Essentially, the urologists wanted proof that cryoablation could kill the entire prostate if necessary, thus duplicating the surgical procedure called the radical prostatectomy, the removal of the prostate.

They were right. It was time for research to produce proof of the claims we were making, that cryoablation was a more effective, less painful, and less dangerous treatment for prostate cancer than traditional surgery. Unfortunately, that led me back to an area of research that was uncomfortable for me—dogs.

The only way we could prove that cryoablation could kill the whole prostate was to do a careful analysis of dog prostate specimens after they had been frozen. I conducted this portion of my research at Wayne State University in 1993. I had taken a position at Wayne State University as an assistant Professor of Radiology and Urology in April of 1991 as it allowed me the opportunity to teach, practice medicine, and do research at the same time.

By working with dogs, I soon had proof that cryoablation with ultrasound guidance allowed excellent

visualization and ice control. Control of the ice determines precisely what region of tissue is killed, thus allowing a physician applying cryoablation to safely "sculpt"
the ice to avoid the rectum, and potentially, even the
nerves. I knew during this research that if we could offer
cryoablation that could thoroughly kill prostate tumors
while preserving urinary continence and perhaps even
sexual potency, we would have a procedure that would
be very desirable for prostate cancer patients. While I
was enthusiastic enough in 1994 to write three protocols
for various aspects of prostate cryoablation that were
approved by the research board of the cancer center and
university, the timing was still too soon for the "male
lumpectomy."

This research on controlling ice ball formation helped
confirm a philosophy that still guides my cryoablation
research today. By approaching the dictum, "What you
see is what you get"; that is, we can accurately deliver
safe kill zones with well-monitored ice formation.

I published an article about this research in the journal, *Urology*, in 1994. I was still young and passionate
about my work, but alas, too naïve.

An editorial came out in *Urology* in conjunction with
my paper. The editorial was a roundabout political dis-
course on prostate cryoablation in general. It did not
criticize the facts of my research. I had presented clear
evidence that we could deliver safe kill zones by following
reproducible freezing techniques. I concluded, therefore,
that the criticism of my article didn't have much to do
with the legitimacy of cryobiology or the science behind
the technology.

I chose to respond in writing to the editorial in a
light—hearted fashion. This was because I believed the

criticism should not be taken seriously, since it was not directed at the science, just the politics.

My response to the editorial began with a humorous and poetic line: "Radical Prostatectomy, Radiation Therapy, and Cryoablation; the Butcher, the Baker and the Ice Cube Maker, each with their own Conflicts of Interest in the Kasbah of Prostate Cancer Therapy."

I intended to draw tongue-in-cheek attention to the economic conflicts of interest going on between *any* advocates of *any* treatment for prostate cancer. I hoped that it would expose the fact there should be an open-minded dialogue about the benefits and potential of cryoablation compared with traditional treatment.

I was aware that as an emerging treatment, cryoablation would need to be adopted and implemented correctly. If the techniques of cryosurgery were not reproduced properly, the potential advantages of cryosurgery would not be realized. At this stage, there was definitely an art to being able to see an ultrasound image and know what was going on inside the patient. This included accurate understanding of the lethal temperatures generated around the cryoprobes according to their spacing and distribution. This knowledge of lethal isotherms has become the cornerstone of safe, effective use of cryoablation in all areas of the body, yet seems to be an abstract concept for many who wish to dismiss the merits of any image-guided therapy. Because it was easy for me, I think I took it for granted that others could learn this skill as well. I didn't think of it as challenging or difficult for someone to learn: I merely thought it was so exciting that we could help patients so much with this new treatment method.

I was too young and too impatient to know that this learning curve, as well as the natural resistance to anything new, combined with the economic threat cryoablation presented to traditional surgeons, would take nearly ten years to overcome. This was my first experience being an inventor and goring someone else's ox and it wasn't pretty!

It is inevitable that every innovation takes business away from someone. The automobile ruined the buggy-whip business. So after my editorial came out, a firestorm of political fist shaking ensued, with furious urologists angrily wanting to crush a "mere *diagnostic* radiologist" who had flippantly called surgeons "butchers."

I'm afraid this was the final straw that led me away from prostate cancer research, especially when a number of prominent urologists scolded me for daring to compare the "new and improved" radical prostatectomy to "butchery." This was never my intent but served as a good political rallying cry at the time.

I had hoped my paper would create *scientific* interest in cryoablation and prompt further work in sculpting lethal isotherms to rapidly expand its use to other areas of the body. Instead, it "killed the messenger"—the passion in me.

One thing became obvious: I was branded a heretic by many urologists at this point in my medical career, the year 1994. To my dismay, it seemed to me that my good intentions and impolitic naïveté set cryoablation further back than any gains I had made with "good science." Back to the drawing board, or should it have been charm school?

Chapter 3: Traditional Medicine Meets the Faith Healer

Laura

2/21/2003

Sunday, late afternoon, Manzanita, Oregon

After returning from Napa Friday evening, we drove down to the coast Saturday morning for the first of Emma's games at the Seaside, Oregon basketball tournament. The girls were all staying at a parent's huge new beach house in Cannon Beach, so Alex and I got to be alone at our cabin in Manzanita.

I watched Emma's first game at Seaside High School, which they handily won (they're so fun to watch). I took off to meet my friend for a massage while Alex and Emma stayed with the team for dinner in Seaside. I let my masseuse know what was going on with my health, and she worked on me with a shamanistic massage for one and a half hours. She said during the first half hour she almost threw up because of all the emotional garbage coming out surrounding the cancer scare issue. She said it was due to the medical handling of everything. She's the third healer now (along with Carlos and Sierra, an energy healer I consulted), who believes I don't have cancer. I'm going to be interested to hear what the lab report says.

***

Alex

Laura and I returned from Napa in a glow after Carlos assured us Laura had no cancer. Flying usually makes life's problems seem simple and small to me, as if life's challenges are far away and reduced to a few details which can be managed easily after landing.

This flight lacked that magic. The nagging worry about cancer invaded my mind at odd moments. Each time created a surge of fear and adrenaline.

This was fight or flight, but unfortunately you can't run from cancer; it's inside and travels with you! So you fight it. But Fight! wants results today, this minute, right now. So your body says, here's some adrenaline to work with!

My emotions said, "Go punch Mr. Cancer and then we can return to a normal life! It's ski season, not cancer season—Laura should be on the slopes exploring the powder in the trees."

However, cancer fighting requires patience, prayer and an alert, inquisitive mind. These every-five-minute bursts of adrenaline were exhausting me, taking me out of the fight.

The first smell of our beach cabin's cedar logs usually brings a flood of fond memories. But as I opened the door and the smell hit me, my first thought was, Laura might have cancer! This happy beach cabin we had built when Emma was little now triggered more distress by reminding me that if Laura died of cancer, she wouldn't be around to keep creating happy memories and instead the cabin would remind me of her and make me lonely.

I felt defeated because the happiest place on earth now made me worried she might die.

Supporting someone with cancer is not easy! It's hard to be cheerful and exude positive energy while enduring inner anxiety.

Emma's game and team celebration dinner afterward was a welcome distraction, taking my mind off cancer for an hour. I dropped Emma off for an overnight with her team and headed out into the dark night. Dark rain and a lonely road brought back the cancer alarms and it made me feel guilty since while I had been enjoying a victory dinner with the other parents, Laura was at our cabin getting a healing massage and dealing with her cancer. I felt terrible that I could escape cancer while she was stuck with it.

Fortunately, a warm and cheery fire greeted me, followed by rain. The gentle sound of the rain on the metal roof gave me the first good night's sleep I'd had since Laura's mammogram found "something suspicious." I woke refreshed and hopeful the biopsy would confirm Carlos's assertion that it had never been a malignant tumor.

***

Laura

2/28/2003, Tuesday

Well, I got "the call" this morning. A doctor taking over for my surgeon called to say the initial lab work shows I have breast cancer . . . "ductal carcinoma." The "good news" is the cells are "well differentiated," meaning they're more like breast cells, not the type that have degenerated, which means spreading. She is still waiting on the hormonal report, which will have more information.

I have an appointment next week with my surgeon. It will take about an hour for her to tell me all of my options. The doctor on the phone said there was a possibility they wouldn't even take the tumor out if I go on chemo.

I was surprised how calmly I took this news. It didn't "hit me in the gut" (most likely because my masseuse had cleaned out my negative energy). I just kept hearing my internal voice saying, "This report is wrong. The tumor is not there anymore. I saw Carlos take it out."

The doctor was concerned and sympathetic. But to give into her sympathy, I would have to give into her belief that I have cancer, and I'm not going, cannot go down, that road.

Even before calling Alex to tell him the bad news, I immediately called Tony, my German naturopath, and got an appointment for Thursday morning. Alex was sad but took it stoically like me. He'd seen the lump Carlos removed. It was a little smaller than a squished pea, with two humps, like a barbell. It was grayish pink. Carlos's opinion was that it wasn't cancer— it was too healthy looking. (He says most cancer tumors he takes out are dark red, even black.) So maybe our quick action seeing Carlos right away was correct. Perhaps he was wrong, it was a tumor, but he had removed it, so what they had biopsied was no longer inside me.

I also called my general internist, and I will see her tomorrow, Wednesday. I'm hoping she will assist me in mapping out a plan for a second opinion, which can check on the work of Carlos, and at the same time help me decide how to proceed with the other doctors. In the end, I want a clean bill of health from them.

***

Alex

What a dilemma! A faith healer said he removed something, but assured us that it was not cancer, just a cyst or something. But science disagrees and says it was a tumor. So if it was cancer and he was wrong about that, did he at least remove it, meaning Laura is now cancer free? Or is the truth that he removed nothing?

The only way to tell was to repeat the biopsy during a second examination of the area.

Radiologist, biopsy, mammogram, hospital, doctor, tumor, I hated all these words! Stage I ductal in situ carcinoma of the left breast. Ductal carcinoma and well differentiated, meaning it probably hadn't spread beyond the duct. As a result, they could infer that it wasn't an aggressive tumor because if it were, at this size, 3 cm, they would see it growing beyond the walls of the milk duct.

Another piece of good news: the tumor was estrogen dependent, so they could treat Laura later with an estrogen blocker and keep the cancer at bay for five years. The tumor was not too large, which was also good, Laura caught it early through regular mammograms. I shouldn't have said regular; she was overdue several months, and only a pleading letter from her primary physician, Dr. Fancher, got Laura to schedule a mammogram in January. Looking back, I think he was psychic, and I appreciated so much his insistence that Laura get a mammogram.

But there was nothing else good about the biopsy. As I had feared, we had should have seen Carlos before the biopsy, not after. Now how would we explain to anyone without them laughing at us that we believed, hoped (I didn't know what to believe now), that Laura needed a second biopsy to prove she didn't have cancer when she'd just had one to prove she did?

Laura scheduled a meeting with her internist to see if she could get another biopsy. I felt like we were punting in football. We hadn't advanced the ball, and now we had to give it up!

We walked through the door of the health clinic the next morning. It was my first visit to this new general practitioner Laura had switched to several years ago. Compared to previous doctor's offices, this was medical heaven! The magazines were current and they offered us coffee. I had never been to such a nice medical clinic.

The plush chairs in the waiting room had built-in writing desks. I noticed all the writing desks were on the right. Did they refuse left-handed patients? Or did left-handed people not get breast cancer?

Note to self: Check breast cancer statistics on left-handed patient incidence of cancer on Internet during morning web research, my mind added to my cancer research list.

I'm going crazy from Laura's cancer, I realized a second later.

"Laura, good to see you. And this is Alex?" Laura's internist is a tall woman with a calming presence and a soothing voice. She settled into her chair as if we were at Starbucks for coffee and she had all the time in the world.

I could see why Laura liked her internist. She behaved like a kindly sister who knows she is smarter than you but treats you politely: highly educated, sympathetic, caring, friendly, patient, someone "on your side."

We soon confessed our Napa Carlos trip and our hope to prove the biopsy was now not current.

"I'll set up the tests if you're convinced Laura was healed," she promised. "They may not be able to fit you in until the middle of March, or the end. But there's no harm in delaying the surgery for a while. And who am I to say that miracles don't occur? Just remember that time is going by and, at some point, if this faith healing is unsuccessful, Laura will need to have the tumor removed."

"When would you say is a good drop-dead date for a surgery?" Laura asked.

"I don't know if I feel comfortable referring to it as a 'drop-dead' date," the internist joked. We laughed, and she said Laura should have the tumor removed before the end of April, given the current size and growth rate. We agreed we had time, but the fear of metastasizing cancer blew a chill wind of urgency.

If this was football, the opposing team had just fumbled our punt and we had recovered. Take that, cancer! We're going to get another biopsy and show you who wins! I prayed the test would show the tumor gone.

Our life settled into an odd routine. Trying to cover all the bases, we are pursuing three alternative cures simultaneously. The first was to continue the quest for a spiritual miracle. Perhaps Laura had lacked enough faith and simply needed to see Carlos again.

The second and third attempts at a cure were alternative, naturopathic treatments from German and Chinese traditions. If the miracle failed and the tumors remained, alternative healing might have an effect. Perhaps the tumors would shrink, giving time to try and knock them back further with alternative healing so Laura could avoid a mastectomy.

Laura received some sort of alternative treatment nearly every other day. Her new job was battling for her breast. I kept rising early, searching the Internet for alternatives and reading obsessively.

Laura was determined to avoid mastectomy but it seemed hopeless because her surgeon had decreed a lumpectomy impractical. There were too many tumors spread around her breast and the lumpectomy protocol demands a safe margin of healthy tissue around each tumor. The bottom line? Given the tumor's configuration, there would be little remaining tissue after establishing safe margins.

Despite feeling defeated, I continued researching cancer. I read about microwave heating of tumors and therapies in other countries. On top of this, a good friend called. She insisted I take Laura to see John of God, a *for real* faith healer in Brazil. I was willing to go anywhere, but the possibility Carlos had failed dampened hope for a miracle from any healer.

All the while, the "Fight or Flight" adrenaline bursts were tearing me apart. After rising early each morning and researching cancer, it was difficult to focus on writing or business. Sometimes the mastectomy alternative seemed welcome—at least we'd be saving her life and things could return to a normal routine.

But I couldn't give up on Laura and her hope for an alternative, so I found myself praying a lot, and hoping that instead of words like "tumor" and "pathologist," I would someday once again hear Laura saying words from earlier winters, like, "This powder is too deep for me! Are you sure we should be skiing here?"

Sleep disappeared. I found myself at the computer Saturday morning March 1 at 3:30 a.m., determined to learn all about cancer. I pored over websites; they are endless. If you Google "breast cancer," you get your choice of 334 million results to review! If you add the word cure, your search drops to 27 million results. It seemed hopeless!

I soon found that most sites offer the same information. One exception I found on that early morning was a website by an Indian doctor. He advised doing nothing about cancer! He argued that cancer usually strikes old people whose time has come to die, and that doing nothing is the kindest treatment. If you cured an old person's cancer you would put them first through surgery, radiation and chemotherapy, a very unpleasant regimen, only to have that old person soon die of some other bodily failure. So why put an old person through agony trying to postpone the inevitable?

However, Laura was barely fifty. None of that "do nothing" stuff for me. We were at war, my enemy was her cancer, and one way or another, I/we were going to win!

Later that morning I received an e-mail from Carlos's wife. He was planning a trip to the Shasta area on the week of the fifteenth of March. When Laura awakened, I mentioned that it wouldn't hurt to see Carlos for a second time.

If the upcoming test scheduled by her internist, it was to be an MRI, showed the tumor was still there, then perhaps another chance at a miracle healing was being offered to us. And if it showed no tumor, we could always cancel.

She agreed, so I scheduled a road trip to Shasta.

Laura

3/11/2003, Tuesday

Last week, I had an MRI to see if Carlos had removed my tumor. It turned out that a third mammogram was not considered safe as it is an X-ray, and even if it is low dose, the exposure would be risky. So I had an MRI and, while waiting for the results, I received alternative healing. Yesterday I had a long morning working with the German naturopath's wife, Sherry Esau. She did a colonic and Reike session.

But today I got a call from my internist. The MRI showed the tumors are still there, two distinct tumors, close but separated. I don't want to give up. I have to try Carlos at least one more time, I'm glad Alex scheduled the trip, it seems a miracle Carlos came back to the West Coast so soon.

***

Alex

On Friday the 14th of March, we began our trip to Shasta in Northern California to visit Carlos a second time. This trip seemed pointless. Laura's MRI had showed Carlos had failed. The tumors were still there despite his claim he removed them.

We traveled because we hoped he could perform a miracle now though he hadn't before. I was going because I didn't want to believe we had failed. But if I were making a bet, it would be that Carlos would fail again. Still we went, canceling a long-planned trip to go see our second son, Louie, play college level lacrosse for Chapman in the national playoffs. He was disappointed we wouldn't come see him play, but he bravely understood.

We loaded up on healthy food for the trip. Laura was determined to avoid foods that might interfere with the treatments of her naturopath. We had a bite to eat in the deli where Laura dove into a mix of rice, eggplants, and noodles. I maintained my carnivorous ways.

"If I get cancer I'll never be able to defeat it with naturopathic medicine," I joked.

"You'd do it if you thought it would help," Laura replied.

"I don't know, I don't think I would pursue alternatives that insisted on vegetables alone."

"Eating vegetables is easier than having chemotherapy."

I'd bought a used Audi A-8 just before all this business of Laura's cancer had started. The purchase seemed extravagant after we learned of the cancer and I had thought of selling the car until we left town in a driving rain. The Audi drove through the rain-slicked surface as if glued to the road. I felt safe, under control, like a jet plane on wheels, motoring down to see Carlos. The control of the car was a welcome contrast to a life dealing with cancer out of control. I felt like it could give me control over all aspects of my life.

We stopped in Eugene. Rain continued the next morning, but when we reached Ashland, in southern Oregon, the midday sun made the drive feel like a family road trip instead of a desperate quest for a miracle healing. We reached Shasta in the afternoon and checked into a lovely ski lodge!

In the urgency of cancer, I'd forgotten Shasta had a ski area. I had always wanted to ski here. It broke my heart realizing we'd come to a ski area not to ski, but to see a faith healer for cancer.

The Audi's control of the road vanished in our room, replaced by cancer, depression, fears and the recent MRI proving cancer. Being at a ski area not to ski but to treat cancer gave me a glimpse of my own future. Someday, no matter how much I wanted to ski, I would hang up my beloved skis and never ride the mountain again.

As we scrambled to unpack and make the late afternoon healing meeting I resolved to myself to die in the summer so my last time skiing would be due to spring's arrival rather than a failing on my part. I want to end my last day spring skiing on corn snow wearing a sweater and getting hot. I want to do my last run in slushy snow, which grabs at your skis and slows you down near the bottom of the hill. I want to be completely exhausted and look up at the hill with the absolute conviction I would return next winter.

The house hosting Carlos lay in deep woods far to the west of Mt. Shasta. Leaden clouds hung over us as sunset drew near. The houses along the country road seemed random and endless, dropped from the sky like giant dice along this road until settling at an opening in the timber.

Just when I became convinced we'd missed the house and were headed for the national forest, we'd round a corner and find another house. And despite all this driving, Mt. Shasta kept looming over us, refusing to recede in the distance no matter how far we traveled, just like Laura's cancer.

All the houses sat far from the road behind pine trees, telling me these folks cherished privacy. We finally arrived. An old truck rested in a side yard. Ponderosa pines towered overhead; their castoff golden needles covered a pale yellow lawn. Snow began falling as we knocked on the door. A woman our age welcomed us inside.

Laura was instantly ushered upstairs to see Carlos and the woman left me alone in the living room. A ticking clock traded sounds with crackling from a wood stove. No music, conversation, or other sound filled the home. A huge dog came into the room, plodded over, sniffed me, lost interest, and then settled by the fire. I realized that as a dog owner, I didn't even notice the house probably smelled of dog. My nose had long ago grown accustomed to our own dogs.

The still, wood-stove heated house gave an impression that surviving winter was the main point of life here. Mt. Shasta loomed out a window, still seeming just as close. The thickening snow and vast forest surrounding the house felt claustrophobic by forbidding civilization from reaching this backwoods dwelling. The cold outside felt the opposite of the vibrant feeling I get in the tropics where nature freely hands out energy.

I soon identified with the sleeping, yellow lab, my only companion. Our common goal, my current definition of a successful life, was to stay warm, eat occasionally, and sleep often. I dozed off, weary from the long drive and worry.

Laura

3/15/2003

Shasta, California

My second meeting with Carlos. We drove down to Shasta to visit Carlos instead of going to Orange to watch Louie play lacrosse for Chapman University. We did this because the MRI showed that I still have two distinct tumors, close but separated. In addition, they saw two new, smaller lesions. This means the first visit to Carlos in Napa was a failure. The cancer is growing rather than vanishing.

After reviewing the results of the MRI, my surgeon's recommendation was to have a mastectomy because she'd have to take off half the breast in a lumpectomy and she didn't think I'd like the results.

I called Carlos after my visit with my surgeon and he said the doctor was wrong: that even if the MRI found lumps, they weren't cancer. My faith was restored by Carlos's confidence and we planned to leave on Friday evening.

On the morning before we left for Shasta, my tall, Chinese, Tuina and Qigong practitioner called. He is essentially a bone-setter/acupuncturist chiropractor. He said I could come over that afternoon. He'd just come back from China and said on the phone that his sister had once had a similar experience. They had wanted to take her breast off, but he worked with her through acupuncture, and she had another biopsy that turned out better, which allowed her to keep her breast. He applied acupuncture in a different way from the other acupuncture clinic that does Chinese medicine—so I've added a fourth alternative treatment technique.

I trust this tall, Chinese man, and his sister's success with cancer as proved by her second biopsy gave me great hope something is going to work.

The drive to Shasta allowed Alex and I to discuss everything. We're betting all our hopes on Carlos and the cure my homeopath is doing through German homeopathy and the Rife machine. If the biopsy I'm to have after the Shasta trip still says it's all failed, well, I guess it will be the mastectomy.

But I'm clear in my goal: I'd like to keep my breast. It's so wired with nerves; it still tingles with the letdown reflex when I see something my heart goes out to, like a cute baby or a puppy wagging its tail.

When I reached Carlos in Shasta, I told him everything that had happened medically after my first visit with him in Napa, and brought him up to date as to who was advising what. He just grunted and didn't comment on my words. Instead, he began healing; he went right to the breast and pulled out tissue with his hands. I am sure it was coming out of my body, I could feel a tugging sensation, but no pain, as he worked. And there was some blood coming from the area where he worked, although just a little and it was runny, not thick. Carlos showed me the tissue as he removed it and dumped it into a plastic tub. The tissue was dark red. When he finished he called down to Alex and asked him to come up and look at it too. Carlos let us pick it up and feel it.

It did feel like clots or tissue and it was not like the tumor he said he had removed on the first visit. That tissue he showed me was grayish-pink, pearly, and hard. He said he could see how the doctors thought they were still there because the MRI picked up this tissue that filled up the hole where the tumors had been.

This made sense, even my surgeon had said that if she did a lumpectomy, tissue would fill up the hole after she takes the tumor out, so for a while, it would look like it was a similar size. This made me feel a lot better and even more hopeful about the next biopsy. It was possible that the recent MRI was just showing scar tissue, because when my homeopath had worked on me, his "Rife machine" had made a circular bruise on my nipple and the MRI had shown that bruise as it is a sensitive machine.

Now I'm waiting for my last biopsy. If it still shows that I have cancer, then it's time for the mastectomy.

But I'm not without hope that the biopsy will be fine, even if Carlos has failed me. After all, I've been on the German medicine for four weeks now. It consists of a catalyst to dump cancer causing toxins and an injection of mistletoe under the stomach skin to stimulate the immune system. This is an accepted practice of medicine in Germany but not something practiced by MDs here in the US. Alex did some research and read that Germans spend about $30 million a year on various forms of mistletoe to fight cancer and that many German doctors recommend therapies for their patients that aren't like those available in the United States. Evidently, mistletoe is one of the most commonly recommended alternatives.

At first, the German medicine gave me waves of fevers and terrific pain in my armpits and groin. I learned to control the pain by stretching, exercising, bathing in saltwater and vinegar, and scrubbing hard with a big stiff bath brush.

I also meditate on white light, running it down my arms and into my hands, which I cup over my breast. Just what Carlos told me to do (I've already been doing it).

I've also been getting weekly colonics from Sherry Esau. She told me to go on a vegan diet and juices twice a day. I was proud to report to her that my wonderful son Sean had helped me get a new Jack Lalane juicer to do just this! And Alex has already found a Rife machine online, which I'm now using twice a week. The electric current is supposed to be able to kill tumors. I don't know if it will work, but I'm doing all I can!

I'm feeling radiantly healthy, except my armpits hurt now and then. I want to chart it all out, so if I'm successful, I'll have a record.

Carlos's parting advice was: don't let them biopsy for at least three days after my treatment. And he also said don't let them cut on you and rush you into a mastectomy; get them to compare apples to apples, the old biopsy and the new one I'll be getting. And ask about the MRI I just had: if the lumps are not gone due to his work, and if the biopsy I now hope to get soon indicates that they are malignant tumors, has their size changed, or has the composition changed? Don't cut, he advises; buy time to keep healing!

After speaking with Carlos when I was in Shasta and having my confidence restored in his healing powers, I called my surgeon when we returned and asked if I could get yet another biopsy. She said yes; she'd set up an ultrasound biopsy, a biopsy done this time using ultrasound so she could locate and sample both tumors. She also said that we could wait for the mastectomy until she was back from her spring break vacation with her kids.

Maybe Carlos removed nothing this last time in Shasta. I don't know but here I am, resting and journaling after seeing him before my surgeon does yet another biopsy.

***

Alex

While Laura was still in with Carlos, I awoke and our host brought coffee and pointed out a TV set I hadn't noticed. I turned it on and the gloom of the forest vanished as CNN reported developing events concerning Iraq. War seemed imminent. Finished with Laura, Carlos called me upstairs and gave me a healing session. I assumed that my treatment method was the same as Laura's and I felt skeptical.

He had me lie on a massage table covered with a sheet. He ran his hands over me, beginning at my feet, seeming to do a combination massage with some "diseased" tissue removal as well. The removal process was in areas that were sore or injured, and not anything I told him of, so that impressed me.

The actual removal felt like he was scratching my skin. If he was removing tissue, there was no pain. At one point he had me lie face down and worked on my neck, again in a place that was sore, and a combination of water and blood flowed down my neck. Later, when I rose from the table, I saw the stains on the white cloth before he removed it.

Was it my blood on the sheet? Before, based on the healings I had from Carlos's mother and other Filipino psychic surgeons I met after my father's experience, I would have said yes. Now? With failures dogging his attempts to heal Laura, I wasn't sure.

I didn't want to jinx Laura's healing by having negative thoughts. But we talked after he was done and he stated that he "got everything" out of Laura today. My radar was screaming fraud. Did he not remember he claimed to have done that last time?

The tests after the Napa trip had proved him wrong the first time. The second biopsy awaiting Laura in Portland after this trip would probably repeat that disappointment. I drove back to the Inn feeling foolish to believe in the possibility of a miracle cure for cancer. I had hoped Carlos would be as successful as the Philippine healer had been with my father.

I felt bitter and wondered if it was possible that some faith healers worked while others didn't. It was frustrating not knowing if one was effective and another not, that there was no AMA listing of miracle healers!

Confused and conflicted, I didn't say anything to Laura; I didn't want to dash her hopes. Besides, the war was depressing enough!

"Carlos took some more stuff out. He says he has the last of it now and not to worry," Laura repeated over dinner. We were eating in a beautiful Swiss-style après ski restaurant. Tables full of young skiers in sweaters bubbled with excitement over the great snow and the promise of good powder tomorrow.

On the one hand, I'd wanted to ski, and on the other, skiing seemed irrelevant. The dog who had kept me company that afternoon didn't ski. He knew the correct way to winter. Stay warm, eat, sleep a lot, and make sure you don't die in the cold. Maybe tomorrow would be sunny.

The weather rewarded that old dog's patience and my own. The morning brought a new, sunny day. As I packed the car, the cool mountain wind filled my lungs while the sunshine gave a warming promise of spring.

The sunshine and soft air promised it was going to be a day of spring skiing, where the fresh snow would be wet, not dry, and it would make a whistling sound as skiers cut fresh tracks. I'd been in those conditions at least a hundred times before and knew all that from the feel of the air.

But our fate was not on the slopes. It was Sunday and people fresh from church packed the Mt. Shasta Black Bear Diner, our favorite breakfast restaurant. The bustle of servers carrying huge trays of food and the animated conversation put cancer and the war in retreat. I drove home confident, renewed, and full of optimism. Perhaps this time the healing had worked. More tests lay ahead for Laura. Brave girl.

***

Laura

3/17, 2003, Monday

After doing grades at Portland State University on the Monday after returning from Shasta, I went to lunch with my department chair. Told him I was sick and might not be able to continue teaching. He supported my decision, especially when I told him of my use of alternative medicine. (I didn't tell him what was wrong with me.) He assured me my job was secure and the most important consideration was my health.

The next day, Tony Esau's tests did not show I had breast cancer. He has a machine from Germany. It requires that I hold two brass electrodes hooked to a computer, which then can diagnose me. It indicated that I have only fibroid tumors, a benign condition. He said this would be a natural condition if the virus that causes breast cancer "transmuted" itself to a new condition. The new tinctures he gave me are for fibroids and scar tissue.

There was a full, bright rainbow outside the clinic's office door. Alex had driven me to my appointment, and as we left, he said it was my good omen. Finally—hope!

***

Alex

On Monday, March 20, 2003, we went to war against Iraq. Operation Iraqi Freedom. I heard later it was going to be called Operation Iraqi Liberation, but someone caught the unfortunate acronym OIL in time and switched the last word to Freedom.

Did Iraq have weapons of mass destruction? Sadaam had threatened to attack America and kill millions of us. While it seemed impossible he could attack us, I had read that he had biological labs for making diseases and some experts worried he could unleash smallpox as an aerosol spray that would go undetected in a shopping mall, or even Disneyland.

I might have been paranoid, or stupid, or too conservative, but I was not happy with Sean and Louie being in Los Angeles, a possible attack site, at the start of this war. Maybe it was simply all the stress of Laura's cancer, but I asked them to come home until the world settled down. They were going to miss some school, but I told them to tell the teachers they were coming home to visit their mother, recently diagnosed with breast cancer, which was an excellent excuse but also the sad truth.

Faith told me Laura didn't have cancer, that Carlos's psychic surgery had worked. Logic told me it hadn't worked and we were just deluding ourselves. I vowed to intensify my breast cancer research on the Internet, although I didn't know if I could.

Between worrying about Laura and the war, I was never asleep past 4:30 a.m., and lately, I had been skipping work and searching obsessively on the Internet all day long for some hope or cure.

I loved all the doctors/counselors/friends who advised, "Calm down, avoid stress!" I'd love to avoid it! Stress grabs you in an unavoidable situation. Stress is not a TV channel that you can change. Stress is a bear rushing at you and no trees in sight, or some men holding you down on a guillotine with your hands tied behind you as an executioner reaches for the blade release.

I think a person's fight or flight response would kick in if he was on a guillotine. That's how cancer, or loving someone with cancer, feels. Avoid stress? Cope with stress? Ha! Good luck. The blade is dropping.

By March 21, the day after the war's beginning, the boys were safely home. It was exciting, calling them on their cell phone as they made their way up I-5 from LA while the bombing was going on in Baghdad. I was filled with so many emotions.

Friends of mine had died in Vietnam. Now my boys were the right age to fight, and their friend was going to Iraq soon as Sean found out a few days earlier. His friend's Marine Reserve Engineering battalion in Portland had been called up.

At the beginning of the year 2000 I had imagined the new millennium would be one of peace and progress. I had my order form ready for my flying car, and money saved for my moon vacation. Instead, the new century brought Vietnam II. A war with vague motives, one you're not to object to because that would be unpatriotic and somehow help the enemy. No amount of protesting the war was going to help the Iraqis. They were toast!

Our boys' energy filled the house. They were home and safe. Safe for now—but how long would this war last, and would they and their friends have to go and fight? And was the war a just cause or a trumped-up excuse to steal oil?

I was pouring my life into getting Laura healthy and didn't dwell on thinking about the war. The anxiety of worrying about her gnawed at me and I couldn't sleep. Seven days a week, I woke up at precisely 4:30 a.m. and went to the computer. I researched breast cancer for several hours before going to work.

At night, it was the same. I became an electronic cancer-information vacuum, sucking up data about percentages of survival, chemotherapy yes or no, Tamoxifen—is it safe? and a million other facts and questions.

Still, after all this, nothing looked promising. Cancer is a controlled crash, a long skid on ice where you steer your best. The best hope is to live long enough that another malady, stroke or heart attack kills you first. Remission is not cure. It is a cessation, a truce, a pause, a bargain with death to return later. We never beat death; we just avoid our appointment as long as possible.

***

Laura

3/23/2003, Sunday

Went to yoga this morning with Sean. He and Louie drove up from LA last Thursday and Friday. They came because the war started Thursday (Disneyland, which is close to Chapman University, is a potential terrorist target), and they came because of me. It is wonderful having them here, their energy and their presence. Just being around them picks me up a lot.

Last Wednesday, I got a shot of catalyst and a shot of mistletoe from Tony Esau. This is a German naturopathic technique. The catalyst is a tincture that Tony formulated. It is designed to help the cells dump toxins that might be stimulating the cancer.

The mistletoe comes from Germany. It is in liquid form and I get it injected just under the skin of my stomach about once every two weeks. These shots are designed to stimulate my immune system. According to Tony, this is an anti-cancer procedure which is well-recognized and accepted in Germany.

Following these shots, I went to Shizeng Yang, my Chinese Tuina and Qigong specialist. He proceeded to load up my breast with needles and then hooked two of them up to electrodes. I was sore that night so I didn't use the Rife machine until the next night, and then I used the Rife electrodes right on the breast. When I woke up Friday morning, something was wrong. I felt heavy and funky and awful. I tried to help Alex with the dishes but couldn't. I think I managed to get some fresh juice made, but then collapsed on the couch. I just felt terrible. Then I remembered that Tony had said that reactions to the Koch medicine come in threes, three days, three weeks, and three months. Now I'm going to have to figure out what kind of reactions he means, but I definitely felt like I didn't want to reside in my body. Dr. Ferrier called to get an update and when I was through telling her, she just said "wow."

She could see why I wanted to give alternative healing my all when she heard the surgeon's recommendation was a mastectomy. She finally finished with telling me that if that was the way it had to go, at least I knew I'd tried everything, I'd given it my all. I can't tell how skeptical she is on all this, but she was glad to hear I'm keeping notes and plan to give her a full report.

By Saturday morning the aches had passed. Actually, they started passing the night before when Alex rubbed my knees and ankles, which were very sore. Also the dinner he gave me felt good—I needed food energy. We walked with backpacks filled with weights up and over Council Crest and it felt wonderful. Later in the day, he and Emma took off for the spring break vacation we had planned at Sun Valley.

They really wanted me along, and we imagined this would be over by then, but my Qigong practitioner said I needed to rest and keep my energy for fighting the cancer and for healing, so I shouldn't go. When I told him I felt relieved that I decided not to go, he explained that deep down inside, I didn't want to go. My body wanted to save its energy for fighting the cancer and until it's confirmed that the cancer is gone, I want to concentrate on doing everything I possibly can to fight it. My goal is to clean my body, be detoxified and healthy. This is the longest time I've had something that my mind has a hard time getting away from. It will start to wander, then is pulled back to the awful words, "You have breast cancer." I better use some energy skills to send those words away.

It's surreal having the war going on. It reminds me of that awful time after my family's accident when the Vietnam War was going on. It seemed like there was no relief from the reality we were in.

No one's in the neighborhood now. Everyone is gone on spring break. There are mostly nature noises outside where I'm sitting on the deck writing this. It's late afternoon and the "Oscars" begin soon, which will be a great diversion. Alex has called from Sun Valley. They've already skied three hours and are exhausted. My heart is with them. The boys are resting, Sean asleep, Louie reading in the recliner massage chair. It's nice to be able to process what's going on.

***

Alex

The days passed quickly until it came down to the last day before Laura, Emma, and I had planned to leave for Sun Valley. Emma announced that at least she and I should go to Sun Valley and try to recreate the fun we had the previous year, even if Laura couldn't go. The boys couldn't come along; they had to leave by the weekend, and we were leaving on Tuesday. Sean and Louie said they'd stay with Laura until the day before we returned, so she wouldn't be lonely.

Emma and I headed for Sun Valley on a dark, rainy, Tuesday night at six. I drove with a heavy heart leaving Laura behind. After all the work I had done trying to find an alternative cure, I could do little now but wait for an ultrasound-guided biopsy which would confirm or deny Carlos's miracle.

I drove hoping the biopsy would prove a miracle cure had occurred while dreading it would prove nothing, no miracle or alternative therapy, had worked. If so, Laura would need a mastectomy; meaning, I had failed.

When you drive east on 84 out of Portland, the city lingers with you for a while. The lights of Troutdale and truck stops extend the cheer and oasis feeling of the city, even on a dark night. I felt fine and confident until we crossed the Sandy River Bridge. After you cross that river all civilization and lights drop away irrevocably, and you swear you are retracing Lewis and Clark's journey back to St. Louis.

Once while elk hunting in Eastern Oregon, I walked on Chief Joseph's winter migration trail from Joseph Lake to Lewiston, Idaho. It is a narrow trail running above a stream and nothing within view displays any sign of the white man's presence. This night felt the same.

Only the thin ribbon of freeway and the warmth of our car reminded us of civilization. Even with those comforts, the rain, the dark, and the cliff walls of the Columbia Gorge loomed over us. The next outpost of civilization waited hours away. The raw, edgy land encouraged the wind to grab our car and shake it. All the while, the cold Columbia ran on our left, waves slapping the banks, corners in the road drawing us to and then turning us away from the water as headlights revealed threatening, white wave crests.

Depression suffocated me. What was I doing? How could I leave Laura with a failing miracle and go off skiing? What if all the alternative therapies had failed as well? Soon she would find they had failed, every one, and the cut of a mastectomy would represent salvation, despite all my efforts to find an alternative.

If not for my love of Emma and not wanting to disappoint her dream of skiing Sun Valley, I would have turned the car around. Only her excitement kept me going. She looked out at the dark and storms, and said, "It feels like we're finally on our way to Sun Valley!"

My leaden sky of no civilization merely proved to Emma that fun was on the way. Beauty is indeed in the eyes of the beholder.

With that note of cheer, she turned on her CD player, put on her earphones, and disappeared from the car. She was right there, of course, but unless I insisted she listen to me, the trip became a lonely grind. Only the sweep of water on the windshield when I passed cars broke the routine. There were moments of occasional cheerful chatter when she grew bored with her music and talked to me.

I sometimes call Emma, Tinkerbell, because one of her little smiles or happy insights is like magic dust that can make a person happy with life for hours. She was right, and I felt better for a while because it did feel like we were finally on our way to a fun break in Sun Valley.

However, as I drove along, my mind dwelled on the whole experience of Laura's cancer. The beginning with the terrible news, the early denial, hope for a Carlos miracle, promise of alternatives from foreign lands, then disappointment after disappointment as nothing worked. Now, when the last inevitable disappointment loomed ahead, I was running away.

I wanted to go back, but I wanted to go to Sun Valley and ski. I wanted Laura to not lose her breast, and I wanted Emma to have a good time skiing. I finally found solace in the thought there was nothing I could do now to alter the results of Laura's pending biopsy, and I'd be back to support her when she went in.

I realized then, I think for the first time, that I might be powerless to help Laura. No matter how much I wanted it, perhaps she had no alternative to the mastectomy, and even worse, maybe even that would not cure her. The only power I had was to fulfill Emma's dream to ski Sun Valley. So, I resolved that was my mission, no matter how miserable I felt; I would see to it that Emma had some fun on her spring break. Inside she had to be hurting as well, and the least I could do was help relieve her pain for a little while.

I warmed to my task of bringing cheer to Emma and realized whatever lay ahead with Laura's cancer, it would take strength. Getting in a few fun days might help with the battle ahead. With that attitude, I settled into the drive and started to enjoy the road-handling abilities and power of the Audi. We got into the high desert past the eastern edge of the Cascades and the skies cleared, revealing beautiful stars and a dry road. Maybe there is hope after all, the desert sky and stars whispered to me. The prelude to Sun Valley and its blue-sky sunshine was always desert dark and stars. Dark before light—possibly a metaphor for Laura's cancer?

I increased the speed and asked Emma how fast she thought we were going.

"I don't know, sixty?"

"Nope, eighty!"

"That's great, Daddy." Back on went the headphones.

"How fast now?" I tugged her on the arm.

"Seventy?"

"Nope, eighty-five."

Headphones and silence.

"Now?"

"Two hundred miles an hour? Daddy, please, I'm trying to listen!"

Alone, I appreciated the joy of the best car I have ever driven. I realized it made me feel like when I go flying and all my problems seem manageable.

I had no control over Laura's cancer, but it felt good to feel in control of the road!

Sun Valley was fun but sad. It felt odd not skiing with Laura; we had skied together for thirty-three years. It was a time of "not's": not having dinner with Laura, not being in the hot tub with Laura, not hearing her cheerful observations on the world. And when Emma joined her pals at night going to the Sun Valley Lodge bowling alley, the room was so lonely.

For the first time in this whole cancer battle, my imagination wandered beyond the operation and the struggle. Is this what I'm in for in a few years? Life as a single dad? After all, Laura's mother had died within two years of her diagnosis of breast cancer. Was this an aggressive cancer? Did Laura even stand a chance? I said many prayers. I didn't want to lose her. There had to be hope somewhere out there!

Sunshine, skiing, and friends filled each day. Nights were much worse, alone in the room, watching TV, my mind obsessing on life without Laura.

I found a movie, *Sun Valley Serenade*, playing 24/7 on one of the lodge cable channels. I watched it every night because Sonja Henie looked so much like Laura, was bubbly like Laura, athletic like Laura. I realized I had first seen Sonja when I was a young boy suffering long bouts of bronchitis and watching old black and white movies during the daytime as I recuperated. Sonja was an Olympic athlete and skater and had a brief film career in the early thirties. Here in Sun Valley, I rediscovered the very woman I had watched at age 10 and had then considered the most beautiful woman in the world.

Until seeing the movie, I didn't realize Laura looked so much like Sonja! Laura acted like Sonja as well. Maybe I fell in love with Laura while watching Sonja as a boy, and it just took another dozen years of searching for me to find her. I decided to name the Audi "Sonja" because I had already planned it would be Laura's car after the operation, if she needed it, so she could be safe driving around on all her upcoming doctor visits.

Emma and I stayed for only three days; it hardly seemed worth it, two and a half days of driving for three days of skiing. But for fourteen-year-old Emma it was all worth it. Her goggle tan guaranteed a triumphant final spring term in the eighth grade because it was proof she had vacationed and skied instead of being stuck in Portland.

I drove fast, wanting to get back to Laura. I felt, irrationally, that if I were there, I could help her fight cancer better. Being away had felt like allowing her to die. We left Sun Valley at noon and got in at one in the morning. I drove thirteen hours straight and never stopped more than ten minutes at any one time. By the time we rolled into Portland, I was in love with Sonja—not the actress, the Audi.

Holding Laura in my arms reaffirmed her life. The next morning, I took her in for her biopsy, this time guided by ultrasound to make sure it was accurate. We returned in time to see Sean and Louie off to college. They'd seen their mom, there hadn't been a terrorist attack on Los Angeles, and it was safe for them to return to their lives. Talk about counting your blessings; they are two huge blessings in our lives.

Laura

3/28/2003, Friday

Alex and Emma got home late Wednesday night so Alex could take me to my biopsy appointment Thursday morning. They skied Wednesday morning at Sun Valley, and then left for home after lunch. A thirteen-hour drive by Alex without anyone to help him! He really loves me and is so supporting me. It gave me such comfort to have him with me at the hospital.

The waiting room had a nasty feel of desperation and a smell of fear. There was a problem with the case before mine, which made it take longer. An attendant called patients in by repeatedly announcing their name. In each case, she greeted the patient with a mechanical sounding "sorry you had to wait." I felt sorry for these patients having to start their appointments in such a disrespected, dehumanizing way.

Finally, it was my turn. However, she called me just as I started heading down the hall to go to the bathroom. I reversed course and reported in. Hearing I needed to visit the restroom first, the technician didn't give the standard, "sorry you had to wait." Instead, we agreed I could use the restroom inside the ultrasound center.

The technician seemed a bit harried and anxious. She told me she had seventeen years of experience but that today a second technician would join us. This new person would be overseeing the procedure and demonstrating a new way to use the ultrasound machine. This second technician was younger and more confident, friendly in a slightly impersonal way. They hurriedly went over what would be going on, telling me in a way that only confused me. I changed and lay on the exam bed. It was cold. Soon I began to shiver. The first technician went to work finding the tumors, two dark spots appeared on the screen, oval shaped, a larger one with a smaller one next to it. She looked for another in the "three o'clock" position but couldn't find it. The surgeon had told me there were two more small spots found by the MRI in addition to the two main tumors.

Carlos had taken took two small lumps out on my second healing treatment in Shasta. He had pointed out that one had a small dark spot on it, so maybe the inability of the technicians to find anything more than the two tumors was proof that Carlos could miraculously remove tissue.

Soon the doctors came in, an older woman and a young man. The male doctor was business-like and professionally brisk. The woman doctor was slower and more thoughtful. She saw red splotches on my neck, which suggested to her I was nervous. She offered for me to hold her fingers, which I was happy to do.

At this point, they asked if I ever got sick at the dentist as the plan was to give me Novocain to numb the pain. I couldn't remember, so they told me I would have remembered if I ever had. When I asked what the reaction usually was, they told me a headache, which I later did get. We began. The male doctor got right to work. He was impressive as his subtle commands made the technicians jump. The older technician seemed to be trying to impress everyone by showing she was still up to par with everything expected of her.

Before he began, the doctor said he needed to make a small incision. I voiced my surprise; this hadn't been explained before. He gave me a placating look, so I didn't object. He was quick, which I appreciated. In less than 15-20 minutes, he'd taken six samples, three at each site. A sharp, clicking sound accompanied the taking of each sample.

Two of them didn't feel numbed by Novocain, but I didn't flinch. I was happy for the doctor's fingers to squeeze. At one point, she left to answer the male doctor's cell phone and I missed her fingers. The last click had a softer sound. I wondered if it was because the sites were soft and not hard. I watched it all on the monitor.

I was happy to have it done. It satisfied me that this process was well documented and witnessed. If a miracle healing had occurred, no one would be able to question it. I fully believe, with this procedure, the worst is behind me.

Being cut into put me into a semi state of shock and I was happy to have Alex's arm to lean on. I was happy to make it to the car and then home, jammies, and the couch with Emma's warm quilt around me.

Emma sweetly took over the entertainment duties. We watched the Ya Ya Sisterhood while I drifted in and out of sleep and Emma filled me in. Then she went downstairs and found Aladdin. At first, I objected, but now I'm so glad she did. Those happy songs keep ringing in my ears.

Friday morning I cleaned and got ready to go to Las Vegas for Emma's soccer game. About two hours before we needed to leave, Alex discovered that he'd lost the tickets. Many phone calls and online computer work later, we decided to go to the airport since they told us that for $300 extra we'd still make our plane.

On the way to the airport, we still couldn't decide if we were doing the right thing, so we pulled over for a family discussion. I said it seemed the flow of events was pointing to us going to the beach instead of a frantic soccer tournament in Las Vegas. How about , I suggested, if one more obstacle got in our way, we'd give up the idea of going to Las Vegas? Everyone agreed.

We got the obstacle. At the airport, we found out it would cost $1,000 each to go. When Emma said she was happy to give up on the soccer trip, we happily gave up on the idea and went to dinner at the airport. Sushi for me. My body was still recovering from the biopsy procedure yesterday. I realized as I ate that my body hadn't wanted Las Vegas, just as it hadn't wanted Sun Valley.

3/29/2003, Saturday

At our Manzanita Beach Cabin

The lazy sun is taking its time to finish the afternoon. I'm up in the loft of the cabin because the sun's shining here and I wouldn't be able to stand the stench on the deck. Both dogs rolled in something nasty and are waiting on the deck until Alex and Emma get home from their bike ride and we'll have enough people for a good dog wash.

The last time I was here with my artist friend from Houston it was pouring rain. It's much nicer to have the weather fair the last weekend of spring break. It seemed so far away at one time. With everything going on, the spring break has crept up in a most unscripted way.

This is a much better, more peaceful environment to recover from my biopsy last Thursday. I'll hear the results next week. While the wait is grueling, I'm getting used to waiting under pressure. Besides, I have a calmness put in place by chi dong treatments and Reike that I had this morning before we left for the beach.

One treatment happened after the other, Reike first from Sherry Esau. Afterward, she said my shoulders had sucked energy like they had the weight of the world on them. We talked and decided it was because I felt I owed the doctors an explanation if the biopsy came up negative or any other hopeful outcome. She assured me I didn't owe the doctors an explanation and that took the burden off me. I did let it go and it felt good. Obviously, the doctors have already bought into the medical paradigm, or they wouldn't be practicing it. Even if a miracle healing happens to me, it will be the exception, not the rule. A miracle isn't going to change the doctor's thinking.

I suppose if more women refuse to get their breast removed and look for alternatives, the doctors may take notice because the flow of money is important. There have to be some better answers (and outcomes), than the medical establishment is offering us. And I guess I hope to show there is.

April 1, Tuesday (April Fools Day!)

Still no word on my biopsy. I had it last Thursday.

April 2, Wednesday

Still no call this morning. The doctor at the biopsy, the male doctor, said that it would take the lab two business days to have the results. I gave all three of my medical doctors' names and addresses to send the results to, so you'd think one of them would at least call me if they had the results.

My sister Kay, who called last night, thinks it's because the results have them stumped. I'd like to think so, too, but I remember it took a full week, Wednesday to Wednesday, to get the results of the MRI. In fact, it might even have been longer.

This week, my surgeon returned from a week on vacation, so she is probably scrambling to catch up. I guess I didn't trust her timeliness so that's why I gave the other doctors our address information. I hope one will call soon.

I had help during my anxious moments yesterday from my older sister. After my framing errand, I tried to nap but the phone kept ringing: first my younger sister, then my older sister. We had a wonderful long talk and discovered, because of her optimism, that my "Sponge Bob-Ness," i.e. naïve optimism, runs in our family. Then a friend from the beach called as well. It's hard keeping all these wonderful supporters in limbo with me. At least I know I'm loved.

The war goes on and I go on. The tension seems almost palpable: I long for a day without tension.

April 2, 2003, Wednesday Evening

What a long strange trip it's become. I'm finally seeing God's guiding hand in my healing. Last Wednesday I got a call from Todd, my yoga teacher, about a mat I'd bought. I let him know what was going on with me, and he was wonderful, encouraging and generous with his thoughts. He closed with the advice that when circumstances look hard and difficult I should "Lean gently into your faith and let it guide you." He reinforced what I already knew, that this was a time to be present and calm and centered, to make all the right decisions.

With that inspiration guiding me, and Alex's encouragement, I made the call to the doctor's office to get my results. The office said they'd just gotten them and were about to call. Unfortunately, the results showed that I still had cancer. I asked if there was any significant improvement and the nurse aide, Kim, said, "None I can see." I asked that she fax this biopsy result and the earlier one to me. I received them, but without a doctor to interpret, I was at a loss to tell the difference. The size wasn't even measured in the new test, even though I had specifically asked the technician to do so. Somehow, discouragement did not overwhelm me. I leaned into my trust of God. Before I made the phone call, I'd asked angels to be with me.

Alex came down to the basement (I had called from downstairs to be private to get the results). He consoled me, and then he left shortly after to jump on the computer as he wanted to follow up a lead on an advertised procedure called "cryosurgery" he'd first seen on a Chicago TV channel carried by our cable system.

I put my head down on the table thinking about how much I'd gotten attached to my breast, and how I wanted a "matched set." I didn't want to lose it. Then, as if a voice was whispering in my ear, I heard the question, "Why are you so sad? You can still have your breast if you want it." I felt a presence, and then the sensation of an arm around my shoulder. Although I was alone and Alex was upstairs making phone calls, I felt calm.

Chapter 4: Dr. Littrup—Life After the Firestorm

Dr. Littrup

I became so discouraged with prostate cancer treatment that I virtually left the field and took up the offer of another surgical colleague. Dr. Donald Weaver of the Karmanos Cancer Institute in Detroit is perhaps one of the most wonderful human beings I've ever met. Beyond his dedication and humanity, he's a superb surgeon, a compassionate practitioner of medicine and, with his subdued, kind ego, he is what we call in medicine "the complete package."

Don sat and listened to my tale of woe; how the people I had offended with my "Butcher Baker" editorial reply were vilifying me. He simply said to me, "Well, Gary Onik started all this cryo in the liver, and we have one of his machines here. Forget about the urologists for awhile and see what you can do with me and Dr. Bouwman in the liver."

The three of us went to work as a team performing cryoablation for liver cancer. At the same time, I was appointed Associate Professor of Radiology, Urology and Radiation Oncology at Wayne State University School of Medicine with my main offices at Harper Hospital in downtown Detroit. Karmanos Cancer Institute, where Don worked, is in the same complex of Harper Hospital's buildings and shares facilities with the hospital.

Ten years passed and, in that time, I did over 200 open liver cryotherapies. By the early 2000s, I had trained Don to the point where he could do all but the most complicated of liver cryotherapies on his own. More importantly, Don had healed my confidence and helped restore my reputation as a solid, proficient radiologist/cryosurgeon. I was a full-time member of the radiology staff at Harper Hospital, doing my duty in traditional radiology, and I worked on the side assisting in liver operations where cryoablation was now a prime treatment modality.

Meanwhile, our early partner in cryoablation, Dr. Bouwman, had gone on to become head of breast cancer surgery at Karmanos Cancer Institute. Although he was still performing general cancer surgeries, he knew what cryoablation could accomplish if adopted and carried out correctly.

In the years after my ill-fated paper, cryoablation had become recognized as a beneficial treatment for prostate cancer, complete with billing codes and acknowledgment by the Centers for Medicare and Medicaid Services (CMS). This had been accomplished primarily through the efforts of my good friend, mentor, and colleague, Dr. Fred Lee, Sr.

While I shrank away from taking the step of going into private practice and offering prostate cryosurgery after the horrible response to my editorial comment regarding prostate treatment in urology, Fred Lee took the opposite course. He struck out on his own and developed a superb cryoablation treatment center. He initially offered it to patients who wanted the benefits of cryoablation and who could afford to pay for it without insurance. His early work opened the door for general acceptance of cryoablation.

One criticism of cryoablation had been that it sometimes failed to kill the entire tumor. Fred did pioneering research in the use of thermocouples (or thermometers), placed along the outer margins of the prostate, which helped control the freezing by multiple cryoprobes spaced evenly throughout the prostate. His research proved that if appropriate temperatures were reached, cryoablation was over 90 percent effective in killing the whole prostate.

In 1999, prostate cryoablation got a huge boost when it was allowed for insurance reimbursement. This caused a boom in the adoption of cryoablation for prostate treatment, especially by urologists who could sometimes collect a better fee than from surgery.

In addition, Gary Onik had demonstrated that a properly controlled freeze could maintain the sexual function of a prostate cancer patient. While I had suggested the feasibility of this procedure based on my research with dogs in an article in the *Seminars of Interventional Radiology in 1994*, it had taken nearly ten years for Dr. Onik to have pioneered and accomplished successful human results. He even wrote a book in 2006 entitled, *The Male Lumpectomy*, which described his tremendous success in healing patients and at the same time sparing potency. This increased even more the appeal of using cryoablation for prostate cancer treatment, as the potential now exists for men receiving cryoablation to kill their tumor, possibly get an immune effect from the freeze process, have less pain and problems with incontinence and, on top of all this, retain their potency.

During this time of progress in prostate cryoablation, I toiled away at KCI doing liver cancer cryoablation. It seemed ironic to me that cryoablation had become well positioned for cancer treatment in the prostate but not for breast cancer. This seemed especially true when one of cryoablation's most recently touted advancements, the saving of potency function, actually borrowed from the term "lumpectomy," which had been coined to describe the removal of the lump from a breast and avoiding a mastectomy.

Even more ironic was the fact that some of the earliest historical uses of cryoablation had been in the field of breast cancer treatment, as is shown later in the chapter on the history of cryoablation. At the same time, laboratory work on the immune effects sometimes occurring after cryoablation had also focused on breast cancer.

The slow adoption of cryoablation for treating breast cancer reminded me of George Santayana's famous quote, "Those who cannot learn from history are doomed to repeat it."

Ignorance regarding the application of cryoablation for breast and other cancers can also be explained by considering a quote from Gustave Flaubert, "Our ignorance of history causes us to slander our own times."

It seemed to me that the ten year's of success treating the prostate with cryoablation had occurred as if in a virtual vacuum when it came to breast cancer treatment. As far as breast cancer was concerned, cryoablation didn't even exist.

No matter what slowed the advancement of cryoablation in breast cancer treatment, looking back I wonder if perhaps as a group we had to apply cryoablation in one of the most difficult organs to freeze, the prostate. This allowed us to eventually use it wisely in an easily treated organ, the breast, which could also benefit the most from its excellent healing properties.

Whatever the reason for the delay in taking up the use of cryoablation for breast cancer treatment, in early 2001 I realized I had entered medicine wanting to make a difference in the world, and I wanted to make a difference in my lifetime. Yet, with a full ten years going by doing trials on liver cancer and working as a general cancer radiologist, I was beginning to lament that cryoablation would never be used on a breast cancer patient in my lifetime.

Sure, research was going on, as I had pioneered the use of cryoablation for benign breast tumors. But other investigators, mainly surgeons, were dutifully freezing cancerous breast tissue with only one cryoprobe at a time, then removing the breast to save it for lab analysis.

We were doing cryoablation, but no one had the courage to say, "Enough documentation of the obvious, let's let the patient keep her breast!"

The infant field of breast cryoablation needed a patient who was willing to take a risk, willing to ignore the conservative advice of those around her, a woman willing to be a pioneer.

Chapter 5: Hope for a Medical Miracle

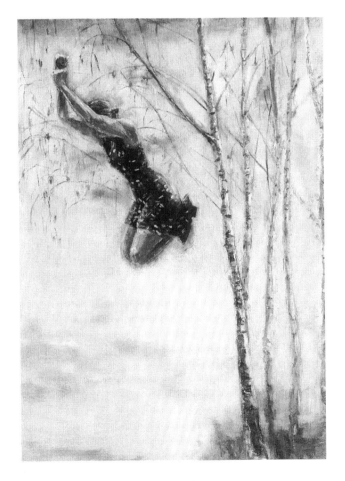

"Leap"

When is appropriate to make a move amid uncertain circumstances? I can't rely on my head to advise me. It seems to caution me to the point of indecision. I can't really decide by trusting my heart either. The emotions my heart reacts to have gotten me into trouble before. However, deciding with my gut feeling...that always seems to work out right. I think this is because when outcomes are uncertain, I can rely on a familiar feeling coming from my gut that propels me into a state of clarity, of be-here-nowness. This is a state where all my senses are hyper-focused, ready to react, adjust, and take advantage for the best possible outcome. Being in this state greatly assists decision-making.

One thing for sure, taking gut feeling-guided action leads me to a place quite different from the stuck place I had been before. That forward, gut-guided, momentum has always made for the moments I've felt most alive.

—Laura Ross-Paul, 2014

Alex

Looking back, if I hadn't lost our airline tickets to Emma's soccer tournament in Las Vegas, I might never have learned about cryoablation as a cancer treatment for Laura's breast. Despite all the research I had done on the Internet, I had never seen any mention of cryoablation for treating breast cancer. I had seen it mentioned a few times but it was always described as an experimental treatment along with exotic breast treat-

116

ment options such as microwave. Oddly, nothing connected it to a possible treatment for breast cancer.

But because we didn't go to Las Vegas, I'd caught up on my work. On Monday morning, I treated myself to an hour of coffee, the paper, and television news running in the background after getting Emma off to school. I ran out of newspaper news and began channel surfing. I landed on a station based in Chicago. And lo and behold, there was an ad promoting a new treatment technique for prostate cancer: cryosurgery.

It caught my attention immediately. It seemed too simple to believe: argon gas run into the prostate and out again though a small tube, the tumor frozen, the surrounding tissue unharmed, the possibility of no loss of sexual function or continence. I scrambled to write down the 800 number. I instantly thought that if this worked on men where bone, muscle and delicate nerves hid the prostate making it hard to get to, it had to be available for treating breast cancer!

After all, the breast hangs completely outside the body cavity and is easy to reach. Even I could do the surgery! Well, probably not; however, the good Lord had put some thought into designing the breast and making it easy to access, or it wouldn't be too useful to a baby looking for milk!

Within hours after writing down the phone number to call about cryosurgery, we received bad news: the second biopsy proved Laura still had cancer—no miracle healing. I consoled her in the basement, and then headed upstairs to the computer. I promised to track down the company that had advertised on TV and find out if they did cryosurgery on the breast.

I called the company. They told me politely but firmly that no, they didn't offer cryoablation for breast cancer, but they could give me a number to call that might have more information. And before I hung up, did I need information on cryoablation for my prostate? I told them politely but firmly, no! As I did this calling, I also searched on the Internet for information on cryosurgery or also called interchangeably, cryoablation.

I placed a call to PCA Cryocare, which turned out to be a volunteer organization, the volunteers being men who had received cryoablation for their prostate cancer, or their grateful wives. I spoke first with a gentleman in Los Angeles, who repeated that he knew of no one doing cryoablation for breast tumors, but he gave me the name and number of a woman in Minnesota who might know more.

I called Minnesota and a woman with a cheerful, twangy Minnesota "don't ya know?" accent greeted me. Her voice and manner on the phone made me think I'd stepped into a warm Minnesota country kitchen with fresh bread just out of the oven; a clean but worn yellow linoleum floor; a spotless, full pantry; and a pot belly stove crackling with a fire in the corner. Karen turned out to be resourceful, happy, capable, optimistic, smart, and grateful that her husband's prostate cryoablation had gone so well, which was why she had become a phone volunteer.

While acknowledging no one was doing breast cryosurgery as a full time practice, Karen did say there was a research doctor at Wayne State University who might do it, a Dr. Littrup, and she gave me the name of the screening physician who handled calls for Dr. Littrup. By this time, it was too late to call, but I let Laura know I was making progress.

I called the next morning at 6 a.m. our time, 8 a.m. in Detroit. The screening physician—I feel terrible I have forgotten his name—had an answering service, which promised he would call back. Later in the day, he called, and I gave him a description of Laura's condition and faxed him all the materials. That afternoon he called back and said he was going to discuss Laura's case with Dr. Littrup, so not to let a phone call surprise us.

While I was waiting for this doctor to call back, I spent most of the day reading about breast cryoablation. Now that I was using the right search terms there was an abundance of information. It's not surprising I'd missed it given those 27 million pages of information I'd tried to sift through!

I found that for ten years, a researcher at University of Michigan in Ann Arbor, a Dr. Sable, had been using cryoablation on volunteers with breast cancer. Two weeks after the cryoablation, he would perform a mastectomy on the volunteer to verify that cryoablation had killed the entire tumor. The researchers never found one case of cancer after the freezing.

Yet cryoablation was not being offered for treating breast cancer. How could ten years of proof not be enough to encourage the medical community to offer breast cancer cryoablation to the public? Why had medicine not released this after three or four years? Ten years and still not available to the public is a glacial pace of advance!

I had always thought that researchers were hard at work trying to find cures to cancer, and when they did, they eagerly rushed them into clinical trials to have them tested and proved. Why hadn't there been more of an advance in the application of cryoablation for breast cancer?

There were no phone numbers on the Ann Arbor website, so I sent an e-mail. By the end of the day, I had not received a reply. Comparing that to the people at Wayne State who were promising to get back to me, I decided to focus my efforts on them. Now we were just waiting on Dr. Littrup.

***

Laura

4/02/2003, Evening

Alex is making progress! He tracked down a screener for a cryosurgery research doctor and was told the doctor would call tomorrow. I have an appointment at Tony Esau's in the morning tomorrow. I am going in for another catalyst shot to fight the breast cancer.

April 4, Friday Evening. We were both hesitant to leave home yesterday, Thursday, since we hadn't heard from the doctor in Detroit. We dragged around as long as we could, but finally we needed to leave to make the forty-minute drive to get to Tony's office on time. Just as we were walking out, the phone rang. It was the doctor—Doctor Littrup is his name. Alex explained why we were calling and then put me on the phone. At first, he seemed reluctant to become involved, saying he didn't want to step on another doctor's protocol if I was being treated.

I assured him we were just trying to make a thoughtful decision that would prevent me from having to have a mastectomy and were looking into every alternative. He took my information and said to fax him a letter explaining why I was seeking this and to include my biopsy and MRI report and he would get back to me.

Happy to have made this hopeful contact, we took off to the appointment. There, right around the corner, blocking the street into and out of our housing project, was a huge moving van that had become stuck. The mover came to the car and told us they were calling for a tow truck, which, he assured us, would take awhile.

There was nothing we could do but cancel my appointment with Dr. Esau and drive home. I was happy because I had the focus and energy to begin my letter to Dr. Littrup. About halfway through that task, Dr. Littrup called back. Excitement filled his voice. He explained that he had bumped into his hospital director and told him about me and asked how to proceed. The director said as long as they followed the clinic's protocol, Dr. Littrup could evaluate my case. If I passed the screening, it was likely they could perform cryoablation on my breast, which would replace the mastectomy!

I would still need to follow up the cryoablation with radiation, which my Portland doctors could provide. He told me ten years of performing breast cryoablation and a follow-up mastectomy two weeks later had provided sufficient proof. The post-mastectomy exam never showed cancer remaining in the breast. This confirmed the research Alex found coming out of Dr. Sable at University of Michigan.

Dr. Littrup said they believed cryoablation alone, while leaving the dead tumors in place for the white blood cells to consume, could potentially train the body to find and fight any tumors elsewhere in the body. He said I was the type of patient they were hoping for. He envisioned patients becoming more responsible and in control of their treatment as the Internet provided more information to the public. He thought that smart and responsible women would begin to choose cryoablation. He said that he had been doing the research for ten years, and he hoped to live long enough for this to be the standard treatment in the future. He told me to call the Karmanos Cancer Institute to set up a protocol meeting with the four doctors involved.

The nurse I called was taken aback, explaining that no meetings with four doctors at once had ever happened there. She said it must be a mistake and that I would need four separate appointments. I told her to talk to Dr. Littrup and get back to me.

Friday morning at 6:30, a call from Detroit jarred me awake. The same nurse was on the phone. This time she was inviting me to a screening meeting with four doctors in one day. I was to meet the head of the research program and hospital administrator, Dr. Henderson; Dr. Littrup, the radiologist working in cryoablation; a surgical oncologist, Dr. Bouwman; and a second radiologist, Dr. Tara Washington. She would consult with me regarding radiation treatment in Portland after my potential cryoablation in Detroit.

***

Alex

What an exciting day Thursday turned out to be! Guardian angels had to be watching over us. We live on a cul de sac and the single road out of our neighborhood has never been closed in the ten years we'd lived here. Yet, on that one day a truck blocking the road had forced us to return home after Laura had a brief phone call with Dr. Littrup, a call that left us feeling he might not help us.

If the truck across the road hadn't forced us back to the house, who knows if all this could have come together? It seemed to me misfortune—losing airline tickets, having the road blocked—was working for us instead of against us.

During the second call I got a chance to speak with Dr. Littrup at length. His voice was every bit as Midwest and cheerful and confidence inspiring as Karen, the lady with the Midwest accent from PCA Cryocare, had been, but in a masculine way. His voice made me feel like I was stepping into an airplane hanger in the thirties filled with pilots, biplanes, and earnest mechanics revving motors and shouting to one another over the noise of the engines. I felt like I was talking not to a doctor but to a mechanic, one who insisted on tidy tools and cleaning oil spills rather than ignoring them.

His hospital administrator had said he could take a look at Laura's mammogram and MR images and see if she'd be a candidate for a trip back there. No, they weren't offering the program yet, but they could do so if Laura was willing.

He seemed so capable. I hung up feeling like Laura's cancer wasn't going to be a big deal. I felt like I owned a Jaguar that had broken down in a small Midwestern town and instead of suffering a long delay, I'd found a mechanic who explained they'd been thinking of offering Jaguar repair services anyway!

After Laura hung up, we screamed, hugged, and skipped around. MRIs, biopsy results, medical records, a torrent of information headed east the rest of Thursday. By Friday morning, Laura's screening invitation became a reality. Time to schedule flights!

Laura

Saturday morning

I got a call from Dr. Fancher. He is my primary physician. The day before, I had hand delivered to Dr. Fancher a copy of the letter I wrote to Dr. Littrup. (I had also delivered it to my internist, and my surgeon). In the letter I stated my request for cryoablation, the reason I wanted it, and information on the procedure. Dr. Fancher said he'd used the Internet and his contacts to check it out. He added that Wayne State was a top cancer facility. They wouldn't proceed unless they were sure they could help me. I had his blessing. My surgeon called Friday, a little more skeptical, but facilitated my getting the films and reports I needed for my meeting in Detroit.

We're ready. We're happy. We're hopeful. We're going to Detroit!

Chapter 6: Detroit and the New Doctors

Alex

At three in the morning, I lay in Detroit, unable to sleep as I listened to a wheezy radiator overheating our international center bedroom. We had just gone through a long day of travel where much went wrong.

We'd arrived early at the Portland airport and every-thing went smoothly (unlike our earlier lost tickets can-celing our flight plans for soccer in Las Vegas). We board-ed the plane in first-class, courtesy of all the miles I'd amassed on American Airlines. To my amazement, one of my old friends from Tae Kwon Do sat two rows ahead.

He told me that sadly, our master had contracted stomach cancer. He did not expect the master to survive.

This wasn't the news I wanted to hear as we left to get cancer treatment for Laura! Master Yom was at least fifteen years younger than me and a bull of a man with a third-degree black belt in Tae Kwon Do. It was always daunting talking to him, knowing he could kill me with his bare hands even though he was a foot shorter.

Thinking of him wasting away from cancer was im-possible. To think I would outlive him was even more disturbing. I wanted everyone with cancer to beat the

125

disease. If someone I knew didn't, it seemed to worsen Laura's odds.

We hadn't eaten much dinner the night before due to excitement, nor eaten breakfast because we had first-class seating on a morning flight and this was the first time we'd flown first-class so we wanted to experience their food service!

Sadly, they ran out of the delicious looking egg and sausage breakfast and could only offer us cereal. We resolved to eat during the St. Louis layover as we munched on a small box of cereal. In St. Louis the connection was tight, so, no time to eat! We promised ourselves that once checked into our room at the Harper International Center we'd eat at a nearby restaurant. The very name international center implied an abundance of surrounding restaurants kind of like a world's fair!

I could tell from the turban and accent that our cab driver in Detroit was probably a Sikh from India, and when I asked him he said he was indeed a Sikh! He became my instant friend, talking about Detroit, the good things to see and do. Then he offered the odd observation that we were not staying in a healthy part of town. He clarified, saying the hospital was fine but the surrounding neighborhood was extremely dangerous.

The Harper nurse had said the Harper International Center was close to restaurants, but there was no one at the front desk to check us in. In fact, we couldn't even get inside because the building was locked. The cab driver grew impatient. It was nearly ten and I was starting to worry not only about getting into the building, but also finding a restaurant at this late hour, so I asked the cabdriver to stay, saying I'd pay him. He said it wasn't necessary, but he kept muttering in a low Indian language what sounded like a secret Punjabi curse.

Finally, a guard came by to let us into the building. At least we would be safe now inside, so Laura said we should let the cab go. My intuition said this was a mistake, but I deferred to her wishes.

Once inside, a clerk appeared to register us after a wait of a few minutes. We asked him directions to the McDonalds we had noticed on our drive in, as we were so famished we were ready for anything warm. He laughed and said even though it was only five blocks away, he wouldn't eat at McDonald's unless an armed guard went with him. In fact, he added, they had an armed guard for escorting people around the hospital campus after dark, but he had left for the day. And they had no food in the building.

Welcome to Detroit! I was now wondering if downtown Baghdad was safer. What had we gotten ourselves into?

I was further upset when we reached the room. It was decent but nothing as nice as places we usually stay. I wanted this trip to be comfortable for Laura. Instead it felt like a refugee's hostel.

Maybe I felt claustrophobic because we couldn't even walk outside. I suggested we pack up our stuff, call a cab, and go to a hotel downtown where we could check in and I could buy her dinner.

But Laura said she brought some food, and that was enough to get us by, and she was too tired to move.

"I have cancer," she explained her fatigue while sounding defeated. My heart melted. She was right, and I felt sad because it seemed as if her spirit was draining away from her. Instead of putting out some more energy to move to a better place and get food like she would have in her healthy days, she was willing to go hungry just so she could lie down and rest.

I was fired up and angry and felt like making an effort to get some food because I was starving! But I gave in because Laura seemed like she was a wounded person who couldn't go on.

So we ate nuts, granola and fruit she'd packed, and decided we'd get up early in the morning before her tests and have a big breakfast!

I lay in bed feeling as if I'd failed Laura and was helpless to do anything about it. Was this International Center a prelude to the treatment we'd receive at the hospital? I fell asleep to the noise of dry, hot air from a wheezing heater doing battle with cold air leaking in around the old, poorly sealed window.

Laura

4/15/2003

Portland, after the trip to Detroit

It's becoming clearer and clearer to me that fulfilling my hopes and desires is a big assignment. It's one I willingly take on, but it will be trying for me, nonetheless. It will be telling my story, relating the new wave of breast cancer treatment to the world from the point of view of a woman who's going through it.

Detroit was wonderful and fatiguing. We landed late and after going to bed I lay awake worrying if the two small additional "suspicious sites" were going to make me ineligible for the cryoablation.

Alex, who didn't get enough to eat at all today, was low on blood sugar and upset this evening. He expressed his desire to be done with all the tension and just get me well. We went over each small step that had brought me this far. At each point, a door was opening just as another one closed.

Yes, Carlos had apparently removed a tumor. Yes, the MRI showed tumors still there. Yes, I had reacted strongly to Dr. Esau's Koch treatment and the homeopaths and the Rife machine, dumping many toxins.

My diet was perfect vegan. Even so, the second biopsy result had come back with me still having a malignancy. This had dashed my hope that a miracle or alternative healing had occurred. But, at that point, a voice had whispered, "I could still have my breast." The cry for help was answered soon after. Our road led to Detroit and cryoablation. Maybe this was an answer to their prayers in Detroit as much as ours. If they were ready to take the next step, so were we.

We woke very early since we were literally starving, and we left plenty of time in the morning to find some food before the appointments began. However, as we were leaving the dorm, my cell phone rang. Gwen Wright called to tell me that Dr. Littrup wanted me to come to the hospital right away to check my breast with ultrasound to see if the two small sites that had showed up on the MRI in addition to the two main tumor sites would pose a problem. Gwen volunteered to come meet us at the dorm, because we had no idea where to go.

Gwen was the nurse who was to be my coordinator and constant companion in Detroit. In her late thirties, early forties, she has the sweetest big smile and a similar disposition. She took us to meet Dr. Littrup, who turned out to be a leaner version of Indiana Jones with a bowl haircut and rimless glasses. He seemed fit, energetic, and sharp as a tack. I recognized a creative disposition and openness to new thinking in him.

Dr. Littrup filled us in on a little of his experience with cryoablation. He'd used it for prostate, liver, lung and breast fibroids. He said he first wanted to check with an ultrasound if the sites were ideal for the procedure. He assured us that he was good with an ultrasound machine, usually being able to see whatever an MRI had found. I had explained that four people, two technicians and two doctors had been unable to find the two additional small sites during my recent biopsy.

After about a half hour of looking, he could only find the two main tumors, and a third small site. A fourth site, referred to as the "fourth area" in Portland, was in all likelihood just a blood vessel. He said he felt I would be a good candidate for cryoablation, as I had two main tumors, with a small adjacent third site that was also a tumor. He said we should proceed with the rest of the meetings scheduled for the day.

I asked him if he could tell whether there was any change in size or other suggestion that my alternative therapies had worked. I gave him the report I'd made about what I was doing to heal the cancer using holistic therapy.

He glanced at it, then commented that all this was good, that he could see I would be probably be very healthy going into this thanks to the alternative therapies. However, he warned me that there are no medical tests which support the claims of the alternative therapies. He assured me that cryoablation was very effective and that it was a scientifically recognized way of killing cancer which would allow me to keep my breast.

***

Alex

I spent the morning in Harper Hospital cafeteria while Laura was being examined by Dr. Littrup. I felt guilty eating a huge breakfast because Laura still hadn't eaten when she went in for her first meeting with Dr. Littrup. I did have a to-go box to bring back to her!

I was grateful for every bite because I'd become lost several times trying to cross the enormous Harper Hospital complex. It was an incredibly busy place, full of doctors, patients, guards, custodial people, elevators, lobbies, research labs and waiting rooms. I felt as if half of Detroit's population was in the hospital seeking treatment while a quarter of the remaining population was nothing but nurses and doctors treating them.

Harper Hospital was a very impressive facility and I felt that if these people couldn't pull off a miracle and save Laura's breast, I didn't know who could.

The afternoon was nothing but meetings, meetings, meetings! We had our meetings individually with the doctors. I think they did this so they could offer their opinion without having to consider someone else's feelings. I felt this was sensible, because if anyone had reservations about Dr. Littrup and the potential of his cryosurgery technique, that opinion could be shared with us in the strictest confidence.

First was Dr. Littrup. He beamed with energy and confidence as he told Laura and me that he had seen

131

only three tumors, which were all close together, and that he had found the suspicious "fourth area," suspected of being cancer in Portland, was nothing more than a duct—not a tumor at all.

I laughed at this point, repeating Arnold Schwarzenegger's line, "It's not a toomah!" and he and Laura both laughed. Dr. Littrup related his confidence that he could successfully treat Laura and that we should talk with the other doctors to get their opinion. But from his point of view, this was a feasible step to take in Laura's treatment.

Dr. Littrup left us in the room alone and, in a few moments, in came Dr. Bouwman, a big guy with a beard and mustache, graying like me, but heavier. I realized that if we were in church together, he'd be Santa Claus at Christmas and I'd be the old elf assistant. Dr. Bouwman would perform the sentinel node surgery, the removal of the lymph node receiving the drainage from the breast tumor.

"You're in uncharted waters with this cryoablation," Dr. Bouwman cautioned. "Sure, it's worked in research for over ten years, but the gold standard for surviving cancer in your situation where the lumpectomy is not possible, is the mastectomy."

Laura looked crestfallen and defeated.

"Is there any reason, though, that if for some reason the cryoablation fails, Laura couldn't just get a mastectomy later?" I asked.

"That's an excellent question," Dr. Bouwman replied. He thought for a moment and then said, "No, not really. If there was a localized recurrence later after the cryoablation and radiation, she could always have a mastectomy."

"Then it seems to me we have something to gain and little to lose," I replied.

We spoke for a short time afterward, discovering that Dr. Bouwman and I shared an interest in boating and he suggested places for us to visit if we decided to come back and pursue the cryoablation treatment.

We were left alone again and, in a few moments, an even taller man, Dr. Henderson, came into the room. He introduced himself as the head of the entire Karmanos Cancer Institute cancer department. His specialty was chemotherapy and hormone therapy, the treatment that typically follows after a mastectomy or lumpectomy.

Dr. Henderson loomed over my six-foot-three inches. As we shook hands, I said, "Each person that comes through the door keeps getting taller. Between the doctors and me, we'd have a heck of a basketball team."

"I actually did play basketball in college," Dr. Henderson replied. "I played center for Cal Berkley during the years Kareem Abdul-Jabbar played for UCLA. Guarding him was an impossible job. We lost every time we played them."

We laughed and settled into a comfortable discussion about Laura's follow-up treatment if she did have cryoablation. Dr. Henderson said it would be identical to that done for a lumpectomy; meaning, she would need chemotherapy followed by radiation.

This rang an alarm bell for me.

"Why does Laura need chemotherapy if she has the benefit of the immune effect triggered by the cryoablation?" I asked.

"No one is sure how or why the immune effect works, and sometimes it doesn't occur at all. To be conservative, one has to use all the treatment options."

"What percentage of time does the breast cancer come back after a traditional mastectomy?" I asked, trying to get a handle on the statistics.

"There's only a 10 percent recurrence rate after a traditional mastectomy if there is no other treatment," Dr. Henderson replied. He was very impressive with his detailed knowledge of the various statistics. However, it just confirmed my sense of dread that treating cancer was a gamble and not a cure.

"A lumpectomy without follow-up therapy has a 20 percent recurrence rate; when combined with radiation, a 17 percent recurrence rate; when combined with chemo, a 12 percent recurrence rate."

It struck me cryosurgery could be compared to a lumpectomy, so it was worth it for Laura to try it as an alternative to mastectomy, which was her only choice. It sounded like she only had a 17 percent chance of a recurrence if she added radiation to the cryoablation. Laura was ineligible for chemotherapy due to liver damage as a teenager. And there was always the potential of the immune effect occurring, reducing even further her odds of recurrence.

I tried to do a "back of the envelope" estimate, being an engineer by training, while Laura continued speaking with Dr. Henderson. Unfortunately, no studies have documented the percentage of occurrence of the immune effect following prostate cryoablation.

I reasoned that at least 10 percent of the time there must be an immune effect because like many things in life, be they customer complaints or praise, the information received is usually only the tip of the iceberg. The truth was that the immune effect probably occurred between 25 to 50 percent of the time and no one had bothered to keep track of the statistics.

Regardless, I was most worried about Laura, so I assumed for the moment that Laura would only have a 10 percent chance of an "immune effect" occurring. In any pool of 100 women, that would mean only 90 women would then be subject to a recurrence.

In her case, chemotherapy was out of the question no matter what treatment she had, mastectomy or lumpectomy. The lumpectomy followed by radiation had a 17 percent recurrence rate according to Dr. Henderson, but in a pool of women receiving cryoablation and enjoying a 10 percent occurrence of the immune effect was equivalent to applying the 17 percent recurrence rate to only 90 percent of the original group.

This meant the rate of recurrence after cryoablation and radiation could be equal to 90 percent times 17 percent, or approximately 15 percent recurrence rate.

This got me excited, because in all likelihood, these statistics meant Laura was going to be safer with the added benefit of an immune effect, even at a low 10 percent immune effect recurrence level, than if she had received a lumpectomy.

It struck me that medical science should really be keeping track of the immune effect's occurrence in prostate surgery cases. If the same rate of immune effect occurrence held true for women during cryosurgery for breast cancer, and the rate of occurrence of the immune effect was around 25 percent, it might be possible that by having cryoablation, women would actually have less chance of recurrence than if they had a mastectomy.

It made me mad to think that I had to estimate and guess on my own when researchers already had years to amass statistics that could prove the additional benefit of the immune effect from cryoablation.

Here's an example of what the statistics might be able to show, if they had been kept.

Breast Cancer Cryoablation, assumed for the moment to have a 25 percent chance of an immune effect occurring. For every 100 women, that would mean only 75 would be in the "recurrence pool." If they then had radiation and chemotherapy, which reduces recurrence to only 12 percent in traditional lumpectomy patients, the chance of recurrence would be only 9 percent, since 75 percent times 12 percent results in only 9 percent recurrence. This number is lower than the recurrence rate for a mastectomy without chemotherapy!

I related all this to Laura in a state of great excitement when Dr. Henderson left us, but she got lost in the math no matter how many times I tried to explain that by having cryosurgery the odds might be better for her survival than they were by getting a mastectomy and that I was surprised Dr. Henderson hadn't "run the numbers" as I just had since he was so focused on making decisions based on statistics.

Laura appreciated my enthusiasm, but in the end, just said that she trusted my brain. I checked my figures several times as we waited for Dr. Washington and could barely contain myself. This was excellent news. Laura was going to save her breast and stood a chance of getting higher odds of survival than by having a mastectomy!

Cryoablation might eventually prove itself to be the new "gold standard" for breast cancer survival if the rate of non-recurrence due to the immune effect could be proven to be at least 25 percentor more. And each

1 percent reduction in overall recurrence means an additional 1,900 breast cancer survivors each year.

I decided I'd research this later when I remembered the wife of a friend of ours who had requested a double mastectomy to improve her odds of survival. The odds might have been better for her to keep both breasts! The statistical possibility of saving thousands of women's lives by combining cryoablation with radiation and chemotherapy than by having a double mastectomy seemed a hugely important addition to the main perceived benefit of cryoablation, that being, keeping the breasts. I wondered why medical researchers had seemingly ignored or overlooked the possibility.

Surely the lives of thousands of women a year deserved a thorough investigation into the benefits of combining cryoablation with radiation and chemotherapy!

Finally, we met Dr. Tara Washington. She seemed the least enthusiastic of the three in explaining what radiation was like.

"The radiation could make the frozen tissue turn into a ball of matter that the body's immune system won't eat up," Tara warned.

My shoulders slumped and I could see a frown developing on Laura's face. This didn't sound good.

"But no one knows!" she said in a bright voice. "All we can do is try and see what happens."

"What happens if we delay the radiation after the cryosurgery?" I asked. "To give Laura's immune system time to absorb the dead tissue?"

"My guess is that she'll have to start radiation sooner than the body has finished absorbing the damaged tissue," Tara replied after a moment's reflection. "But at least a large amount of it would be eaten already."

"Meaning that if the part where the tumor lies is absorbed, I'd have a chance at the immune effect occurring before starting radiation," Laura asked.

"Well, yes, that's true," Tara reflected.

Bingo, I thought. I married a very, very smart girl. I don't know what she was talking about earlier about not understanding. Laura got the message. Stimulating the immune effect was the big reward adding to the odds of survival.

Tara left and was soon replaced by Dr. Littrup. He said that overall, his team was prepared to offer the cryoablation to Laura if she wanted it. We said that we'd like to have a chance to think it all over before Laura made her decision.

The cab ride back to the airport and the flight home remain a blur. We talked and talked unless we were sleeping. When we landed, Laura and I agreed, she would have the cryoablation. We arrived home late, exhausted yet hopeful. Laura would keep her breast! And if my math was right, she had at worst, close to the same odds of survival as if she had had a mastectomy. And the odds might even be better!

One thing Dr. Littrup had added to the mix in his second visit was that if Laura did have a recurrence in the breast, he could do a "touch-up"—a refreeze. This sounded excellent to us. If the immune effect didn't happen the first time, we could "reset the clock" with a refreeze and up the odds even higher. And very worst case? She could have a mastectomy.

To an engineer and businessman, this sounded good. We were playing the odds the right way. As a husband, I still wished old Carlos had been successful. But maybe the cryosurgery was the miracle we'd prayed for, delivered in a different package.

Chapter 7: Dr. Littrup—I Meet Laura

Dr. Littrup

My first interview on the phone with Laura and Alex was positive. They seemed like decent people who were motivated to find a cure for Laura's cancer without using a traditional mastectomy.

I raised the issue of offering this treatment to Laura with Dr. Richard Bouwman, Chief Surgeon at Karmanos Cancer Center, where I was working as a radiologist. I gave Dr. Bouwman the specifics regarding Laura's background after her charts arrived. His first reaction was, "Are you sure that you want to have such a difficult cancer as your first patient?"

Laura's cancer was multifocal, with three confirmed—and possibly a fourth—tumor sites, and the three tumors were all over one centimeter. I knew the ideal candidate for a first cryoablation was a patient with a single site under one centimeter. This is because, if I didn't get all the cancer, there could be a recurrence, and that would give cryoablation a bad reputation.

However, I pointed out to Dr. Bouwman that I felt confident I could create a freeze ball large enough to envelop all of the cancer. If we took out the core of the tumors with a mammotome and then took biopsies all around the freeze ball, we would know that we had achieved clean margins.

Then if Laura followed up with radiation and possibly chemotherapy, I felt confident that her chances of a recurrence were no greater, and possibly better than, those of a person having a mastectomy.

There is still a suspicion today that cryoablation doesn't kill cancer cells. This is despite the fact that it is a Medicare-approved treatment methodology for prostate cancer. Ten years of liver cryoablation at Wayne State proved that in each case, freezing destroyed the cancer as reliably as surgically removing large portions of the liver.

Given my success in treating prostate cancer and my experience ablating non-cancerous fibrous adenomas in the breast, I felt confident I could treat Laura. The big question, though, was what kind of patient would she be?

Laura and her husband traveled for the first time to Karmanos in early April, 2003. I wanted to examine her breast using ultrasound and confirm my ability to freeze the tumors. The first thing I determined, much to our mutual delight, was the fact that the suspicious fourth tumor site was a false reading. The tumors, although there were three, had concentrated in one, treatable quadrant of the breast, a good candidate for a successful freeze.

My colleagues and I at Karmanos wanted to make sure the Paul's gave informed consent. In one day, they met with a surgeon, Dr. Bouwman; an oncologist and the Chief Medical Officer of Karmanos, Dr. Henderson; and a radiation oncologist, Dr. Washington, who was the expert on radiation therapy. We insisted on radiation as a follow-up since we were treating the cryoablation like a lumpectomy. The follow-up protocol would require that Laura have radiation just as if she'd had a lumpectomy.

Our meetings with the Pauls were surprising. Both Alex and Laura had come with a long list of questions that they shared with all the experts. I learned later that at one point Dr. Bouwman complimented Alex for asking intelligent questions. And Laura was obviously motivated to be treated and have her breast conserved. She proved to be very stable, not emotional, very informed and prepared to take the risk of being the first patient in the United States to receive cryoablation without a mastectomy as a breast cancer treatment without additional surgery.

They both agreed that if there was a recurrence, they still had the option of "touching up" the breast. This meant I could go back in and freeze the small area of recurrence. And at the worst, Laura could still have a mastectomy, so she was not endangering herself by trying the cryoablation.

We agreed on a surgery date in late April, and they returned home as we prepared for the operation.

Chapter 8: The Cryolumpectomy in Detroit

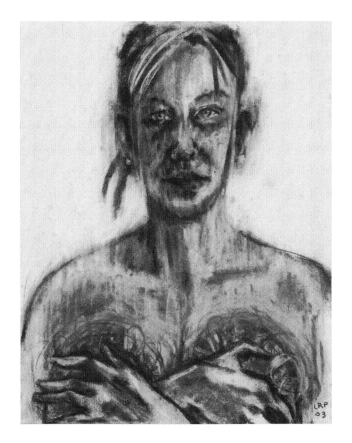

"Self Portrait"

"Laura Ross-Paul made this series of charcoal drawings at an introspective time, during a period of serious illness that cut into her time for painting. In these drawings, nature is replaced by the elemental energy that goes awry and is reclaimed in illness and recovery."

—Catalog essay by Camela Raymond for the exhibit "Draw," curated by Malia Jensen for the 2003 exhibit, "CORE SAMPLE: Portland Painting Now"

Laura

April 21, Morning

Somewhere over the Rockies. We are flying to Detroit for my operation. I am nervous but resolved and trusting in God's will. I was so blessed by all the events yesterday. It was Easter Sunday. We went to First Baptist church with Sean and Emma, for the first time in a long while. It was so sweet seeing all our old church friends. Everyone seemed so genuinely happy to see us. The new pastor had a clever and quick wit and playful sense of humor, which complemented his fervent faith. We liked his message.

While I didn't let anyone in on my medical condition, it was so nurturing to be with these gentle, God-loving people. After church, we went to "Uncle Bill" Brock's farm to join the Sauter family's Easter celebration. Brock Farm was full of potluck dinner; laughter; and friendly, constantly interrupted conversation. I told Marilee, Rachael, and Rebecca about going to Detroit soon for the cryoablation. Then songs outside around a fire—hymns about resurrection and redemption, testimonials and Easter lessons for the kids. Mothers asked questions of their boys' girlfriends, putting them on the spot to test their faith.

A testimony followed around the fire from an African man picked up by Bill. This large man attended their church for the first time that morning. He had come to America searching for a long-lost brother who came here for college but never returned to Africa and rarely wrote.

Then after prayers, dismissal to recreate. Chaos! Kids went everywhere, jumping on the trampoline, running in the fields, teenage boys playing touch football, middle-schoolers riding madly around on mini-motor bikes.

I mostly sat and talked in the house with Rebecca and Rachael about my cancer. Soon Rachael's son came in and reported that the whole gang was up at the field shooting clay pigeons and targets.

It was the finale that brought the activities to a close. As we gathered for our good-byes, the whole group gathered around me for a prayer circle with all their hands laid on me. It was wonderful. I loved my cousin's strong, confident prayer, and could feel their energy penetrate me. Therefore, I was ready for my journey to Detroit.

The next night, Monday night before we left today, I received even more support. Fifteen women from our wonderful neighborhood gathered at my friend Martha's house. I filled them in on what I was going to do in Detroit. I needed their help because although Grandma Emily, Alex's mom, was going to stay with Emma while we were gone, she no longer drove. They not only offered to drive, but set up a dinner preparation schedule so Emily wouldn't have to cook. What a wonderful, sympathetic group. I didn't worry at all about Emma while I was gone.

***

Alex

On April 21, Laura and I flew to Detroit for the second time. This time we checked into a lovely downtown Marriott Hotel. No more hunger, we had dinner in the evening after we arrived! Laura ate light, because the surgery was the next day. We had to wake at 5:30 a.m.— 2:30 a.m. our time. The next day was going to be a long day so we tried to get to bed early, but it was difficult getting to sleep. We finally dropped off, only to have the phone wake us. The alarm clock read 2:30 a.m., Detroit time.

"Daddy? It's Emma!" With only one daughter, I pretty much know a young girl calling me Daddy is my daughter Emma, but I didn't correct her grammar.

"What is it, sweetie?"

"Taffy ran outside the electric fence and went over to Sarah's yard."

Our neighbor Sarah has three female Jack Russell terriers. When they bark, they sound like pigs squealing and fighting over food. I know this sound because I worked on a farm as a boy. And after hearing this sound late at night, our male dog ran out. After all, it was spring!

Even though our male dog is "fixed," when Sarah's dogs are in heat (she breeds them), our male dog knows that, "SOMETHING IS GOING ON NEXT DOOR!" Our male dog runs through our invisible electric fence despite his high-voltage shock collar. He can only sniff and visit the female in heat, and possibly feel sad about what he can't do. It is obviously worth the pain of the electric fence.

"So anyway I ran and got him," Emma continued. "But to get him back through the fence, I had to take off his collar and carry him. When I walked over the wire, the collar shocked my hand, so am I going to have a heart attack or something?"

I had once told her a story of a man in Lake Oswego, Oregon who had bought a training collar. Not wanting to subject his favorite pet to undue pain, he placed the collar on his own neck and asked his wife to press the button to see how badly it hurt him. She hit the button and he dropped to the ground in convulsions, all bodily functions losing control. This his eyes rolled up into his head and he lay still as if he were dead. Supposedly, this is a true story.

The firefighters were prepared to start his heart, but when they arrived from the 9-1-1 call, he was sitting up and drinking water. So Emma must have been thinking about the fellow in the story I had told her. By this time, I was wide awake.

"Emma, listen to me carefully! You only have two minutes left to live, there's no hope!"

The line was silent for a few seconds, and then:

"Oh Daddy . . . Do I really only have two minutes?"

"Yes, it's called a delayed heart attack!"

"But it's been more than two minutes since it happened!"

"Maybe it's ten minutes," I teased. "I can't remember."

"Oh, that's not true!"

"I know you know, but I'm glad you called anyway."

And there it was. Poor little Emma was fourteen going on

four, reduced to sadness and loneliness by her mother's battle with cancer. Emma had been staying home with Grandma and had no contact with us all day. She was upset but brave and giving off that tough, I-play-soccer exterior. I knew inside she was upset and probably crying herself to sleep every night.

"Well, I'm sorry I woke you. But you did tell me about the heart attack guy and the collar and stuff."

"Yes I did. I'm glad you called and it's good to hear your voice."

"Can I talk to momma?"

"I'm sorry, she's out cold. She didn't wake up with me talking, so maybe I shouldn't wake her now cause she is pretty tired. It's 2:30 in the morning here and we have to get up early."

Pause.

"But it's only 11:30 here, so it's not that late!"

"It is when you have to get up at 5:30 Detroit time."

"Oh. I see your point. Well, I better go!"

"I'm glad you called. I'm sorry we didn't call when we got here. Momma's fine. She's going to be okay."

"I know."

"I love you, sweetie."

"Love you, Daddy."

I looked over at Laura. She remained asleep. How could she? I was worried about the operation, hoping this would turn out all right and I wasn't even the patient! I'd had a premonition that it would be successful two days before when we were trap and target shooting at Bill's farm.

I had brought some two-inch round, stick-on, exploding targets. I stuck them on a rotating metal silhouette squirrel target that I'd placed in the ground fifty yards from the firing line. Then I'd given all the relatives' kids my scoped Ruger 10-22, and they had been blasting away for an hour, none of them able to hit the target and blow it up.

When we finished skeet shooting, I came over. They had shot all the ammo, but as everyone was cleaning up, one of the kids found a single .22 shell on the ground.

"Shoot the target, Uncle Alex," the kids cried. I cleaned the shell and chambered the round, then stood freehand and aimed, keeping in mind that they had all failed to hit it shooting prone. I am not normally superstitious, but I said to myself, *If I hit the bull's-eye, Laura is going to be just fine.*

From standing, I shot and the target exploded into flame. Everyone clapped for me. I knew Detroit would go well!

I rolled over to sleep, trusting the omen of my good shot.

We woke to a cold spring morning and were on the streets by 6:30 a.m. There was not a soul on the streets of downtown Detroit, not a car. Newspapers and trash skidded into the curbs, borne by a stiff wind off the lake. Detroit: lonely, gray, windy, with hard-etched surfaces of concrete and a neon sign flashing the lures of Greek Town casino and restaurant, the last sign of life in an abandoned urban core that looked post-apocalyptic.

We arrived at Harper at seven, right on time, and spent a long time signing forms. They asked for advance payment because our insurance company had not approved anything yet, even though Dr. Fancher gave us a referral and said Laura should have the cryosurgery.

Since our insurance company didn't offer cryoablation in Oregon, he had assured me we would have some coverage, so I didn't worry. I assumed it was just taking a while to process Dr. Fancher's request, because we let him know we were going back just a few days earlier.

So Harper's staff took a prepayment from my Citibank American Airlines card, and I consoled myself that at least I was building miles for future visits here if needed.

The nurse warned me the operation might cost over $30,000. I had been prepared for spending far less, about half the cost. What could we do at this point? We're here; Laura needs treatment, I thought. Even if we had to pay and charge it on credit cards, it was worth it. I knew this was important to Laura and I didn't want her to have the scars and defeat of losing her breast like her mother. And if this immune effect worked, this cryoablation would save Laura's breast and life. Like the Mastercard ads say, "Priceless!"

After financial matters were concluded, we headed to the Barbara Karmanos Breast Cancer Center in the back part of the hospital. The walls morphed from old Detroit to renaissance Detroit: marble, light, an atrium, fountains. And a line?

There was a line to sign up for breast cancer treatment at 7:30 in the morning. It was a long line, twelve women deep, and more came in as others headed for their operations. I listened as they registered and found that all these women were having breast cancer procedures—lumpectomies or mastectomies.

The horror of the breast cancer statistics struck me as I waited in line while Laura rested. I imagined a line of one year's worth of patients somehow all coming here on one morning, their line extending out the door. Hundreds of thousands of women lined up and down that long Detroit street all the way back to our hotel across the river and into Canada. In my mind, all these women waiting in a line to get a mastectomy or a lumpectomy that morning had all been left behind by society, Medicare, insurance companies and the medical profession.

I felt angry standing there. I had not walked in these women's shoes; I didn't have breast cancer, but I had stood in line with them. It was a cold, uncaring line that should not exist. It was not the fault of Harper; I was sure this line formed most weekday mornings in hospitals all over the country.

Yet, it was so sad. These women deserved more dignified treatment. Many were going to lose their breast on this day, because in cases where a lumpectomy is not feasible, a mastectomy is still the gold standard. Mastectomy—a removal of the breast: a symbol of sexuality, fertility, suckler of babes, nourishment guaranteeing the survival of the human race until the so-recent invention of bottles and rubber.

It is an event of consequence to lose a breast, to lose this connection to life and the ability to provide life. There should be an acknowledgment, a ritual mourning this event. Somewhere in Detroit or at the hospital, I felt, there should be incense burning and a holy man or woman offering a blessing and prayers mourning this loss and acknowledging the pain and suffering each woman was about to go through.

Native Americans would have a ceremony for this; they are far more sensitive to passages in life. I knew this because once they had come out to the airport and greeted some buddies of mine who had come back from a trip to Vietnam. They pounded on their drums and chanted a chant for the return of warriors. It was very moving and cleansing.

If not drums and chanting in mourning, each one of these lovely women deserved at least a warm lobby where a concierge discussed their situation, asked if they needed to use a restroom or a phone and handed them a preregistration packet that eliminated any line.

Medicine; our country; and in the end, all of us have ignored the help that women could get from cryoablation. Men have had cryoablation available to them since the 90s to treat their prostate cancer. The art of the treatment has advanced to the point where in many cases erectile dysfunction can be prevented. And with cryoablation, some percentage of men treated get an immune effect from it. If all this can be done for men, then why not give cryoablation to women?

And there are so many women. One in eight women get breast cancer during their lifetime, and if cryoablation was offered, they wouldn't have to have a breast removed. As I stood in line, I also thought that more women might stay alive as well, given the possibility of the immune effect.

Breast cancer is not an isolated illness. It's an epidemic! If a flu virus was going around that infected one in nine people and killed, eventually, a minimum of 10 percent of them, we'd be up in arms demanding a vaccine. Why aren't we—men and women—up in arms, demanding cryoablation for breast cancer treatment?

As I stood in line, I realized it would be ironic if all the cancer research into chemicals, DNA, genetic engineering, and everything else ended up being eclipsed by a technique more typical of a naturopath, one that harnessed the body's natural defenses. To quote Dr. Littrup:

"We freeze the tumor, and then the body learns the tumor is a foreign entity because the cancer can't mask itself from the body any longer. Then the immune system goes out and kills the cancer everywhere else that it has spread."

This is simplicity itself, working with the body's immune system. Medicine knew in the 1850s that freezing the outside of the breast tumor could sometimes cure cancer, according to Dr. Littrup's history of cryoablation. A promising cure for breast cancer in 1850 and nothing done to make use of that knowledge by 2003! One hundred fifty-three years later and Laura was going to be the first!

I so prayed this would work! If it did, it would be the miracle we had prayed for and, even better, it wouldn't be a fickle miracle by a healer, working on one person but not another. No, this could work every time and be available to anyone. I vowed then and there to be like the women volunteers at PCA Cryocare who staff the phone banks to spread the word about the miracle of cryoablation for prostate cancer, because they're so happy to have a whole and healthy husband. Only I was going to have a whole and healthy wife!

I resolved then to do more than just help Laura save her breast. I decided to write a book and spread the word about this miracle treatment. If I was Laura's knight in shining armor coming to her rescue, then I could do the same for all the other women without the option of cryoablation all across America on this chilly Detroit morning.

Out there somewhere women are walking around with breast cancer and not even knowing it. Others face it in their future. Some are hearing a diagnosis this very second.

All will be told that mastectomy is the gold standard of treatment if a lumpectomy is not possible, and that a lumpectomy with follow-up treatment is an equally good alternative if it is feasible. However, none will hear of the power their immune system might have if they froze the tumor instead. I resolved then to help change that, to spread the word.

After check-in, Laura settled into a wheelchair. She was now, officially, a patient, and no longer allowed to walk. We headed for the basement and the radiation department. Heavy metal elevator doors opened onto a different world.

I sniffed a faint odor of ozone, or something electrical, in the air. There was no noise here, no contact from the outside world. What life there was in the cold wind above did not reach here. Here the air was warm and technicians scurried around in light, white coats, passing through heavy doors with yellow and black radiation symbol signs: WARNING!

It felt like we had journeyed to a Strategic Air Command bunker. Laura was at DefCon 4, Defense Condition Four. Somewhere B–52s were scrambling, missile doors opening in Nebraska, and Laura had come to an underground bunker to wage war on her cancer.

We were here to hunt for the sentinel node.

The sentinel node is a tiny lymph node and it's where the tumor discharges fluids and wastes. Blood nourishes the tumor, but the theory is that cancer spreads throughout the body by using the lymphatic system. So the sentinel node is where you will find the first spread of cancer. If they find any tumors in the nodes over two millimeters, doctors recommend the removal of the entire node. Otherwise, they are left alone, and the cancer can be killed by radiation.

As I waited, I recalled from my Internet studies that some researchers believe cancer spreads not in the lymph system but in the bloodstream, all at once everywhere. This means that cancer is a systemic, or system-wide disease, rather than a localized one that spreads from the first tumor through the lymph system. Oddly, even though the blood might carry cancer, the first place cancer typically begins forming outside the original tumor site is in the sentinel node. Maybe both models are true. Maybe it is in the blood as well as the lymph.

At the moment, theory didn't matter. Laura rested on a table with marking dye injected in her breast, a seven-foot tall, five-foot long massively heavy arm pointed directly at her chest. It resembled the long-range Martian super weapon used in the film, *Mars Attacks!* I wondered if the director of the film had seen this machine during his wife's cancer treatment. Then I thought I should research this on the Internet and find out how his wife had done with her treatment.

Once again, I realized I was going half-crazy from lack of sleep and worry about Laura's cancer. I was constantly trying to find something more I could do to get her healthy. It then crossed my mind that now there was no more need to obsessively surf the Internet for answers. The decision had been made; the doctors were in charge and my work as a medical researcher was done.

A large TV screen hung on the wall behind Laura. It displayed little ghost dots with stuff bubbling along white lines between them.

"There's just one node you can see there." The technician pointed at the screen. He was a wiry, cheerful, mustached younger man in his forties with black glasses and no fat.

I nodded politely, though to me the screen mostly resembled a live-action shot of my grandmother's lace tablecloth during English teatime just after someone spilled milk on it. For all I knew, there could be 100 nodes on the screen, but I was glad to hear that with only one sentinel node, Laura's procedure would be simple; they would just remove it and send it off for a biopsy. Then the cryoablation would continue.

The scope analysis was to take some time so I went into the hallway and found a gurney to nap on. I didn't sleep much. Well-meaning nurses kept asking me if I was all right just as I would drop off. I thought of replying that I get heart attacks if people wake me from a nap to ask me if I'm okay. I didn't. But who knows? They might have wheeled me off for emergency treatment! I gave up on napping.

Soon Laura whizzed out on a nurse-piloted wheelchair and we headed upstairs. Then, too quickly for me to say a proper good luck with a kiss and a cheerful wave, she was whisked away by the nurse and disappeared behind massive double doors. I felt a gut-wrenching sadness and joy at the same time. The doors had shut and the fight against her cancer had begun.

There was nothing more I could do. At least I felt confident we had decided on the right treatment. Although Laura's surgeon in Portland had objected to the cryosurgery, I felt no fear over electing to do this. *This was not risking Laura's life; this was going to save her.*

The waiting room TV shouted out the squeals and clapping of an early morning game show. No one in this crowded room was squealing, clapping or watching. Everyone here had a friend or relative of a woman in that operation registration line. We were all waiting for a loved one's operation to end.

I felt slightly guilty—and privileged too—that Laura was going to be able to keep her breast while many of the mothers and sisters and wives of those here today would not be so lucky. I retreated to the restaurant and my laptop computer to write about the radiation room and its resemblance to SAC HQ.

I spent hours in the cafeteria until my computer ran out of power. Then hours more back in the waiting room. There were over fifty people in here when I left in the morning. Now there were only two others. A game show lulled me to sleep.

Dr. Littrup finally came out. He was so kind and enthusiastic, and almost a dead ringer for the guy who played the Rocketeer. I imagined Dr. Littrup with a leather jacket and flying goggles back in the twenties. I'm sure he would have been an aviator, not a doctor.

As Dr. Littrup crossed the waiting room, my thoughts drifted to a young protégé of Henry Ford, Harry Brooks. He flew every morning in a miniature plane from Bloomfield to Ford's Dearborn factory, showing the potential for a future commuter plane for the average person, the Air Flivver, the Model T of the skies. One day, he crashed and died, and Ford in his grief canceled production of the air flivver.

I saw a Harry Brooks in Dr. Littrup; here was a man of courage and nerves of steel.

"Laura's doing just fine," he began. "She's in post-op and recovering. The procedure went well. We used a mammotome to scoop out most of the first two tumors, then we froze everything and got good coverage. We had to put in a large quantity of saline solution to lift the skin to make sure it didn't freeze. Oh, and good news, your insurance called and said you're covered."

This was great news! They had healed Laura, and our insurance company had agreed to pay.

Dr. Littrup then made an odd remark.

"Some people! I can't believe your insurance company."

"What do you mean?"

"We had Laura anesthetized, unconscious. Then we got a call saying there was no coverage and that your insurance company wanted us to stop the procedure until we faxed a bunch of information to them. But we refused because we didn't want to risk putting Laura under anesthetics twice, and told our staff to fax the information as quickly as possible. They did, and later your insurance company said they would cover the surgery."

I was grateful that they didn't do anything that could have endangered Laura, and told him so, and then I went into the recovery room to see her.

The recovery room had a long bank of windows facing west. Laura's bed was near the center of the room, but I could see through the window. Outside, a cold wind blew while clouds streaked across the sky. The sun was low and ready to set, and Laura was barely conscious. They had tubes going into her nose for oxygen plus tubes in her arm. Wires ran to her from various monitors. One monitor chirped with her heartbeat and showed her blood pressure in red numbers.

"How are you doing?" I whispered. Laura mumbled, she was barely awake, and asked me to give her some ice chips.

"Is it over?" She glanced around the room.

"All done. The tumors are gone. You're healed," I replied.

"Thank God!"

Laura shifted around and her blood pressure monitor buzzed. A nurse rushed over and felt Laura's pulse. I read the numbers and became alarmed. 173 over 125!

"Is blood pressure normally this high after an operation?" I asked.

"Not always, she's right on the edge, though, of having to give her something."

But Laura drifted back into sleep and the alarm stopped. The nurse walked away, so I guessed everything was all right.

"What was that sound?" Laura woke up a few minutes later.

"Your blood pressure alarm." Laura has had problems with blood pressure the last few years. I hated how we were having multiple crises interacting with one another.

"Is it all right now?" she asked.

"Yeah, just relax and rest."

She drifted off, so I went to the window and watched the sunset. It was glorious, with rays of gold from the West Coast reaching us here in cold, freezing Detroit.

"Soon, before you know it, you'll be back in the ocean, boogie boarding," I promised her later as she awakened.

"Not too soon," she joked. "I'll need to get my bandages off." Our beach cabin is only five minutes away from one of the best surf beaches in northern Oregon. We try to live down at the beach as much as possible in the summer and surf nearly every day we're there. Laura loves to boogie board, which entails lying down on a three-inch-thick piece of shaped foam that's about three feet long and two feet wide. It gives a person enough buoyancy to catch a breaking wave if they paddle hard with swim fins and push the nose of the board down the wave just as it breaks. Surfers condescendingly describe boogie boarders as sponge riders, though I am the first to admit they often ride waves I don't have the guts to tackle.

Laura doesn't go out in deep water. She waits in chest-deep water and jumps into whitewater or foam-broken waves that shove her along until she's almost beached on the sand. I tease her and call this foam sponging. She ignores my teasing because it's a lot of fun and, to be honest, I usually join her at the end of a surf session because I enjoy it too.

Between the cold of Detroit; the distance from our playmate, the Pacific Ocean; and Laura's condition, boogie boarding in the ocean seemed far away. But I held onto the promise of that mental image. I wanted Laura out of here, laughing on the beach and healthy, not hooked up to a machine which buzzed a warning of her high blood pressure.

By mid-morning of the next day, Laura was recovering in her hospital room, and I was enjoying my new favorite restaurant, Harper Hospital cafeteria. I came to pick up Laura early, but they weren't ready to discharge her yet, so I came down for some breakfast, only to find out they stopped serving breakfast at 10 am. It only added to my suspicion that the word Detroit really means, "No breakfast served here!" in Algonquin or Mohican or whatever Detroit dialect might apply.

I visited Laura's room at noon. What a surprise! Her poor breast was enormous. She had a special Iron Maiden bra on because they had to fill her breast up with saline solution to protect the skin from freezing. As Dr. Littrup had told me, which I could now see, the saline solution lifted the skin away from the tissue as they froze the tumor underneath. With all that water still inside, Laura had a hard time moving around. For the first time, I felt sorry for certain well-endowed personalities.

Laura roomed last night with a charming woman, Pat, also in for cancer treatment, and they had held a prayer vigil. They were fortunate to have each other because they are both devout Christians. Pat's daughter came to pick her up while we were in the room. It turned out that they were all big fans of the Detroit Lions and Joey Harrington. They were amazed when Laura said she was a sorority sister of Joey Harrington's mom while at Oregon State. Now Laura was a celebrity as Pat explained the new procedure to her family. She spoke glowingly that Laura was the first woman in the country treated with cryoablation without a planned, follow-up mastectomy. This combined with the fact that Laura was friends with Joey Harrington's mom was too much and the room started to feel like Christmas. We became lifelong friends and I knew Laura would keep her promise of writing.

Dr. Henderson came in just before we left, and he was happy and positive for Laura. It was a great send-off for Laura's recuperation in Detroit.

Every little bounce or jiggle of the car caused Laura pain. We were going to be in for a rough time at the downtown Marriott. She could barely walk across the lobby.

Thank goodness our room wasn't far from the elevator, because she almost fell over in the elevator, I had to grab her by the shoulders to keep her upright. Where was that wheelchair now that Laura actually needed it?

Laura

April 24, Midday

Marriott Downtown Detroit

It's over. It's done. My tumors are gone. I haven't felt like writing until this evening. Discharged on Wednesday, I had to go right back in on Thursday for another exam.

It's funny how a little detail will catch your eye. On Wednesday, in the afternoon, I checked out of my room in Harper after my overnight, and they wheeled me down to Dr. Bouwman's office in the Karmanos Breast Cancer Institute for my discharge exam.

After my exam with Dr. Bouwman, I used the bathroom at the cancer center. I glanced over at a silver bowl next to the sink. Made of open scrollwork, it was more decorative than functional, and it held nothing. The bathroom was a generous size, floored in deep blue tile that went up the walls, with a long white sink faced with teak. The silver bowl didn't fit with the modern look of the sink, but seeing it brought joy to my heart.

At first, I couldn't think why, and then I remembered the moment, ten days before. I'd used the same bathroom after Dr. Littrup's exam the first time we came to Detroit, the exam that would determine my eligibility as a candidate for cryoablation. He had been positive that I could have cryoablation, but when I used this bathroom, that final decision was still pending.

164

They measured the tumors, then, and he could find no evidence of them getting any larger. In fact, the largest one that measured 1.2 cm in my first MRI, he had found to be just 1 cm or slightly under. The smaller, new, suspicious spot picked up by the MRI in Portland could be found in a line with the other two tumors. He hunted for the fourth, small, suspicious spot, but was unable to find anything. His comment was, "They certainly haven't grown. I feel sure I can get these."

Being alone in the bathroom with my eye landing on the scrolled bowl, I finally got a chance for it to sink in. When I was first here, the operation was in the future. I was going to have my tumors cryogenically killed, and we were going to make history. If I survived longer than the statistical expectation, there would be no reason not to let cryoablation replace a mastectomy. Women like me with multiple tumors could have the choice of keeping their breast because a lumpectomy wouldn't leave enough breast tissue. A significant change in cancer treatment would occur.

I would contribute to this scientific breakthrough in a big way. God would answer my prayer to help find a treatment for this horrible disease that took my mother. But the answer arrived in a way I never intended. However, I was making a significant sacrifice and effort to bring it about, even though I had not imagined this.

Now it's over! As I sit here in the hotel room, writing in my journal, I feel a stinging pain in my armpit. After suffering two bloody nights with my huge, seeping breast, I thank God for leading me to this place. I found out from Dr. Littrup today that it will be three months before the huge swelling goes down, then three more before the hard dense part inside is eaten. It will be a year until it dries up entirely. Then he will be ready to "make it known and call it a victory."

Dr. Henderson, the 6-foot-8-inch medical administrator, came into my Harper hospital room the morning after the operation to congratulate me just before I checked out. He told me Dr. Bouwman (who did the sentinel node removal) expressed great pleasure at how normal the node looked, and that Dr. Littrup "was skipping around saying it went perfectly."

Next Monday, before we leave, we will find out the information from the sentinel node biopsies, but it sounds as if there has been no spread of the cancer to the node.

I bled so much Wednesday night after coming home from the hospital that Alex called Dr. Bouwman at home. After giving instructions to clean the wound, they told me to come in for an examination, which we did today, Thursday.

I saw Dr. Littrup first. He said the bleeding was actually only leaking saline solution and that I shouldn't worry. The successful freezing of the tumors concerned him the most, so he checked with an ultrasound, and said, "Everything looks great. The tumor area's holes have filled with fluid."

Then I saw Dr. Bouwman. I found out he is of Dutch descent. He is large, at least 6-foot-2-inches," with upturned gray eyebrows and curly gray hair and an ample stomach. The night before he had watched the tape I had given him of the Art Beat program about me, which had originally been broadcast on Oregon Public Broadcasting. I'd offered to donate a painting to Karmanos when I'd given him the tape. He said he enjoyed the program.

He agreed that the leakage from my breast was saline solution injected to protect my skin and surrounding tissue from the freeze. Mixed with a little blood, it looked bad. His exam revealed it did not consist of fresh blood. The leakage pleased him, since it was the easiest way out for this unneeded liquid.

He said to get feminine pads to use as a dressing because anything with the word "surgical" included in the name would just cost more money. Alex remarked that it worked the same way with boats: anything with the word "marine" in it costs more money as well. Dr. Bouwman laughed and admitted that he was a boater like Alex and, as it turned out, in his spare time, Dr. Bouwman likes to make and captain speedy, modern boats.

He also shared suggestions for tourist highlights of Detroit, both artistic and natural wonders of Michigan, as well as his enjoyment over the years of the nearness of Canada and the Great Lakes.

His manner was calm and easy. I felt blessed to have him as part of my team of men who are caring for me. All of them—Drs. Littrup, Bouwman and Henderson—have worked hard to save me, and especially my wonderful Alex, who hasn't faltered a moment and has gone beyond the greatest husbandly duties imaginable. This great team of men has championed my keeping my breast—the removal of which my female surgeon was so easily ready to do. She felt I was easily curable and cryoablation made her nervous. "You're not the best candidate."

But the psychological impact, without breasts, to me meant that I'd have never been "normal" again and that cancer would have won. A mastectomy would have scarred my body and my life. But now, I still have my brave little breast. I'm weak, but I'll get strong again. I will be cancer free and two-breasted. Never in my life have breasts looked so good!

Alex bought me a fashion magazines to celebrate. How could I ever be feminine without my breast? Sexy? Nature has given me the perfect design and the route I've taken honors my creator's most beautiful form. It's a "design worth preserving." I've gone through the valley of the shadow of death, and I feared no evil. Thy rod and thy staff, they were with me. I will dwell in the house—my two-breasted house—of the Lord forever! Amen!

***

Alex

In the late afternoon, while Laura was asleep after journaling, I watched anglers far below us in the river and wondered what they were after. I didn't feel like fishing, though. What a night last night! Laura had decided she needed a shower, and needed my help getting in and out. Once she was in, though, the hole where they inserted the mammotome and took out the tumor started weeping blood. A great deal of blood it looked like to me. Blood was flowing out around the dressing. She felt so weak she had to put her head down to keep from fainting. I called Dr. Bouwman in a panic and asked if Laura needed to go into the hospital emergency room. I imagined a major blood vessel had burst, because she was bleeding so badly.

He asked me in a calm voice to describe the volume of blood escaping.

"Well, it's hard to say, but I've seen deer I've shot bleed less. And that's just before they died."

"It's probably nothing."

"Nothing?" I asked. "It was gushing out all over the shower!"

"Was the shower water running over the bandage?" Dr. Bouwman asked.

"Yes, it was, actually."

"That's it, then. When water mixes with blood, the blood can make it red and seem like there's a large quantity of blood coming out. But really, you're just getting blood from the bandage. Just put a Kotex on it and keep it dry and you'll see that it's not bleeding that badly."

Well, he was right; blood and water had mixed. No severe bleeding. It wasn't pretty! This cryoablation isn't all a piece of cake. To be honest, I wished they'd kept Laura in the hospital for a couple of nights. All this blood-soaked saline solution was now coming out into the dressing and, honestly, it was not pleasant. This was one part of the operation I was not prepared for. I've had no nurse's training!

Fortunately, I've had hunting training, and the sights and smells there are far worse. I figured if I could stand that without complaint for the joy of the hunt and bringing healthy meat home to the family, I could certainly put up with a temporary blood and odor problem.

What was funny, though, was that Laura couldn't smell anything. Her nose was turned off to smelling it. If anyone else plans to do this in the future, be forewarned. I don't know if you can prevent it, but at least knowing it's coming might help any future nurse, male or female.

It was a small price to pay to help Laura. So, every time Laura went to the bathroom, I supported her support bra. I became a support person for a support bra!

By evening we were getting into a routine. It revolved around the bathroom, helping her get there. Then she'd come back, drink water and then either sleep, eat or watch TV. Thank God for in-room movies! We were gradually working our way through every decent movie they offered. Fortunately, they had a great assortment.

I gave up being even remotely concerned about budgeting money on this trip. The movies were $12 each; split two ways that was only $6 each and we were bored in our little room. I think I finally knew what was meant by the phrase, "captive audience." I did find the hotel gym and worked out on the elliptical trainer for over an hour each day; it was great to get a workout. I recommend it for anyone planning to be a support-bra support person.

On Friday, April 26, Laura had more energy. We had originally talked about a road trip to go see Niagara Falls. Laura had even brought watercolors to paint them. What a joke, though. She barely had the strength to go see the doctors. At least they assured us everything was going fine.

On Saturday, we went to a great museum, Detroit Institute of Art. They had everything: suits of armor to great art to a Medici collection on display. Fascinating— and Laura made it through with flying colors. Each day she grew stronger.

On Sunday, a beautiful sunny day, we went to the Ford Museum. I knew spring was here. What a cool place Detroit is! First, we walked down to a waterfront fund-raising concert. Laura said she felt strong enough afterwards to go to the museum, so out we drove to Dearborn, not far from downtown Detroit. The Ford Museum is cars, cars, cars! They have the limousine that held Churchill and Roosevelt when they met in Malta during World War II and a bunch of camping trucks that Edison and Henry Ford used to go camping with around America. We saw plaster casts of Abraham Lincoln's hands—they are enormous—and George Washington's actual wooden false teeth. It struck me that Henry Ford had collected an odd combination of curios and history during his life.

I wandered through a part of the museum where there were only a few people. I saw a collection of some of Ford's first factory power generators, enormous machines stacked together, generators, steam generators, pumps and huge valves. I began to realize that Henry Ford was the Bill Gates of his time.

My cell phone rang. It was Laura. She was feeling weak so she stayed in a little movie theater about the history of the car. She was feeling faint and had seen the film seven times.

I rushed past the first Mustang, the biggest steam locomotive ever built, a Volkswagen and I gathered up Laura. I say gather up because she leaned against the armrest of the chair as if she was coming apart with fatigue. We walked past the Omnimax theater, and I looked with hope at Laura to see if she was up for the Lewis & Clark film.

No, and I agreed; she was not looking well. I was disappointed. After all these years of going with Laura to art museums, I had found a museum that made me smile. Then I realized with a start that instead of worrying that Laura was dying of cancer, I was worried about not getting to see all of a museum.

What a great feeling that was as I drove Laura to our little home away from home in the hotel. After dinner, we settled into a movie and sleep. Life was getting back to a good routine. Even if it was one of nursing and recovery, the cancer was gone! Hallelujah!

Laura

4/28/2003, Saturday

Writing after collapsing after an adventure to the Detroit Institute of Art. There was a huge display of artwork sponsored by the Medicis, including works by Michelangelo. My mind was willing and active, but my body collapsed. Inspiring, though; maybe there is a will to get back to work bubbling up. We went to the Ford Museum afterward. It was too much.

After each trip I have a rest, then a simple meal if we haven't eaten on the trip—maybe room service or a salad from the second floor Greek deli. Finally, we watch a movie, and then Jay Leno or the late night news. It has been hard for me to give in to rest. I have been pushing myself to walk every day, sometimes on the ninth-floor track around the tennis courts to the point of exhaustion. Sadly, this is sometimes only a ten-minute walk, but I am getting stronger each day. I don't think I am a good patient.

Alex is a good nurse, however. He has become a champ at changing my dressings, which happens at least three or more times a day.

We are staying on the nineteenth floor of the Courtyard Marriott and have a magnificent view of the Detroit River. The landscape is flat with big sky. Canada and wilderness is to the left, the city's buildings to our right. It is open for at least a block all around us so the view is far-reaching—an eagle's nest view. The twilight is long, lasting from 6 to 9 p.m. with the pale pink above the horizon subtly changing in the most gradual, restful way. We have settled into a routine of sleeping in, at least me—Alex gets up early to write. Then taking our time to shower and change my dressing. On our first day out, Thursday, we ventured to a health food store in the suburbs to find some supplements to help me heal (plus Chinese dinner afterward). One day, there was a trip to the hospital to check my drainage. On other days we visited the second-floor shopping plaza and GM Center.

More recollections of April 22, 2003, the day of the operation, after I've had some recovery time.

I liked the whole Detroit team. They seemed to get along together so well. The radiologist in the nuclear medicine department needed to pinpoint and mark my tumors exactly for the core removal and the freezing margins after. It would be a tricky procedure because I had three tumors. The doctors extracted the core of the tumors with a mammotome, a small tube. Then they froze the area around the tumor twice, with a warming in between. During the operation, saline solution circulated under my skin to protect it from freezing. The whole procedure took about three hours. I was so grateful to wake up and still have my breast there. The swelling and bruising were more than I could have ever possibly imagined. Dolly Parton had nothing on me!

Bloody discharge soaked my support bra, gown, and bed after the operation. We eventually had to use Kotex to soak up all the blood.

The woman in the hospital bed next to me was an older woman named Pat. She was from the Detroit area and this was her third bout with cancer, the other two being for lung and colon cancer. She was friendly and talkative. She told me about her challenging life and her trust in Jesus. We ended our evening holding hands and praying. She was a good prayer warrior. I was a lot more swollen and bruised and wiped out than I thought I'd be.

I'd brought art supplies to work on but just couldn't do it while I was recuperating from the operation. At first, I managed to get out once or twice a day, holding onto Alex while walking around the track of the hotel. We were on the twenty-second floor and had a beautiful view of the river and a lit bridge with the flame from an oil or gas refinery beyond it and green Canada on the other side. I watched the sky change color as the day drifted into night. Alex wrote a lot and read to me. I like his young adult adventure book. I longed for my family but appreciated the quiet. I slept a lot and watched the news and movies. Read some but not much.

Finally, we went back to the hospital for the pathology report. It turns out a small malignant tumor was in the sentinel node Dr. Bouwman removed. The tumor is over 2 mm in diameter, but is less than 3 mm. Less than 2 mm is considered clear, in the sense that if the tumor is less than 2 mm, it has typically not spread to the next lymph nodes. Once it is over that size, there is a possibility cancer has reached those nodes.

What a dilemma! Dr. Bouwman says that it would be wise for me to stay and have three or four more nodes removed and checked, just to make sure that they are clear. Alex points out that my Portland surgeon could do this in just a few weeks after I have recovered. Dr. Bouwman agrees, so we decide to wait. This will need addressing soon after we get back to Portland, however, so I am not as cancer free after this operation as I hoped I'd be.

Since I have a tumor in the sentinel node, Dr. Henderson states that I need chemotherapy after radiation. Not the harsh kind that makes your hair fall out, but something that can reduce the chance of recurrence further.

While I don't know it yet, I have a huge job ahead of me meeting with doctors in Portland. Some will be supportive; some will not. In the end, the decision to go to Detroit will prove to be the most important decision of all. Unlike in dying, I'm fortunate in being able to find out how much I'm loved while I'm still alive. Somehow, now I will learn to plug back into life.

Chapter 9: Difficulty Getting Radiation at Home

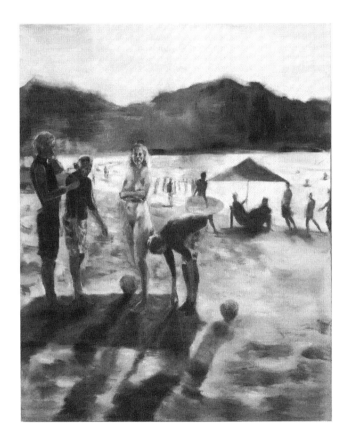

"Drop"

> *"Here she is also naked but is now*
> *surrounded by others in one of those*
> *gatherings common to the Oregon beaches*
> *that Ross-Paul frequents with her family.*
> *In this painting, young people gather in the*
> *foreground taking a break from their*
> *activities in the surf. They pay little*
> *attention to the naked woman in their*
> *midst and she pays little attention to them.*
> *Some experience has separated her from*
> *the lives of those around her. She may*
> *be exposed but they do not see her. She*
> *makes eye contact with the viewer, but her*
> *steady gaze does not create a bond and in-*
> *stead establishes her distance. She is very*
> *much alone."*

> —Teri Hopkins, curator for the Marylhurst
> Art Gym, writing for the catalog for the
> 2006 exhibit, "Naked" Froelick Gallery,
> Portland, Oregon

Laura

5/1/2003, May Day

Oh happy day! Oh happy day! Last evening, I got a phone call from my surgeon. She has spoken with Dr. Bouwman in Detroit. She says it isn't necessary to remove more lymph nodes. She said her experience of doing follow-up surgery on a sentinel node as small as mine has always been to find no more cancer. Instead, she recommends moving on to radiation, and making sure they also radiate the auxiliary area (armpit node area). This will take care of any minute problem that might be there as indicated by the 2 mm plus-sized tumor in the sentinel node.

178

Even better, this means that I am considered "clear" and I won't have to have chemotherapy!

No more surgery and no chemotherapy! Yay! I was so incredibly relieved. I called Alex on his cell phone (he was getting a haircut with Emma). He was delighted.

Oh happy day. On May Day! On this day, a beautiful, sunny, flower-filled perfect day, I am perfect. And perfectly happy. I'm sure I'm an idiot to be thinking this way, but I'm happy about all the growth and lessons this cancer journey brought me.

May 3, Saturday evening

Out in the world tonight, my artwork is opening in San Francisco and in Tacoma at the new Museum for Northwest Art. Both openings are happening without me; I just don't have the energy to attend an opening yet, especially out of town. Charles, my Portland gallery dealer, surprised me with a visit this morning. He told me while I was convalescing in Detroit, the Seattle newspapers prominently featured my work. The openings I can't attend yet are a world beyond cancer. I have a part in it, but tonight, I'm home nursing a flu-ridden husband and allowing a socially starved daughter to regroup with her friends. It's a contrast; what could have been and what is.

And while the worst is over, it's not over. While I'm getting stronger, I'm not strong. I spent the day tidying the house and putting out the flowers Charles gave me. The house is clean, perfect, and welcoming, yet I sit alone. But I have been friend-filled in the past and am buoyant with goodwill and good wishes. No one sees it, but tonight I am perfect.

May 6, 2003

My mom's birthday. She would have been seventy-nine. It's impossible to think of my mom as so old. Somehow, on this day, I think she knows about what I've done and she would be proud. I had a long talk last night with the woman, Karen, who gave us Dr. Littrup's name. She heads an organization that spreads information about cryoablation. She said medicine needs people like me to try out and test new procedures so they can move into the mainstream practice. Happy Birthday, Mom! And tonight is an anniversary for me. I figured out that tonight is the anniversary of my conception. Fifty-three years ago, the sperm and egg got together. All directed by a higher force.

I need that powerful force now, on the anniversary of its bringing me into the world. There are so many energies of the day that need correcting. I woke up to a dream of being in the city, our city, the part we lived in for so long, one time modern but now aging, with business (busyness) going on. I take a break at the edge of the building, Alex comes into the dream and, suddenly, we turn into termites with huge teeth. We devour the foundation of the whole building. In seconds, it comes crashing down. I can feel the soft wood; it's nothing. Foundations are crashing. The busyness around us stops at the crash. Surprised. The big blue sky swallows the dust.

Midmorning, conscious, real-time now; I'm at Dr. Fancher's appointment. He thinks the results of the operation are great--they are! But, he thinks I need to talk to an oncologist and rethink the chemo decision. I hate this. But I tell him I'll do it. He gives me a list of names.

May 7, 2003

Appointment with my surgeon. She says nothing about how beautiful and free of mutilation my breast looks. Instead, she probes all around it with her fingers, deeply, especially in the armpit node area. Ouch! Days later, it still hurts. She talked again about the decision process for me to go to Detroit. She seems offended in some way that I decided to go there and not have a mastectomy under her supervision.

I can feel the emotion in her voice. This has left me shaken after the appointment. I tried to be calm and explained our thinking, and I think I grounded her a bit and gave her more confidence in my decision. She tells me there would be less morbidity for me if I do not do chemo. She gives me good advice that we should carefully decide, and then don't look back down the line. I believe this is just what we did with the cryoablation. I have no regrets now and expect none in the future.

Later, I called Gwen Wright in Detroit and requested that Dr. Henderson call my surgeon in Portland and assure her that the team in Detroit took all the proper considerations and that I'm getting, and got, the best care possible.

Later in the day, my neighbor came to talk. In all this journaling, I have failed to mention that she has breast cancer as well. The diagnosis is almost the same, although she only had one small tumor and was able to have a lumpectomy. It is amazing that we both have almost the same cancer and pathology. We're both worried about micro metastases in our nodes and trying to decide on chemo. She has become something of an expert by now, reading almost every up-to-the-minute paper or study posted on the Internet.

We go over the pluses and minuses of chemotherapy. She feels for me it probably wouldn't be a good idea. I can't tell where she might go with it for her, but I can tell that she's comfortable that nobody (doctor, researcher, nobody), is able to tell her if it will make a difference or not. Statistically, they can prove that fewer women die of breast cancer if they get chemo. But the improved chance of survival is low.

Unlike Ellie, I have the potential of the "immune response," meaning that my white blood cells are learning to find and fight cancer by eating my frozen tissue ball. For me, this could be hugely more important than chemo. To increase this effect, I'm taking vitamins and herbs prescribed by Tori Hudson, a Portland naturopath renowned for helping women deal with post breast-cancer-operation treatments.

My friend Fawn shares an office with her in Manzanita, Oregon, and Fawn called Tori to see if I could squeeze into her long waiting list. Tori put me right in an after-office-hour's appointment last Wednesday. I explained clearly and intelligently my whole situation, which impressed her. She chose specific herbs and vitamins to help me through radiation. They will support my connective tissue and prevent it from breaking down. I'm worried the combination of cryoablation and radiation may have an effect which would kill the connective tissue and leave me with a big hole where the tumor and freeze ball was/ is.

The vitamins and herbs protect against abnormal cell division and support the immune system and help build the killer "T cells." This is the most important work going on in my body to help with the crucial immune response, maybe more important than chemo ever would be.

Later that evening, we got a call from Karen, the woman running the PCA Cryocare website. She was the link, from Alex's call, that led to Dr. Littrup. She assured me the cryoablation immune response is nothing minor.

She said that anecdotal evidence suggests prostate cancer patients almost double their chances of non-recurrence. The actual statistics still need to be gathered. I'm beginning to think that this time between surgery and radiation, which is letting my immune system work, might be as important as the time some people devote to chemotherapy before having radiation.

Back to the visit with my neighbor, Ellie. After we exhausted her scientific knowledge, I was able to help turn her attention to more intuitive matters. I told her the more spiritual side of my story; how I have a long history of trusting the Holy Spirit to guide me. I even told her about how we found this house and about the flowing female presence exuding unconditional love who guided me here in a dream vision.

I told my neighbor about hearing the voice whispering to me that I could keep my breast if I wanted it on the afternoon I got the second pathology report, which confirmed there had been no miracle healing. I confided that I felt led to Detroit and the cryoablation and, as a result, a feeling of faith and trust had taken away my sense of worry.

My friend was amazed, and I think it may have sparked some trust in God for her. She already has a deep belief system. I just want the chemotherapy decision to be right for each of us no matter what we choose to do.

The Sunday Oregonian's review of the Tacoma exhibit gave me a favorable mention. I wish I'd gotten to see it.

The museum used my image for its advertising, the only painting they used from the show.

Aye Yi Yi! It's been a great year and an awful year, an intense one and a learning one. Not boring, almost overwhelming, sometimes exciting, sometimes the opposite; I feel the weight of dead air.

I want to impregnate it and move into life again. My art will lead me to it. I'm ready to get back to work.

May 17, 2003, Saturday

It's a rainy, cold, late afternoon. I've just awakened from a nap but still feel woozy. Sarah and Barbara, my neighbors, treated me to brunch today. It was great to have "girl time." Then I had to go to the gallery to pick up a painting to show a couple of curators who will dine with fellow artists Sherrie, Katherine and me on Monday night as we discuss next year's museum show. Was wonderful to see Charles at the gallery, see the new show, wonderful to just drink in a world other than cancer.

Earlier this week, I moderated a panel of art professionals—a gallery dealer; curator; critic and artists just starting, mid-career and established—for students who were about to graduate and go out on their own. Afterward, the panel all went out to Higgins Bar together. I was so high from the meeting's excitement that I stayed out until midnight. I'm probably still paying for it now with my current fatigue, but it was worth it to re-engage with the world. I'd gotten out with my girlfriends the night before to see the Mark Morris Dancers, which somehow stimulated my creative juices—aah, a world beyond cancer.

May 18, Sunday

It's a beautiful, sunny afternoon and I'm sitting outside on the veranda in my favorite chair and spot, catching the sun's last long rays. Taffy, our dog, is with me. Last night, we had dinner with our neighbors, Corbett and Peter, and with each social event, I escape further into a non-cancer existence where I savor and appreciate my life. I took my friend Linda for lunch last Friday. She demanded I immediately go down to Brazil to see "John of God," for a healing and ignore additional medical treatment. "Don't let them do chemo! Don't let them do radiation! Women need to demand spiritual healing. The next ten years will bring about massive changes in healing."

I gently explained that I have felt spiritually led to be doing what I'm doing in choosing a path which involved doctors and the medical community. John of God may well give me a cure, but I feel I may be able to help the majority of mainstream women dealing with this disease who would never consider visiting such a healer. After all, cryoablation is a new way of dealing with cancer, which also uses the body's own immune system, and the doctors are willing and enthusiastically participating.

Linda finally understood what I was telling her and even backed off and apologized for coming on so strong. My task is going to be hard dealing with all types of people who want to mold my experience into their belief system.

My Unicorn Dream

Last night I had a powerful dream about a unicorn. A beautifully dressed, handsome young man with a hidden, sinister look had taken me into his modern long house to be his bride. The house was mostly a long wall with big windows facing a garden on either side, rather institutional looking. He was trying to charm me, treating me as if I were being honored, but I got the feeling I was trapped and this was not my choice. Something outside the house in a side yard kept distracting him, and when he left, I had a chance to look around. Lining the long hall were big glass cabinets containing hundreds of dried remains that looked uniformly organic, like dried skins or something that had been alive. However, I couldn't quite make out what they were. At any rate, they looked like they had died awfully, by neglect, and that I was likely to be one of them soon if I wasn't careful.

I went to spy on my "husband" and found him attending a beautiful white unicorn in a pasture right outside the door. The unicorn was pacing and obviously unhappy to have its freedom taken. My "husband" was controlling it to tap its powers of immortality. The "husband's" face shone with a mad evil, which made him ugly, where he had been handsome before. He was so occupied with his task that he didn't notice me spying. I also saw he had left a gun lying next to the fence unattended. If ever there was a chance to save myself, I had to take it now. I grabbed the gun, a rifle, and started blasting away. I shot him in the stomach, the chest, and full on in his face. I wanted to be sure I fully destroyed him.

Just at my moment of victory, as I was starting to relax, he raised his head and came back to life. I could see his evil face even though there was a hole through it. It was like he was transparent.

"You fool!" he cried. "You can't kill me! What do you think I was doing with the unicorn?"

He reached for me and I was terrified for my life. I knew my moment had come and I was a goner. Just then, the long tusk of the beautiful white animal jutted through his stomach, and his eyes went wide as true death overtook him. The beautiful eyes of the unicorn locked with mine knowingly. I knew only this magical animal could truly kill the one who must have been the devil. The devil that brings cancer. As our eyes locked, the unicorn's and mine, I knew we were both free. I also knew he was my new ally. I knew I only needed him, my white blood cell immune system, and no chemo, ever.

May 25, 2003, Sunday

Memorial Day Weekend, the beach

I am waiting for everyone to get ready to go to a friend's fiftieth birthday party. It's at the Pine Grove Community Center in the middle of town. It should be fun, as most of my beach friends will be there. A girlfriend brought a beautiful new flower blue top for me to wear and I feel feminine and pretty.

Alex and I have our usual kids camp going at our cabin. Emma and Louie brought friends and Emma's boyfriend and his friend have also been spending most of their time with us. The weather's been great and it's been a renewing getaway. Time to put things in perspective. Today, the boys posed for the cover of Alex's book. Emma's boyfriend posed for the character Arken while his friend posed for Asher, with Louie and his buddy posing as Neanderthals.

Now we're home from surfing, and everyone looks cleaned up, suntanned and healthy. Except everyone's tired! Hope the party wakes us up.

Last Tuesday, we went to see the oncologist, Dr. Takahashi. He agreed with my surgeon, saying that more node dissection wasn't necessary. He added that chemo would cause "morbidity." He encouraged me to consider Tamoxifen after I've finished radiation; however, he didn't seriously suggest it. We asked him to do blood work to see where I was in my menopause hormone levels so we could consider Arimidex or something with fewer side effects. He said that I'll have to get shots, actually a hormone capsule implant just under the stomach skin, that will throw me into menopause, which means I may have bled my last.

Dr. Takahashi was brilliant scientifically. He explained about cytokines, saying they give directions to the white blood cells about what to attach to. He said dead cells stimulate them to do this, just as the dead microscopic cancer cells left in my hematoma. He really understands and appreciates the theory behind the immune response.

Although he called it crude and simple, he also seems to appreciate there's so much about the immune system we don't know or understand. He feels it's better to support it and perhaps this is why he didn't push chemo—because it could wreck my immune system without much benefit.

Dr. Takahashi is in his forties. While calm and relaxed, he seemed on the busy side. Overbooked but wanting to get me in again sooner rather than later, he moved his schedule around so my next appointment is Wednesday, after getting back from SF. In fact, we have to fly home early.

He remarked about how healthy my breast was looking. I tried to give some credit to the herbs that Tori Hudson was giving me, and he even photocopied her notes from my folder. (I guess she's respected among the local doctors.) I think the non-mutilating benefits of cryoablation have impressed him. He made a passing comment about my throwing my surgeon off by doing this cryoablation. However, I got the impression the cryoablation was a positive treatment to him, rather than a negative, and I believe he understands and supports my wanting to keep my breast.

My radiologist, who works out of our local hospital, whom I met next on Thursday, did not. I'm not sure what my surgeon had told her, but this radiologist seemed irritated that I was now her problem. I thought this meeting would be routine. She is the radiologist, and this is standardized therapy. Because I thought this would be a routine meeting, I went alone without Alex.

The radiologist began by attacking my decision to have cryoablation. She also expressed her lack of faith in the immune response therapy. In fact, she said she had made a note in my chart stating her opinion that I was in the 40 percent cancer recurrence rate group! I told her about the immune response possibly doubling the non-recurrence rate in cases of prostate cancer, which it does, according to Karen, the contact volunteer for the PCA Cryocare website.

However, the radiologist said this didn't apply because the way prostate cancer is treated is not comparable. I realized I should not have repeated what Karen had told me, even though my oncologist, Dr. Takahashi, had also voiced his belief that the immune effect may well be significant.

In the middle of our argument, my radiologist kept getting called out of the room, and it was hard to stay on track with her. Getting called out was fine with me, though, because I was able to use meditation techniques to enforce boundaries between her and me. My radiologist seemed as if she was scolding me when I first came in, like I was a hostile patient that needed to be put under control. I wondered where she had gained this impression of me since this was our first meeting. Or perhaps she treated all her patients this way. Regardless, as the meeting went on, she warmed to me.

She quit interrupting me so much and started listening. She had so many assumptions going it was hard to make progress regarding my concerns. I needed to know how the radiation was going to affect the cryoablation-damaged collagen. Also, would the radiation stop the tumor absorption process, a necessary part of the immune effect? She decided to give me three more weeks to heal. She warned me that the radiation may even make the healing stop, either temporarily or altogether, and I may have a permanent bruise ball.

I felt she added this to scare me, which is a technique of asserting control. Instead, it simply displayed her ignorance about healing and the body. I was not surprised when I heard later from our neighbor that she was very non-impressed with my radiologist's knowledge of the latest up-to-date information on cancer innovations and statistical information. Our neighbor made a good point later, saying that doctors involved in research and innovation are worlds away from the day-to-day practicing doctors. My radiologist said nothing about how the breast looked. She didn't seem to have any understanding or sympathy for my happiness at being able to keep it. My comments about those feelings didn't even register on her face! Why are all the men doctors so much more sympathetic than some of the women doctors? Oh well, I'll get by her, finish what I have to do, and move on.

She has ordered a CAT scan, MRI and bone scan, so more wait-and-see and hope for the best.

Summary of My Cancer Treatment: Partial tumor removal through mammotome, followed by the cryoablation lumpectomy by freezing the tumor out to safe margins.

Femara and Zolodex to turn off and block estrogen—not Tamoxifen, thank goodness! According to Alex's research, Femara doesn't weaken the bones. It also does not lead to uterine cancer, which might be a problem with Tamoxifen. I will move on to radiation of the left breast, including the node area.

Alternative treatments I have also had:

- Calendula gel on my breast where I was irradiated, homeopathic and Koch catalyst given with a "push" shot (a vitamin IV) in my left arm
- Vitamin E, buffered C, pectin, IC# QEMz10, Rhodiola, antioxidants, melatonin
- Solvent cleanse
- Chlorophyll, rice protein powder

May 4, 2003

Dr. Littrup called this morning just as I was about to leave for my MRI. In fact, he was calling to see if I'd had it done yet because the National Cancer Institute was after him to get a paper written about using cryoablation to treat breast cancer. Apparently, it would be in response to a paper the French had come out with about a study where sixteen women had used cryoablation for their breast tumors. I am probably not the first one on the planet, but I'm still the first in the US to have cryoablation and keep my breast. It was comforting to hear his voice. It carries with it so much intelligence and confidence and somehow elicits trust. I got his opinion on if I should just have my ovaries out instead of using Tamoxifen (if I can't do Femara and Zolodex).

He said the ovary removal sounds reasonable and said I should wait to begin radiation (at the three-month mark, things really seem to open up and happen; the hematoma begins to go down very quickly). I will pursue exploring my options.

I am so glad I thought to have Edie Vickers (the oncologic Chinese medicine doctor) advise me on what I should do. She is a great, clear thinker, and while I don't look forward to another operation, it appears getting your ovaries out increases your chances of survival as much as six months of chemotherapy. My neighbor helped me find some studies that said so. She also helped me find some great studies that say postponing radiation for up to seven months doesn't seem to reduce its effectiveness. We are concerned because, if the radiation adversely affects the absorption/healing process of the hematoma, it could calcify and I would have to have it removed. I'd have a huge hole in my breast! Just the thing I was hoping to avoid.

I'll know more after the appointment next week.

May 6, 2003

My radiologist called this morning to discuss the MRI, which I had earlier in the week. She said that it looked like the tumors are still there! This confused me because I was told that they were taken out. She said a core biopsy doesn't get all the tumors, just the core. Now they want to go in and use MRI to either needle biopsy the tumors or stick a wire in, then have my surgeon surgically remove the tumors. She said she'd shown my pictures to the tumor board to reach this recommendation.

I told her the films were being sent to Dr. Littrup and that he was an expert in reading them. She asked how he could be an expert when I was the first patient. I told her that he'd read hundreds of films for all the liver and lung and cyst operations he's done and that he had warned me these MRIs would look different. I said I'd talk to her again after I'd heard from him. A very, very unsettling phone call!

Alex became angry when I told him. He said, of course, that the MRI showed that some of the tumor remained; after all, that was how the cryoablation was planned. Some of the tumor was removed by mammotome and the rest was killed in place by freezing. Those dead cells remained; first to conserve my breast tissue, otherwise I would just have had a lumpectomy; and second, so that my white blood cells could eat them up and train the immune system.

He said if they took the "remaining tumor cells" out and examined the tissue on the slide, they would show up as dead cancer cells because that's what they are! And perhaps they wouldn't even be able to tell if they'd been killed by freezing, or from being removed by my surgeon's biopsy. So they could actually remove them and then triumphantly point to dead cancer cells, which they think are dead because they have been removed from the body, but in fact were dead already before they were removed. With their assumption that they were alive in the body, they could show these remaining cancer cells to be "proof" the cryoablation didn't kill the tumor, because these cells, though dead, were still in my body!

Alex also said anything puncturing my hematoma could endanger it by giving it an infection, even gangrene, which might endanger my life. He said there was no way he was going to allow anyone to stick me. Now he has a call in to my radiologist, so we'll see what comes of it. This war of the doctors is hard to be in the middle of. Being the first at something is really hard, I'm learning.

***

Alex

The phone conversation with Laura's radiologist was very frustrating. First, when I called, her office related she would not discuss Laura's case with me without written permission from Laura. I faxed a signed letter five minutes later.

The radiologist accepted my second call and was very rude. I tried to explain my understanding that there could be new, healthy tissue growth in the old tumor area, which was replacing the tissue killed by the cryoablation, and in this new growth tissue, there probably was still an area of dead cancer cells. As well, I patiently explained the fourth lesion area had already been identified as not being a tumor by Dr. Littrup.

She astounded me by replying in a very condescending voice that she understood how, as Laura's husband, I would want to believe in the cryoablation, but the fact of the matter was, "The cryoablation was just like the faith healers we had visited, and that it hadn't worked!"

I asked how she could possibly compare some of the best doctors in the world at Karmanos Cancer Institute to a faith healer? I also wondered how she even knew we had sought help from a healer, because Laura hadn't told her, meaning that one of her other physicians had passed this on.

She replied that it was her "professional opinion that cryoablation didn't work and that, frankly, the Karmanos people didn't know what they were doing!"

At that point, I told her that I could no longer continue my conversation with her, as there was no basis for any discussion if she began it with those beliefs. I told her that regardless of her opinions, we would return to Detroit for any further examinations and let the decision to start Laura on radiation be up to them.

After hanging up the phone, gently, I related my frustration and anger to Laura. She looked downcast, and I could see that this "battle of the doctors," or should I say, the attack by the radiologist, was very upsetting to her. So I just said we would go back to Detroit to get this resolved and left it at that. At that moment, I appreciated my Tae Kwon Do training, which helped me control my emotions because my frustration with this radiologist was compounded by a letter from our insurance company I found in our enormous mail pile waiting for us after arriving home from Detroit.

The insurance company told Harper Hospital they would pay for everything except possibly the cryoablation on the day of the surgery. However, in writing they had now decided not to pay for one penny of expenses incurred in Detroit.

They did agree to pay for all expenses incurred treating Laura in Portland, which seemed ludicrous, because they were proceeding as if Laura had an effective lumpectomy by offering to treat it with radiation and chemo. On the other hand, they were saying they wouldn't pay anything at all for the operation in Detroit.

Why? You'd think they'd pay something, because there has to be some operating cost they'd have paid during an operation in Portland. Surely if they paid an equivalent "Portland operation" amount as even partial coverage for our expenses in Detroit, it would not be asking too much.

We decided to appeal their ruling.

***

Laura

5/20/2003

Last night, my cousin came to visit with a friend. Her friend might partner with me on a product we have discussed manufacturing: acupuncture charts that use characters that I paint. The friend is a whiz at marketing and she called to make the arrangements. It necessitated making dinner for them. They didn't offer to buy or bring food; only to come at that time. My cousin didn't ask about my condition or prognosis. She seemed to want to reinforce how healthy she was, which she repeatedly brought into the conversation. Somehow, my having come down with cancer has upset her. Inside, I think she worries that she might get breast cancer as well, that it might run in the family. I don't know what to say to her, and, after awhile, I realized I'm too tired. I have to take care of myself, so I excuse myself and go to bed exhausted. Thank goodness Alex is able to stay awake and talk to them into the night.

June 16, 2003

It's a perfect June day. Not too hot, light breezes, lots of bird noises. The kind of day I could get lots done if I were working properly. But I'm not working. I'm almost paralyzed. Today, I should have heard from Dr. Littrup; but so far, nothing. I had to go to St. Vincent by myself late Friday to pick up the "dupes," or duplicates of my films. After daily checking, the hospital finally concluded they made a mistake and never sent them! It cost me $70 to make sure they'd arrive in Detroit first thing Monday morning by sending them US Express at 5:45 p.m. on Friday.

I needed a break! We hiked one and a half hours with weight-filled backpacks on Saturday morning. We saw "The Italian Job" Friday night and drove up to see the new Tacoma Art Museum on Sunday. My painting there looked wonderful! Charles says the curator wants to come down to talk to me.

Tuesday, June 17, 2003

Still no word from Detroit. Dr. Littrup did send a quick e-mail last night saying he did get the films and will be going over them with an expert today. I don't know if I need to be concerned or not. Meanwhile I am moving forward as if everything is going to be okay: doing errands, paperwork, getting organized. I'm about to do a huge closet sorting out.

Today, when I got home, there was a phone message waiting for me from the curator of the Tacoma Art Museum, Rock Hushka, who had heard I'd been up. He wanted to know how I liked the museum. Yesterday, he sent me a very sweet card, wishing me well. There is a wonderful life waiting for me outside of cancer.

Wednesday, June 18, 2003

A sleepy overcast day. After walking, I finally got the e-mail I'd been waiting for. Dr. Littrup says it's all fine. He will detail it out for me later, but the main points are: the cryoablation-treated, live cancer is gone (dead cells remain in the hematoma to be consumed). The 5 mm kidney-shaped small mass on the other side of the breast is still there, but hasn't grown and is findable on ultrasound, a sign that it's benign.

Hallelujah! It's hard to let it sink in. Like everything's been all along, there's still a hurdle. Dr. Littrup will leave it up to my radiologist to decide if the presence of the small lesion—the "fourth tumor" that is possibly a growth, though benign since its size has not increased—will hold up radiation. He will be glad to take it out and I will be more than willing to let him, so it's possible a trip to Detroit is imminent.

Tuesday, June 20, 2003

Last night we visited Emma at her basketball camp at Lewis and Clark College. I had the pleasure of showing Louie around the grounds where so many of the summertime adventures of my youth happened. I'd attended picnics of our community church and worked there in food service in high school. Later, I taught in the art department. Louie, unlike Emma, who had gotten the tour a few days before, totally appreciated the grandeur, the intimacy, and pure horticultural spectacle the main grounds offered.

We stopped at the viewpoint of the final terrace, the scene of Louie's trauma as a toddler when water balloons were attached to him by our Japanese houseguest, Jidaicho. Louie laughed at my description of the scene;

he barely remembers that tearful summer day so many years ago now.

Standing on the terrace and looking back to the Manor home, Louie rightly said, "Versailles has nothing over this place except size."

The tour brought me back to all the inspiration the Lewis and Clark gardens had given me as a youth with their beautiful symmetry and the texture, richness and color of the flora found there. It is probably one of the main reasons I cannot leave nature out of my paintings.

Friday, June 27, 2003

Peggy's birthday (my sister who died in a car accident at the age of 13). I'm going back to Detroit. Dr. Ferrier called a little while ago to tell me she had talked to my surgeon and Dr. Littrup. My surgeon said the way she would handle the distressing fourth lesion (possible tumor site), would be to cut it out with margins. She admitted this might not be to my liking because of the efforts I've gone to trying to conserve my breast. Dr. Littrup said he'd like to do a mammotome procedure if it proves necessary, more than a needle, less than an operation. We're headed for Detroit. Again!

He also wants to be the one to handle the needle biopsy of the growth surrounding the hematoma, and I want to let him. It's odd to have this fear of a return of cancer when other things in my life are going so well. Emma was making a big thing about the fat on my stomach going away because I'm losing weight. I'm not dieting. The only thing different is the Femara and the solvent cleanse, chemicals to remove solvents from my body that Tony has put me on. Something's working!

I had a lovely visit with a dressmaker friend from New York out at her mom's place a few days ago. She gave me a beautiful ring she brought me from Mexico, a very magical opal.

July 1, I got an e-mail from Dr. Littrup. He said to be prepared when I come back. I may have to be re-treated with more cryoablation, this time only with one probe at the edge of the hematoma because of the multi-focus nature of my disease. He doesn't think this will be the case, but I need to prepare for it to be. Somehow, I'm worried. I want my family with me when I go there.

I want to go to the Henry Ford Museum with them. Will I have stamina and be able to see it all? Or will I have to sit a lot and maybe not even go, because I'll be weak and recovering like last time? I think I'll get to see it but with lots of internal emotions going on. I'm going into the Fourth of July weekend with the need for another surgery looming over me!

Saturday, July 5, 2003

The fireworks came through the filter of the trees beyond my deck last night where I watched them alone. The lacy dark silhouette of the fir trees was a beautiful natural contrast to the bright, shiny, intense patterns. We had a lovely dinner party at our house with elk barbecued hamburgers that were supposed to be cooked by Alex, but he had a good excuse. He helped save two teenagers from a cliff. And he was interviewed on the evening news!

Alex was surfing at Short Sands Beach with Sean, Louie and all their friends. He had gone to the far south end of the break and heard someone calling for help. He couldn't see anyone, and he could barely hear their yelling over the sound of the surf. But he asked them if they were joking or if they were serious, and they said they were serious. They were trapped on a shale cliff, unable to climb up, with a sheer drop off just below them. Alex paddled in and ran up the beach, asking for a cell phone until someone had one. Then he called 911 and directed the firefighters who arrived first on the scene. They were unable to reach the teenagers, who had evidently wandered off the walkway and slipped to the edge of the cliff, so the firefighters called the Coast Guard. Alex could have left then, but he stayed for the exciting airborne rescue by basket sling. So we forgave him for not cooking the barbecue this year. At least he contributed by getting the elk!

The evening ended with lovely fireworks on the beach. I was too exhausted to go down and mix with the crowd, so we watched from our deck. Another great Fourth of July on the Oregon coast! I hope there are no fireworks waiting for me in Detroit.

Chapter 10: Return to Detroit—Do I Still Have Cancer?

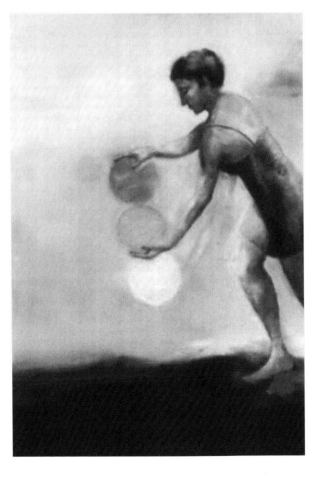

"Juggle #3"

"Her 2003 painting, 'Juggle #3' depicts a woman running with zest and vigor as she balances three balls on top of each other. Their colors are orange-red, blue, and white. The blue and the red could represent healthy and unhealthy breasts (they are breast size) while the white could represent the "ice ball" that was used for surgery. Interestingly, this was the last painting Ross-Paul created before she found out she had breast cancer, and it was an 'ice ball' that eventually saved her breast."

—Roberta Carasson, Artist Profile, Art Ltd. Magazine November/December 2009

Laura

July 13, 2003

Starting a new journal today. This could be called the cancer journal for sure. It's been a very trying season in what has been an interesting and challenging time. I'm such the "cancer expert" now. While I'll never really know for sure, I strongly think the nasty, painful, double mammogram from last April, the one that took weeks to recover from, probably triggered a growth of my breast cancer cells. I believe they were otherwise lying dormant. My liver might have prevented this if it hadn't been compromised by long hours in the studio around solvents. That's my suspicion, but who knows. If they knew how cancer started, they would be preventing it by now.

Regardless of how I came about this cancer, I've accepted my fate, embraced it and learned by it. My choices may help thousands, even millions, of women after me to keep their breasts. I've grown and been tested and persevered.

July 17, 2003

Sitka Center, Otis, Oregon. There's a warm, muggy breeze blowing through the window of the upstairs loft of our cabin here at Sitka Center. Alex is at the landing desk, looking out the big round window, finishing the last touches to his novel.

Not a bad place for me to begin a new journal. I didn't think I was going to make it to Sitka and teach my watercolor workshop again this year. I thought I'd be doing radiation by now. But my last MRI showed areas of growth around my hematoma and a small node-looking area, which was suspicious enough to cause my cautious Portland radiologist to hold out for a biopsy before proceeding with radiation. That biopsy will take place next week, in Detroit.

I will be going back to the scene of my cryolumpectomy, the first performed in the US where a woman has been allowed to avoid a follow-up mastectomy. This time, the National Cancer Institute will help pick up some of the tab as Dr. Littrup is writing a national protocol for the procedure. His PowerPoint presentation will star my brave little breast.

Dr. Littrup has assured me he thinks the suspicious "fourth area" is just a lymph node and the biopsy—if he has to do it—will be very breast conserving and not too "morbid."

If they find anything suspicious, they may refreeze the area if the biopsy shows there's cancer there. They'll only freeze using a single probe, so it won't be as involved as the three-probe original procedure. That one took more than a week to recover from.

I'm happy to be going back to Detroit. I'm glad I'll again see that happy hospital family. But I'm nervous too. My body's memory of what happened before is kicking in. My eye twitches. I can't rest it. It's a good thing I'm teaching, because I have to be strong, focused, and present. The last few weeks were hard; there were several funerals.

First, my dear friend Dianna's mom, whom I had just seen in San Francisco, died of cancer, at about the same time I was diagnosed. She had been my mom's best friend. Then, my beloved art history teacher, Claire Kelly, who taught me medieval art and the coming together of Eastern symbolism and Western realism, died, though not unexpectedly. She had Alzheimer's. She was young—only sixty-four. The beautiful funeral in a Catholic church with Madonna statuary was just what she would have wanted. But the Portland State crowd of my era was too close to home. My own funeral started to haunt me, and I needed to move away from the thought of it.

An event and a project have helped. Last weekend, we went to Camp Namanu, a Campire Girl's camp nestled along the Sandy River on Mt. Hood's flank, for a fundraising dinner. Dazzle (my old camp pal), joined my son Louie and I. Louie was our perfect date, all young and handsome and full of sunshine (as he always is). He kept engaging with the current camp staff in age-appropriate ways, like high-fiving and shouting out camp names (his is "Moog"). He flirted; he joked; he made us feel important just to be with him. At one point, we three snuck away and went up to the cathedral of Ferny Glen, a natural amphitheater of firs and ferns, to just meditate on what camp meant to us; how it had transformed each of us into something that was more confident and whole than we'd been before. The three-way conversation made each of us realize that what we thought had been a personal, private conversion was really a universal experience but only because we had allowed its magic to work on us.

It was good having a chance to visit with Dazzle, as she has had her own struggle with breast cancer, which began six months before mine. Luckily, she only needed a lumpectomy and radiation to treat it. She is on hor- mone- suppressor medication as well. She's been a ter- rific support person and champion of all I've done and been through.

Then there was the fellowship application. The Regional Arts and Cultural Commission's "Master Artist Grant" was due, and I asked Grants Writer Donna Milrany to help me with it. I also asked former Museum Curator Prudence Roberts, and Modern Art History Professor and Art in America Author Sue Taylor to write me letters of recommendation. Three powerful women all affirm- ing the importance of my candidacy helped me to affirm myself. It helped me turn my eyes away from cancer to see my way back to my artist self.

Friday, July 25, 2003

Detroit, Michigan

It's over! Though tired, I'm intact, and no re-freezing required! Yesterday at Harper Hospital they gave me two MR images and about six to eight needle biopsies, done with ultrasound guidance.

Dr. Littrup was wonderful. It was great to see him again. A very sweet, former Pakistani named "Z" did the

MRI on the hospital's new machine. Then Dr. Littrup and a confident no-nonsense woman named Dr. Soulin (the hospital's MRI breast specialist), looked the films over for anything that might be a candidate for a biopsy. The suspicious fourth area was seen again, but it was not as prominent. Dr. Littrup explained it was behaving much like a node, coming and going, but definitely not like a tumor, which would have shown some growth by now. He said part of the problem with MR images is that they show up questionable, mysterious things that aren't necessarily abnormal, just unknown.

He also said that to take out this fourth node area would unnecessarily cause me morbidity.

In the hematoma area as well, they confirmed that the new growth is not cancer but new healthy tissue growing back in (just as Alex had suspected). To remove this tissue now would be a higher standard of cautiousness that I would never be submitted to, even if I'd only had a lumpectomy in Portland and not cryoablation in Detroit. So, no cancer, and no more operations!

At 1:15 in the afternoon, he decided to let me leave. He said he'd do the biopsy work on Friday, after Dr. Soulin and he had a good chance to study the films.

Alex, the kids, and I had just gotten on our way; I hadn't even been able to tell them what happened when the hospital called me to come back. Things couldn't be scheduled for the following day, so everyone was staying late to finish with me.

A very sweet ultrasound technician named Dianna Hatch was coordinating our schedules at this point. Dr. Littrup handled the ultrasound machine with her assistance. He stuck the spring-loaded biopsy needle in at least six times, but it could have been eight to ten. At one point, he removed fluid pockets that he felt caused some of the suspicious areas around the hematoma. I'm afraid to look at my breast now. It probably looks like a pincushion! He searched for the node area but couldn't find it. It was close to a rib, he felt, but impossible to find and biopsy.

Then they bandaged me up. Dianna had told me of an aunt of hers who had contracted breast cancer at twenty-eight when she was pregnant. Because of the baby, they could not treat her. She died when the baby was only six months old. Both Dianna and I said we were so glad about Dr. Littrup's development of cryolumpectomies. A freeze might have put the breast cancer into remission so that the mother could have been alive longer for her baby. Dianna told me Dr. Littrup had taught someone at the Mayo Clinic how to do cryoablation and now the Discovery Channel was doing a story there.

Dr. Littrup told me that he had taught a colleague, Dr. Fred Lee, how to do cryoablation on the prostate. That doctor then unleashed a public relations blitz, only to be railed upon by the urology community for advertising cryoablation, which they claimed was still unsound and untested.

He said that's why he's working with the National Cancer Institute to give them a protocol, and with the FDA, Blue-Cross and Medicare. He then told me that Karmanos is building a ten-million-dollar machine that he co-invented, which will make ultrasound as useful and exact as MRIs are now. It is going to be called CURE technology, which stands for Computerized Ultrasound Risk Evaluation. There are already several patents covering the machine, and more coming out soon. What an incredible mind! Dianna tells me he comes in almost every day with new ideas, and they have to slow him down as the staff can't keep up with him. He told me they were on the verge of getting something going that was very big, and that I was being helpful to that cause more than I'd ever know.

I'd given him a framed reproduction of my painting, "Waterfall," which he'd liked. On the card was a reproduction of "Dorsal," a young boy with juxtaposed wings/ clouds, which he also liked. I told him it was because he was my angel. I'd written a message about how my paintings often depicted figures in precarious, even dangerous situations, yet they have body language full of confidence. They're unclear where they'll land, but they show trust that they'll land all right. I thought it illustrated my situation with him.

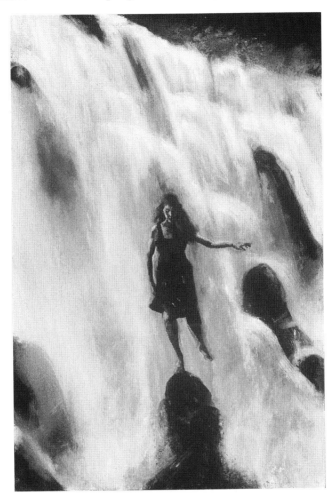

"Waterfall"

Finding a state of "balance" has been a common theme in my paintings, especially those done during the years when my husband was working long hours developing his company and I was raising our three young children while being a university adjunct professor and a multiple gallery represented artist.

211

*I've often felt I've had more courage than
confidence. This has led me into situations that require confident action to move
forward. Do I do this to myself as a trick,
a sort of "now what" situation that forces
action over complacency?*

—Laura Ross-Paul 2014

After the biopsy, I went back to "Z" for at least another hour in the MRI machine. The last test they gave me
showed all the chemicals present in my body. Evidently,
if cancer were present, it would leave trace chemicals that
would show up on the machine. It is a spectrographic
MRI machine. Three very interesting doctors sat at the
computers in the control room to analyze the readings.
They told me that the preliminary results showed none of
these chemicals to be present. We finally finished at 7:30
p.m.—I'd arrived at 7:30 a.m.!

Z took me back to my family, who had been waiting
over two hours in the waiting room. I hadn't wanted them
to leave this time, and they had kindly agreed to wait.

After we got back, Emma watched a movie with me
while Louie and Alex brought us back a salmon dinner.
It was delicious.

July 27, 2003

We spent the day at the Ford Museum after sleeping
in until 2 p.m. Eastern time. Alex finally got his dream of
revisiting the museum with his kids to his heart's content.

While we were there, I called Dianna Hatch, who said
Dr. Littrup was trying to get a pathologist to read my
slides before I left for Portland. She said that I'd made
a big impression on her and that Dr. Littrup called me

212

a real sweetheart. He called me later to say he'd arrived just after we'd left the hospital the evening before and was sorry we hadn't gotten a chance to say good-bye. Then he told me that he'd talked to the pathologist, and just as he thought, no cancer was found in the biopsies taken from the "suspicious" areas of the hematoma.

He was very excited and said he'd now be turning in a protocol to the NCI, the National Cancer Institute. He will send me a letter to present to my radiologist in Portland to begin radiation. We will have to make a specific request to get the pathology report from the hospital, but that is just a matter of forms. He also asked me to write the chief CEO of the hospital in Detroit who has supported his work. I'm already thinking about what I will write. My phone died as we were talking, so he left a good-bye message, which I retrieved later.

Wednesday, July 30, 2003

Manzanita, OR

Back from Detroit. Went to see *Seabiscuit*, a story of an underdog winning. Alex and I are at the beach. Emma's at a basketball camp with Ashley. Louie is at home running the painting crew at Beaverton Lodge. I'm here to "process." Alex is finishing his young adult book, *Arken Freeth and the Adventure of the Neanderthals*.

So many wonderful, poignant emails awaited me when I got back in response to my group e-mail sent from Detroit saying I was in the clear—no more cancer. I spent most of yesterday visiting or phoning friends, sharing the latest news and allowing them to help me get what I've been through in perspective. It almost seems like a dream now.

But I still have a big hematoma in my breast telling me it's real. Maybe the most amazing thing of all is that I still have a breast! There is such beauty and symmetry in the balance of the body: single head, two shoulders, double eyes, single nose, and so it goes down the body, a rhythmic cadence between duality and singularity. The total package a balanced whole. Any missing body part breaks that rhythm, that symmetry, that perfection. I don't want to be double breasted because I am cleavage oriented or a sexpot. I'm not, but I do appreciate the beautiful way God put us together. I didn't want a constant visual reminder of my body's one-time failing. It's been corrected; the mental and emotional scars are enough. I can heal from those, but breasts don't glue back on so easily.

An artificial one, even one made of my own stomach fat, sporting a tattoo nipple, wouldn't have served me. It would be like a badly done drawing, an ugly reminder that it wasn't the original. Oh, I appreciate the way God made me and my experience has made me want to work hard to maintain that perfection.

When my course was set and I knew I was going back to Detroit to have my operation, and I was fully aware of the risks and fear a new technique brings, I had a distant reminder that comforted me. Years ago, after my mother died of breast cancer, when the wound was fresh, I said a fervent prayer. It was to let me be significant in the search for a cure. Of course, I thought that would mean a career in research, much like Dr Littrup's. But, I struggled with my science courses in college and soon gave way to the career my natural skills made me destined for, being an artist.

Perhaps I could heal through painting. The dream of making a significant difference drifted away. But what I'm finding out about prayers is, the answers have their own way of working themselves out. Mysterious forces that come from a more encompassing viewpoint have a way of coordinating energies in the most unexpected ways. Because I've grown to trust these forces, I've allowed myself to be picked up by that energy and ride with it without judgment. The conclusion of the ride can be humbling when the recognition comes that it was all done so much more encompassing than a single vision could have imagined. I wanted to help in significant cancer research. I have; not in a way I would have chosen, but that doesn't diminish the contribution.

Perhaps it was the only way my non-scientific brain could have participated. I don't have a scientist's smarts or genius, like Dr. Littrup, but I do have an artist's awareness to think outside the box. I'm comfortable with bringing into physical form that which is a mere idea. I trust cause and effect.

I went to Michigan, the land of ideologists, innovators and inventors. I came from Oregon, the land of pioneers. I had motive. I had unwavering trust in my guidance system, trust that lifted me up above fear. Perhaps I was the perfect candidate to begin on. Although it was hard, I never wavered.

And now, now that the results are so conclusively positive, now I can revel in the amazing way that God works. I've seen it firsthand. It works only if we trust and believe in both our guidance and ourselves. If we each do our jobs, it works. The faith to get us through is there, if we open ourselves up to it. This experience has added to my courage. My attitude is one of curiosity.

When we were in Detroit, the car had a guidance machine on it, a Hertz Never Lost system. If we made a wrong turn it rang out, "Recalculating Route," but it always got us to the intended destination. I could never have guessed this route, but my guidance system got me to where I wanted to go.

July 30, 2003

I am amazed at how much energy I have now that I know there's no cancer! Was I depressed before? Yesterday, at the beach, Alex and I went for a two-hour walk with weighted backpacks. Then we drove home to Portland and hosted a swim and barbecue party for visiting friends from Germany. This party went late into the night. Today, I've already done a lot and will probably do more before the evening is out. When I was down at the beach, I got a chance to read over the whole journal experience of the cancer trial. I had left out so many stories, such as Emma's comment after we first returned from Detroit. She had just seen *The Matrix*, something we never got to do because of the timing of the operation.

She told me there was a scene where Neo sticks his hands into Trinity after she has died and brings her back to life. "That's what happened with you and Daddy. He took you back to Detroit and brought you back to life! You two are my heroes!"

Also missing is the statement I said so many times: "What woman wouldn't want this operation? It is almost like a miracle. You get to keep your breast and get an immune response to your cancer. All you have to put up with is a hematoma in your breast for six months to a year. Not a bad place to have to carry one."

There's more, and I'll add it as I can.

Tuesday morning, a gallery dealer from back east called to express interest in representing my work. I'm going to check out his gallery, but during my time at Short Sands, I got a beautiful lesson from the waves. As I floated on my boogie board, I just enjoyed watching the sets roll in and the surfers playing on them. It was great watching the waves jack up suddenly, the mere sight sending a flash of excitement down my spine.

So much potential—should I go for this wave? Will it hold? What experience will it bring? Some waves that are gone for work out! Some are way more exciting a ride than expected; some aren't. Some dissipate too soon, or are slowed by the shore break rushing back. But the really wonderful thing is that there are always more waves. More sets. Lulls in between, yes, but always more sets.

August 16, 2003

Short Sands

It's the time of the end of the daylight when the sun shines over the north end rocks. Today the air is warm and golden, the water smooth and welcoming. I am full of happy exhaustion from my fun rides with Emma through the foam on our boogie boards. My skin is salty and brown; everyone gives an endorphin smile. One of these days, I might be feeble and no longer vital. We might all end up that way. But not today. Today I am alive. I am alive to the fullest. Peter, Marshal and Fawn share in Alex, Sean, Emma and my aliveness. I am too happy to indulge in thoughts of not ever being this way again.

August 27, 2003

Mars closest to us since prehistory, 60,000 years ago, and my little sister's birthday! Labor Day weekend is ahead, traditionally our last weekend at the beach. We always promise that we'll come back for some of the glorious September weekends, but school and sports seem to take over and we don't get down too often after Labor Day. I am sad to see the summer go, but I am happy to have been able to spend part of the summer here.

Chapter 11: Radiation

Laura

9/2/2003

Saw my new radiologist who replaced the original woman so opposed to my cryoablation. My new radiologist did my simulation, the set up for radiation. She answered all our questions and assured me radiation won't be so bad.

Earlier that morning a Dr. Lars from Atlanta, who hosts a medically oriented talk show, called regarding an upcoming program she wants Alex and I to be guests on. The program will be about cryoablation and will feature us in our own half hour to tell the patient's experience. She was interested in the viewpoint of a patient's advocacy just as much as the new procedure. Talking with her gave me calm about my upcoming radiation as well. Her voice was low, soft and steady, with a real clarity and intelligence. When I told her that I was wondering why I still had to have radiation after my tests came back negative, she said, "I can see you're smart enough to know the answer to that one."

Later in the day I got a call from a woman named Maria, a friend of Schizen Yang, who wanted to thank me for recommending Dr. Peterson's Ray Gel. The gel is applied before radiation and protects the skin. Maria was half way through radiation and had been hit by fatigue from the first session. ("It feels like the worst sunburn you ever had and wipes you out totally!") It was her earlier report that had put me off radiation, and I was so happy to find out about the change of reaction with the gel.

Then the next day I visited Edie Vickers, my Chinese medicine doctor and acupuncturist. She told me to put freshly sliced aloe vera plant on my skin at night and use Calendula gel right after a treatment. She also gave me herbs to keep my energy up and signed me up for weekly acupuncture, which was said to be the most effective thing to combat radiation fatigue.

September 3, 2003

Or is it the 4th? I don't know! It's wonderful to not really know the date! I know it's a Wednesday, however; Emma gets back from school camp today. Went to see my sculptor friend this morning, she gave me an ochre-colored marble sculpture she carved. It was an abstracted torso of two breasts and it is lovely. She said it was my reward. It was great she thought this way. She recognized hundreds, thousands, maybe millions of women will benefit from this new procedure. My courage helped make it happen. It's humbling to get such a gift when the ones who deserve it are Dr. Littrup and the team at Karmanos.

Later in the day, we ran into a friend who is a local news anchor. She joined us for lunch and cried after hearing the whole story. She was so happy because her sister had to have a mastectomy at thirty-six. Then she started talking "Oprah." (My little sister has done this to me too.)

The terrifying thing is that something like this could actually be Oprah worthy. When I went through it, it was real life. But now that it's over. . . well, it happened and I can't undo that! So it is history now. My history. Will it be noteworthy? I certainly hope the treatment is, whether my part in it is or not. The option is just such a wonderful one to have. I feel it is practically my duty to sell it, to put a face and feelings on the concept, on the actual experience.

When we got home from Detroit the first time, the most wonderful cards started coming. I have a box of them by my bed (a heart-shaped box, my stepmother's gift—a coffee mug came in it). The cards offered such great encouragement. It was so touching and uplifting. Having recently looked at the box of cards left from my mother's death, I was struck by the similarity.

Then it hit me. These are the people who would have written if I had died. I had the fortune of being affirmed by those very ones who would be mourning me if things hadn't worked out. I got to glimpse my own death and step back away from it into the arms of the ones I live my life with. I can't begin to express the way it has lifted me up. Now it's on to radiation.

I called my neighbor the other night, full of my Detroit happiness. She soon had my exuberance pulled up short as she mentioned her recent visit with her radiologist. It seems I run the risk of my aorta being damaged. "You'll have to make sure they don't burn your aorta." How do I do that? Will I have gone through all this only to have my heart kill me prematurely?

I will go through it and I will endure! I'm tough; I've proved that. I can get through this.

I walked with a friend this morning down to the point where the Nehalem River mouth meets the ocean. There we saw a pod of seals swimming quietly out to sea. They were in a v-shaped pod just like a flock of geese.

September 5, 2003

Today, I had a friend over to help design a ventilation system for my studio. It will be nice to be working around such a sweet, sensitive soul. He reminds me of a male version of my beach friend with his big brown eyes and soft-spoken manner. Our goal is to have the studio ready to go for oil paints at the end of October. I should be done with radiation by Halloween! (I will be giving out great candy!)

September 9, 2003

It was one of those big days yesterday. Jordan Schnitzer invited Alex and me to go along with him and Annette Dickson, the museum print curator, and Candace Nunn, the director of his foundation, to Pendleton to see the "Pressure Point" exhibition curated from his collection, in which I have several prints. It is installed in a museum in Pendleton.

After the museum tour and lunch we met with Don Sampson, the current CEO of the Umatilla tribe. We had time for all this due to Jordan's private jet, which turned a long three-hour drive into a half-hour flight. Don gave us a tour of the reservation and told us about plans and goals that the tribe had for future development.

We then attended an opening of more prints from Jordan's collection, which were in a show at Crow's

Shadow, the print shop Jim Lavador started on the Umatilla reservation. There I gave a short talk and afterwards received a compliment from none other than Jim Dine, who was visiting a foundry in the area and had come to the reception as well.

After a visit to James Lavador's studio at Crow's Shadow, we moved on to Sen. Ron Wyden's fundraising dinner at the Umatilla tribe's museum. As the sun set, illuminating the beautiful rolling hills to the east with the moon rising over them, the senator filled us in on his current interests and legislation.

Jordan, who is chair of the senator's fundraising committee, introduced the senator to Alex and me as we said our good-byes in the parking lot with the open fields all around. I was able to succinctly get out the basics of breast cryoablation and asked for his support in the future when Medicare is asked to fund it. He chairs the Medicare Oversight Committee. Whew! It would be wonderful if this chance meeting resulted in Medicare funding cryoablation for breast cancer treatment as it already does for prostate cancer.

September 12, 2003

Back to the beach, a last weekend stay, before we seal up the cabin for winter. We got a call from the insurance company about an upcoming hearing to decide my claims. Since it is in nine days, I had to scramble to assemble records before we were to meet my grade school friend Dianna Taylor at the cabin. We made it by the meeting time, but she had to cancel because of a need to visit relatives in town. I was relieved in a way; we went to Seaside to the cove where Emma and I had a fun surf session with a beautiful late afternoon sky full of big tropical clouds in the background. Then the Pig and Pancake for dinner and home. Emma and Louie enjoyed each other's company.

September 13, 2003

Got going on cancer drawings, transposing to larger paper, small drawing book renderings I've been doing throughout my treatment. Malia Jensen is curating a "Core" exhibit of established artists that have influenced her. She wants their raw drawings. These certainly are that; I think she's looking at how an artist thinks.

Wednesday, September 17, 2003

My third day of radiation. Returned from Texas on Sunday where I gave a talk at the opening of the "Pressure Point" show at the University of Texas in El Paso. Following the show we had gone on to Houston to visit an artist friend of mine, Terrel James, and her husband.

Terrel is a contemporary artist who also shows at Froelick Gallery in Portland. They had traveled to Portland for a show in the fall of 2001. The events of 9/11 left them unable to fly home and we became friends forever during the week they were stranded at our home.

I received my diagnosis of cancer when she visited Oregon last year. She helped me make my decisions. Then she received a diagnosis of breast cancer when I was having my operation in Detroit.

Last weekend when we visited in Houston, she had just come home from the hospital following her lumpectomy. Now radiation and chemo lie ahead of her. This is the third friend of mine who has come down with breast cancer around the same time as me, and all of us are in our mid-50s.

On Monday, I made cookies in the morning for Louie to take to college at Oregon State. I took part of the batch to my radiation team and they appreciated them too. They all seemed to be starving! My appointment was at 11:30 a.m. and the cookies helped us get off to a good start. After my appointment, I did a great drawing of Louie. Then I helped him pack and Alex drove his stuff down in the van while I rode with Louie in his Audi. He had fixed it up to give it a sportier look, including a big SAE (his fraternity) decal on the back.

What a flash to the past to see Alex's old fraternity house with my son moving into Alex's old room! His roommate looks just like his dad, also from our era and a member of the house. The roommate's birthday is the same day as Louie's, only a year earlier. A party was going on with "girls" and "beer." The "brothers" looked far too young to be fraternity boys. I will miss Louie. I called the next day, but he was too busy to talk and the promised call back never came.

It had taken Alex and me until after midnight to drive home after helping Louie. I was exhausted on Tuesday. After radiation, I went to Tony Esau's office to be checked. He gave me something to protect my cells, but not interfere with the radiation. I also looked over Dr. Littrup's report and photos of my operation. I wasn't prepared for that— made me more nauseated than I already was.

Made a big chicken soup for dinner but couldn't eat it as my stomach was upset. Couldn't sleep at night. I was relieved to be going to see Edie Vickers today. Her needles really did put energy in my body, and I even had a big tuna sandwich when I met Alex to do shopping afterward.

Charles is traveling to Houston today. I hope he can help with my artist friend—I'm so worried about her— she looked so frail when we saw her last weekend in Houston.

Sunday, September 27, 2003

Walked with Alex in Forest Park for forty-five min- utes with twenty-five pounds of weight in my backpack. We then picked up Emma from soccer practice and had lunch at New Seasons afterward. For being in my third week of radiation, that's not too bad!

It's been a hard week, though. Also, I'm worried that I haven't heard from Dr. Littrup for a while now. He hasn't responded to my e-mails telling him how I'm doing in radiation. I guess he's just too busy.

Chapter 12: Dr. Littrup—Breast Cancer Cryo Program Cancelled

Alex

Laura's surgery went well, even better than I expected. It seemed to me that this would be the first of many breast cancer cryoablations, or cryolumpectomies, that could now occur at Karmanos. Little did I know that fate had another plan for me.

The first discouraging news was that the Pauls were unable to secure any medical insurance coverage for their operation. This, despite assurances by phone by the insurance company personnel to our staff on the day of the operation that they would try to cover everything that was standard besides the cryoablation. Their reversal of position and their refusal to pay for anything created a huge cloud over the potential for using cryoablation at Karmanos because, without insurance, future patients would have to pay for the entire procedure.

This payment method is called "boutique medicine," where the rich choose their treatment, regardless of their insurance status. This is how my mentor, Fred Lee, pioneered cryoablation for prostate cancer. However, I knew the rocky road he had traveled on and the criticism he

227

suffered when patients left their urologists and tried the new, radical cryoablation, with great success. His success was so great that eventually urologists took up cryoablation as a standard tool.

I had hoped that breast cryoablation would not have to repeat this difficult initial struggle with acceptance. However, the refusal to pay for the slightest expenses in Laura's case dashed my hopes. The Pauls were appealing the case, but it seems they have little chance of getting any reimbursement.

The refusal of their insurance company to pay for any of the expenses created a big problem for us at Karmanos, since we are an affiliate of Harper Hospital. Harper is in the middle of Detroit and provides medical care for various people of lesser means typically covered by Medicare or Medicaid.

The problem was that if we offered cryoablation to wealthy individuals, and Medicare/Medicaid didn't pay for cryoablation, then an indigent patient could legally demand that we provide cryoablation for their breast cancer. Instead of Medicare paying for it, Harper would have to pay for it!

This potential legal burden of treatment cost would have been catastrophic for the hospital and Karmanos. As a result, Karmanos placed my much-hoped-for, cryoablation-for-breast-cancer-treatment protocol on hold.

My only hope for breast cancer cryoablation to get going at this point was that Sanarus, the maker of the cryoablation equipment, would pay for clinical trials for breast cancer.

However, I contacted Sanarus and, to my dismay, they displayed no interest in offering clinical trials. This was frustrating, as was their company policy of manufacturing a single probe cryoablation machine (something I also had hoped I could convince them to change).

The machine I used to perform Laura's surgery was actually a prostate cancer treatment machine with eight probes and manufactured by another company. This company, called Endocare, holds the original patents for argon gas cryoablation machines. They licensed all breast applications to Sanarus, but kept the technology themselves for other medical uses, and wisely made a multi-probe machine for those applications.

I used three probes in Laura's operation, coming in from different angles to get a good freeze ball that completely covered the tumor and provided clean margins around the tumor. One of the biggest concerns when using cryosurgery is killing the entire tumor. The only way to insure the tumor's destruction is to use multiple probes while monitoring the ice ball's development on ultrasound. If a certain area requires more freezing, then the second or third probe is deployed to achieve freezing.

When Sanarus received a license to use the technology to treat breast conditions, they decided to focus their efforts on freezing fibrous, nonmalignant tumors (fibroadenomas) rather than breast cancer. The upshot of this decision was their machine was inadequate and unsafe for performing cryoablation on nearly any breast cancer over 1 cm.

So, to operate on Laura, I used a prostate machine. Sanarus found out about this soon after Laura's operation and contacted me, and I told them what I had done. They were upset. I told them I felt it was irresponsible of them to build a single probe machine that was inadequate for treating breast cancer. This was especially true because they had the commercial use of the cryoablation locked up by patent and license agreement.

Essentially, this meant that currently, any doctor wanting to perform a safe breast cancer cryoablation by using a multi-probe machine, has to "secretly" use a multi-probe machine from Endocare equipped with at least two cryoprobes. This is at the doctor's discretion since Endocare cannot sell cryoprobes for breast use without violating its agreement with Sanarus to let Sanarus supply cryoablation equipment for the breast. If Endocare did so, they would open themselves up to a lawsuit from Sanarus, their licensee.

When I first began working with Sanarus, I couldn't understand their refusal to build a multi-probe machine that could be used for breast cancer treatment. I was even more puzzled by their unwillingness to fund a clinical trial to prove that cryoablation can safely treat breast cancer! Cryoablation seems to me the logical next advancement in treating breast cancer. Many women who now get lumpectomies or mastectomies could receive satisfactory cryoablation treatment if they had insurance coverage for the procedure. There is now insurance coverage for prostate cancer treatment, so I believe coverage will someday inevitably extend to breast cancer treatment, although I believe that this safe, new option in treating cancer could spare women the removal of their breast and therefore should not be delayed. However, in Sanarus' defense, small, struggling, start-up companies have a difficult time getting funding for a large cancer trial to secure insurance approval.

Before Laura's operation in 2003, I traveled to China in the fall of 2002 and during that trip, I thought long and hard about the roadblock that Sanarus had unwittingly created for the use of cryoablation in breast cancer treatment. I had traveled to China to consult with Chinese physicians about lung cryoablation. My first trip to China had occurred in 1999. However, when I returned to China in 2002, I admit to traveling there in a state of trepidation due to an incident that had upset me during my earlier visit.

In 1999, the Chinese doctors I met insisted that I teach them how to use cryoablation to treat liver cancer. I pointed out the standard operation was simple; they just had to open the patient under anesthesia and freeze the tumor. However, for some reason, they didn't want to open the patient. Through the confusion of interpreters, it took a while for me to understand.

I finally realized they wanted me to perform cryoablation percutaneously, meaning, inserting the probe through the skin, relying on CT and ultrasound to guide me to the tumor. They also wanted me to do this without giving the patient anesthetic, or at least only a local on the skin! I said no, that this was too risky, especially for the large tumors they were showing me. They said they understood that I had already used CT and ultrasound to guide liver cryoablation in animal research. So they could treat it by pushing a probe under the skin into the liver. Simple.

They insisted that I try to do this on large liver tumors and I kept refusing, saying that it was too aggressive and that an ill patient might come to harm in trying such a procedure. The doctors—there were about ten of them in the conference room—had a huge discussion among themselves. After this discussion, the interpreter came back to me and asked, "How about a healthy person?"

They wanted me to perform a percutaneous cryoablation on a perfectly healthy person! I could only hope that it was a volunteer for the operation (it flashed in my mind that may well not be the case). I wondered exactly what I had gotten myself into by traveling to China. They had assumed there would be no hesitation on my part about treating only part of a big tumor, but since I was reluctant, they'd get me a healthy one to use as a guinea pig to test a small ablation!

At this point, I realized that no amount of objecting would ever convince them that I was not going to perform percutaneous liver surgery. I politely told them that my back was hurting and since I was feeling ill, I should return to my hotel until my condition, partially faked of course, improved.

After several days of ignoring their pleas to perform cryoablation percutaneously, they finally showed me a CT of a patient with a smaller tumor near the liver surface that could be easily reached. After getting their thorough assurances that the patient was giving informed, written consent to the procedure and its risks, we performed the first CT-guided liver-tumor cryoablation in October, 1999.

Despite my concern that a second journey might hold new and disturbing surprises for me, the trip in 2002 turned out to be both fascinating and prescient. The Chinese are working hard to enter the modern world. In some ways, they have an advantage, because they don't have the history or investment in some of the existing technology we use in the West. They are therefore able to pick and choose from our technology. I have found the Chinese government to be blunt in stating that they don't have the financial wherewithal to consider treating cancer with radiation, even though it has proven to be successful in treating many cancers. For them, it is just not cost-effective, and they are looking for far more efficient and low cost ways of curing cancer.

This is one reason they were so interested in using cryoablation to treat liver and lung cancer. They perceived, correctly, that it is a low-cost treatment of the disease.

The three years that had gone by since that time had seen the expansion of the use of cryoablation to several centers throughout China. After some media reports about my first lung cryoablation in the US, in September 2000, a Doctor Hongwu Wang in Beijing began a very scientific, well-monitored trial of the use of cryoablation in China to treat lung cancer tumors. When I visited Dr. Wang in October of 2002, he showed me superb data from the treatment of over 200 patients. I realized this needed to get into US medical literature. It was ironic that on this second trip to China, the student had become the master, but that was the case, and I followed through and helped Dr. Wang publish his landmark series in Radiology a few years later.

It was disheartening to see how quickly the Chinese had adopted this superb treatment tool compared to the glacial pace of advance in the US. In fact, in the case of breast cancer cryoablation, an absolute roadblock to the use of cryoablation had been created in the US by Endocare, the only manufacturer of viable cryoablation equipment, because they had licensed all breast treatment to Sanarus, a company with no desire to pursue breast cancer treatment!

However, seeing the use of the large argon gas tanks in China on a regular basis made me realize that there was a need for smaller, less cumbersome equipment to generate the cold temperatures necessary for cryoablation. Frankly, it was a little scary seeing the difficulties of using cryoablation in limited medical facilities because they had to use large, high pressure, argon gas tanks. I reflected then that if there was an earthquake, the 6000 psi tank could be knocked over. If this caused the valve head to break off, the sudden release of gas could propel the tank like a rocket with enough force to pass through a foot-thick concrete wall!

The potential danger of using high-pressure argon gas as a freezing agent was in my mind when I passed through Moscow on my return from China. Dr. Alex Babkin, a Russian-American colleague from the University of New Mexico had also traveled to Moscow at the time to work with partners at the University of Moscow. He had e-mailed to say that he and his associate from the University of New Mexico, Dr. Robert Duncan, would be in Moscow and suggested we meet. Babkin and Duncan are both world-class, low-temperature, physicists. During our meetings in Moscow, I related the danger of using high-pressure argon gas in the primitive settings I had observed in China.

I lamented that the argon machine was unwieldy and impractical in general since to hold the gas it required a huge pressure vessel about five feet tall like a welding tank. The tank is made of thick steel and weighs up to four hundred pounds. In Japan, they are very worried about earthquakes, so they chain the tank down so heavily it looks like a cartoon villain. It is humorous to see this tank chained to a square, four-wheeled base that prevents it from tipping over and turning itself into a missile. Despite the humorous look, their concern is valid.

Alex and Bob explained that this would not be the case if one could use liquid nitrogen as the freezing medium because it can be stored at relatively low pressure compared to Argon. However, I explained the difficulties I had encountered while using liquid nitrogen for cryosurgery. By the end of my explanation, they could see that nitrogen's expansion and vapor-lock problems had led to the development of the argon machine.

My friends said they thought they could design a probe that could use nitrogen and not suffer the problems of vapor lock. They said the only problem was holding the nitrogen at the correct pressure so the gas stayed at what is known as the critical point. They stunned me with their idea. If they could develop such a machine, it would prove to be a breakthrough in the delivery of cryoablation.

Nitrogen gas is cheap to produce; it is the most abundant gas in the atmosphere. And in liquid nitrogen form, it takes up very little space. If we could develop a multiple probe, liquid nitrogen machine, cryoablation could become a widely accepted, clinical operating tool. The enormous size and expense of the argon tank makes it a tool only a hospital could house or afford. A small nitrogen machine—I imagined a unit the size of a water cooler—could easily fit in a clinic and be very inexpensive. This would dramatically reduce the cost of providing cryoablation.

It was frustrating to come from China, a place so willing to become an advanced and practical country that it bordered on the unethical, and return to the US, where corporate decision-making hampered progress so severely. Sanarus had the only technology available to legally perform breast cancer cryoablation. In the fall of 2002, it appeared I had no alternative but to wait for my friends to invent a machine that would break the deadlock. I went back to my old routine of being a typical radiologist, reading x-rays, CAT scans and MRIs while biding my time.

However, when Laura requested treatment in the Spring of 2003, I decided to proceed with the cryoablation using a multi-probe prostate machine in the hopes of demonstrating to Sanarus what I already knew to be true due to years of research: that multi-probe cryoablation was eminently successful in treating breast cancer. However, despite the success of Laura's treatment, Sanarus still refused to participate in treating breast cancer, and even worse, with the insurance company refusing to pay for any of the treatment, Karmanos reluctantly had to stop offering cryoablation as well. As if that weren't discouraging enough, soon after, disaster struck in the fall of 2003.

Chapter 13: Dr. Littrup—Silenced by a Torn Aorta

In September 2003, just three months after I had seen Laura in Detroit for her follow-up exams that preceded radiation, I was in Chicago visiting my college friend and roommate, Dr. Seth Kaplan, and giving some talks. I was staying at a resort that had a lap pool. Swimming had resurfaced in my life as a great stress reducer, and I had put in a mile on Thursday and again on Friday. But Seth encouraged me to stay the rest of the weekend at his home near Lincoln Park until I had to return home on Sunday. I agreed.

Before giving another talk on Saturday afternoon, I enjoyed a leisurely morning of reading in Seth's kitchen. An article about the tragedy of John Ritter grabbed my attention. The *Chicago Tribune* highlighted the shocking effect his sudden death had on all who knew him. Other articles described the rare, sometimes confusing symptoms of aortic dissection. Many patients didn't make it to the hospital. Others, like Ritter, died on the operating table from complications of the massive, yet delicate surgery. Of those who survived, many experienced some form of brain and heart damage.

Being a radiologist, I hadn't thought much about this deadly condition. The humanity of the article and never knowing when "your time may be up" resonated within me. These thoughts were soon to become the basis of some crucial decisions.

When I woke Sunday morning and sat up, a searing pain deep inside my chest ripped up to my throat. It subsided a little, so I tried to shake it off by taking a shower. The pain lessened and I thought I should be a good jock and "walk it off." After all, morning pains get more common after forty! But I became so dizzy in the shower I had to sit down.

Something was wrong. I dressed and then an overwhelming weakness forced me to the floor. I could barely move. I put my head between my knees and called for help. Seth's son Justin was already awake, watching TV on the next story of their brownstone.

The next thing I knew, Seth was there. I asked him how long it might take for an ambulance to arrive. He said, "It might take up to forty-five minutes." "I don't think I have forty-five minutes," I told him. Seth and his wife whisked me into their car despite me being just shy of deadweight. The original plan was to go to Northwestern Hospital, but when Seth saw my gray color in daylight, he decided on the closest, level 1 trauma center, Illinois Masonic.

Seth is a practicing ophthalmologist, but I trusted his decision. He had originally received board certification as an emergency room physician and had trained in Chicago. I didn't recognize the hospital, so I just asked Seth to try to get the best surgeons to come in on that Sunday morning. I had a premonition that aortic dissection was causing my pain.

When we arrived, Seth transformed into Super Doc. He doesn't want to hear it, but he certainly seemed like my "hero" at the time. He parked right at the entrance, grabbed a wheelchair, and got me inside. He blew through security and triage saying, "I'm an ER doc and my friend is having a massive MI. I'm taking him right to a cardiology bay!"

I wanted to tell him it felt more like a dissection, but hey, he was the guy who knew how to score the grades in college, so I said nothing.

He certainly primed the staff and got them moving! My blood pressure hovered in the seventies and they couldn't get an initial temperature. The cardiac surgeons appeared after an echocardiogram showed an aortic dissection, complete aortic insufficiency, and pericardial fluid. My condition had progressed into partial rupture, and my blood pressure was becoming unstable.

Seth told me not to worry since the lead surgeon, Donald Thomas (M.D. 1986), was also a Michigan-man just a year behind us. I didn't know it at the time, but his partner, Alvaro Montoya, had thirty years experience and had led the cardiac transplant service at Loyola. These guys turned out to be my Dream Team.

Somehow, I remained conscious through the pre-op frenzy and even selected a biological over a mechanical aortic valve in a power-chat with Dr. Thomas. From having seen complications on CT, I wanted to avoid the powerful anticoagulant Coumadin required by the mechanical valve. But time was running out.

Seth displayed character traits that I will be eternally grateful for in a physician and a friend—love and compassion. He held my hand so often during this entire ordeal that he kept my sheer terror at bay long enough for me to talk to my son since Seth couldn't reach my wife,

Martha. He managed to contact my oldest son, Gerrit, who was fifteen.

When I heard Gerrit's voice on the phone, the ugly facts of operative mortality and morbidity choked me up. I could tell him only that I was truly scared because I was going into a big operation. I regretted telling him even that, but I wanted to be honest. My thoughts were getting foggier as the sustained hypotension took it's toll. I was finally able to talk to Martha, but the fog was getting thicker and all I could manage was, "I love you."

I felt like I was literally clinging to life. I focused on holding the hands of Seth and a wonderful nurse, Meredith. I even asked the surgeons to pray for me. Meredith got a hospital chaplain to say a prayer before they wheeled me off to the operating room.

Only an hour-and-a-half had passed since the first ripping pain. I continued holding Seth's hand down the hallway to surgery, quietly praying. I promised myself that it was not going to be the last conversation I would have with my son! My skin color had faded to a mottled blue-gray and my pressure was dropping. My neck veins bulged in an ominous sign of impending death from tamponade—when the blood can no longer enter a heart being squeezed like a boa constrictor by the surrounding blood in the pericardium. I told those around me that I was getting even dizzier. The last thing I heard was, "Pressure sixty and dropping. We gotta go *now!*"

According to the OR records, after they sedated me they emergently "cracked my chest." A large amount of bluish blood had gathered around my heart, preventing it from beating effectively. Dr. Thomas later told me at that point I didn't have minutes left, only moments. My aorta was torn and dilated up to six centimeters while my otherwise clean coronary arteries were just hanging off this damaged piece of aorta.

Curiously, the tear stopped before the carotid arteries and didn't wrap around the aortic arch, limiting the extent of the repair needed. Better yet, they removed the blood and clots found in and around the carotid vessels of the aortic arch without causing stroke or significant side effects.

The surgeons installed the new "pig" valve in a long and difficult surgery that saved my life. Had it not been for my swimming and my anaerobic interval training, I might not have come out of the ordeal without obvious heart or brain damage. As it was, I recovered fully.

Seth said later he knew I was going to be all right when I focused my combativeness after surgery on wanting an alphabet board hanging on the wall in the intensive care unit. Despite being intubated and groggy, I wanted to tap out the message, "I M-A-D-E I-T!" Maybe I believed my wife and sons could hear it too. But the best thing I ever heard a surgeon say came from Dr. Montoya the next morning. He told me the repair that he and Thomas had done looked "gorrrrgeous!" I was going to be fine.

I'm not sure why my life was saved that day. Time can only be my friend in solving that mystery; every day is now a precious reminder of my second chance. All I know is that it took a miracle to avert a catastrophe. When I analyze it, a catastrophe and a miracle seem to be diametric opposites on a probability scale. Both are rare, unforeseen events. The odds for everything going right that day seem incalculable, inexplicable, and divine.

My survival left me with a strong feeling of appreciation for all the people who helped me live, for my friends and family. It also amplified my desire to live and watch over my sons, as someone had for me during my operation.

After I came home and began my recovery, Gerrit was diagnosed with mild hypertension and a dilated aortic root. My Michigan cardiologist, Kim Eagle, perhaps gave me the most profound insight: "If you're wondering why you made it through this incredible event, perhaps it's so you have the chance to be your son's guardian angel."

As I look back on my survival now that time has passed, I feel more and more that this incredible defying of death somehow parallels my birth. My arrival on this planet could so easily never have happened, and my existence on earth could have ended that Sunday without me ever seeing my efforts to spread cryoablation come to fruition. If my mother gave me an initial impetus toward wanting to make a difference while I was here, my survival has given me the feeling that I must be working on something important. It was a miracle that I survived.

For some strange reason, I was not able to read for almost two months after my operation. No one is sure why this is the case; I could speak and hear easily and felt my brain was working properly, but reading was impossible. The letters made no sense to me.

Shortly after my operation, I received a detailed technical report from Dr. Robert Duncan and Dr. Alex Babkin. It was their first work on our new cryoablation machine that we had discussed nearly a year earlier in Moscow. They had solved the problems and had proven mathematically that it was possible to use liquid nitrogen to perform cryoablation without the problem of vapor lock. More importantly, they even had a crude but working prototype in Alex's garage! This was a revolutionary breakthrough. But I felt so embarrassed about not being able to read all that, I did nothing with their study for over six weeks. Each day I thought I would be able to read and get on with my work, and each day brought frustration.

But after six weeks, suddenly, reading was possible again, and their study was one of the first projects I dove into. The brilliance of their work astounded me. I called Robert and Alex when I was done.

They told me on the phone that they thought they had done good work but had decided that for some reason I thought their invention was impractical for surgery, and I must have been too embarrassed to tell them the truth. They felt relieved when I told them that I was the one suffering embarrassment, because I should have told them of my inability to read. I think I didn't tell them because I worried deep down that I might never read again. I didn't want to confront that possibility.

Regardless, the result of their work was that we applied for and received a patent on this device. The next step was to secure funding for developing a clinical prototype of the machine. During the next several years we proceeded with our project and finally produced a prototype and, soon after, were delighted to license our device to Endocare. However, after further trials and construction of more advanced machines, we finally determined that the technology offered by the near-critical nitrogen device was not commercially viable.

After this roadblock, Dr. Robert Duncan dropped out of our research efforts and Dr. Babkin and I were joined by William Nydam, a former executive of Endocare. We formed a new company called CryoMedix and continued with our research until we were able to come up with a completely different approach to creating cold which we determined to be commercially viable. This device we call a Single Phase Liquid Cooling system and we have applied for patent protection. This device uses a closed loop concept that "pumps" liquid refrigerant into the cooling tip and then back out to be re-cooled. This keeps the tip cold enough, down to -190 centigrade if needed, and also allows for low operating pressures and quicker freeze-thaw cycles. In addition, the unit can use propane or several other liquids and is highly portable; only 10 inches by 10 inches by 25 inches high. Another benefit of this device is that we are able to cauterize the probe track as the probe is removed if so desired.

Armed with our new patent application and working prototype we have formed a separate company dedicated to female applications called CryoFem Inc. It is estimated that more than half of the women in the U.S. will see a doctor about a breast abnormality sometime during their life. Most of these physician visits are the result of a woman's self-examination in which they discover a lump in their breast. While the majority of these masses are non-cancerous or benign tumors referred to as a fibroadenomas, they generally cause significant anxiety for the women. Fibroadenomas are usually solid, round, non-cancerous tumors that feel like a marble within the breast.

The first application of CryoFem Inc. will be the treatment of benign breast tumors, followed by the treatment of cancerous breast tumors. Additionally, CryoFem Inc. will be working with the various insurance companies and Medicare to get reimbursement for fibroadenomas in the remaining parts of the country where is it not currently reimbursed as well as reimbursement for cancerous breast tumors. Since cryoablation is a more cost effective approach, it is expected that reimbursement will be obtained.

It is expected that there will still be a place for the mastectomy in certain cases; however, the Chinese, who have become the true pioneers in this field, have applied cryoablation to some rather remarkable cases, cases considered untreatable here in the US but treated by cryoablation in China with the cancer going into remission. One specific example that comes to mind is a reported case of a woman with advanced breast cancer that had actually become gangrenous. The diseased areas were frozen and, incredibly, the gangrene was cured while the cancer went into remission! The potential for cryoablation is tremendous and I am so pleased that I am seeing this tool being used to treat breast cancer in my lifetime. I truly feel I was blessed by my opportunity to stay alive and continue my work.

Chapter 14: A Renewed Commitment to Spread the Word

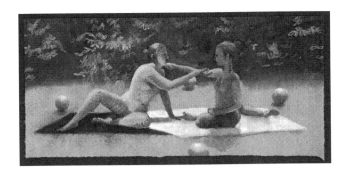

"Yellow"

"In a broader symbolic sense, the geometric patterns in her paintings refer to the belief in transformation that provides the foundation of Ross-Paul's philosophy."

—Jessica Hunter-Larsen, curator for the 2007 exhibit, "The Allusive Self," Colburn Gallery, Colorado College, writing for the exhibition catalog

Laura

Friday, October 2, 2003

On Wednesday, Alex and I were on an East Coast radio program, "House Calls," out of Atlanta. Dr. Littrup was on, too, as the subject was cryoablation and especially its new application to breasts. During the ads, Dr. Littrup told me he'd just gotten out of the hospital. I called him on his cell phone later and found out he'd had his aorta blow out! John Ritter died of the same condition only a few days before! Dr. Littrup was more fortunate, however, as he was with a friend of his that was a former ER trauma center doc. He had Dr. Littrup to the emergency room within minutes where two heart specialists happened to be free. As he was trying to talk to his fifteen-year-old son, the emergency staff whisked him into the operating room to have his valve replaced. Afterward, while he was still unable to speak, he pointed to the letters on his alphabet sheet that spelled, "I made it!" Wow, what a dramatic story.

I guess I came close to being the one and only cryo-lumpectomy ever given! The radio program had given me some insights into my own role and Alex's in getting the operation to become an alternative for me. Dr. Littrup revealed that our preparation and knowledge in our meeting played a big part in the decision to take on my cryosurgery. And I was glad to hear my second trip to Detroit had been helpful to the NCI report.

The close brush with death had Dr. Littrup saying that he was, "only ten days old," meaning, the operation had given him a new life. He said he had been rethinking his purpose and that starting the center for cryoablation was much more on his front burner. He even brought up the possibility of writing a book with Alex and me. I'm going to send him Betty Eadie's book, *Embraced by the Light*.

Sunday, October 5 2003

Just dropped Alex, Emma and Louie off at the Civic Stadium to see the USA women's soccer finals: America vs. Germany. I gave my ticket to Louie. I went last Sunday to see US versus Ghana and Russia versus Canada play and needed to leave early because of fatigue. Also, the crowd bothered me. Guess I'm feeling vulnerable.

Today's already been a big day. We got up early to take Emma's friend Ashley boating on Haag Lake. Louie was home from school, and he used his new wakeboard behind the ski boat. He was awesome! He got right up and then he started jumping waves. His muscles are huge! He's been rock climbing and weight lifting at school. He wanted to come home this weekend to see Emma's homecoming soccer game Friday night. She did great and OES won 3-0. We went out with some friends who've just moved back to town from years on the East Coast.

Saturday morning I had a studio visit from a curator at the Tacoma Art Museum. He just wanted to meet me even though I didn't have much new work to show him, having just sent most of the spare inventory back east to my new gallery in Philadelphia. I did have the new drawings including my self-portraits to show him and much of our talk was about how I transform experience in my life to imagery. I related how my brain has started working differently since I started radiation. I told him about the strange symbolism that looks like it could have

249

eastern or ancient roots that I keep drawing like doodles. It's as if below the level of hand-eye coordination there is a type of seeing that recognizes rhythm and pattern and symmetry. I think the doodles might have something to do with energy, energy intersections, like mandalas or life force in general, but somehow they feel to me as if they link us to nature.

I told him how I'm struggling to integrate these in my regular figurative work and how right now I just don't know how that will work. I just feel I need to process it. He seemed like an interesting curator. He's currently putting together a fascinating show involving Lewis and Clark as the theme, but will feature contemporary artists and Native Americans dealing currently with the Lewis and Clark "myth." This should get some attention. People will either love it or hate it. He told me that my piece was about his favorite from the recent show, and that he'll look for ways for me to get more of my paintings on Tacoma Art Museum's walls. Wish I wasn't so tired; I want to get back to painting!

October 8, 2003

Arnold Schwarzenegger won the governorship of California!

Alex and I went to see some attorneys. We are organizing legal representation for our insurance company hearing on Friday. They refused to pay for any of the cryoablation and related surgery in Detroit, so we are appealing their decision.

I spent most of yesterday getting a package ready for Dr. Littrup. In it is Betty Eadie's book, *Embraced by the Light*, about her near-death experience. I thought Dr. Littrup would relate to this after his aorta experience.

I sent Dr. Littrup a letter, a handmade card, and excerpts from my journal about the time I was in Detroit. I also included reproductions of some of my recent drawings, including the self-portrait illustration.

October 16, 2003

Fifth week of radiation and very tired. I could hardly make it around the opening of the multiple location art show called Core Sample last Saturday night. We made it to three of the venues in the Pearl District, including the one I'm in, "Draw," curated by Malia Jensen.

Malia did a wonderful job transforming the former office space into a gallery. The drawings were mostly strong, although there weren't many women; it featured mostly male art. The range of artists makes it interesting. The exhibition displayed older ones like Hank Pander, Harry Widman and Mel Katz alongside younger ones like Patrick Long and some I didn't even know.

The idea for this comprehensive Portland Exhibit originated with Randy Gragg. He wanted to echo, on a Portland scale, the survey show put on by West Coast curators called "From Baja to Vancouver," going on now at the Seattle Art Museum. He asked about twenty people (thirty to fortyish active movers in the Portland art scene) to curate shows of their own devising. I felt flattered to be in Malia's show in which she wanted to reveal private perception, close observation and interpretation in works not done for marketing. I first showed her my cancer drawings, which she recognized as raw and personal. She gently suggested I should go back to working with models, which I did, and was able to integrate the energy imagery from earlier studies with the figurative studies. These works are beginning to point the way back to painting.

The audience appreciated the drawings, and I received some heartfelt compliments as I moved about the exhibits through the evening. Some great stuff was going on with plenty of energy. It reminded me of the NAW, Northwest Artist's Workshop, days. I didn't go to the artist's night-clubbing parties afterwards. I'm not into a scene like that just now with the fatigue of radiation going on. Instead, we went with friends to a lively dinner in NW Portland at Lucy's Table and had a wonderful visit. Went to an east side "Core Sample" venue with an artist friend yesterday. Thank God she drove! This radiation fatigue is getting to me. It's hard to focus on anything.

This morning Charles called (he loved my drawings). He told me some artists and a local writer had called to complain about the "Core Sample" show. They complained about "artistic elitism." I'm sorry for this. This feels like the heyday of Paris: jealousies, breakaway shows, big egos, big personalities—but mostly, artistic energy.

October 23, 2003

A beautiful fall day, crisp but sunny, with long golden shadows. For the first time, I didn't feel "leaden" after radiation this morning. They began my "boost" today, which means that they are only radiating my tumor area and not the three other surrounding areas.

I brought cookies to the valet staff, the office staff and the women technicians to celebrate. One of the girls drew a circle on me where the radiation hit so I'd know where to put the calendula gel afterwards. As I treated myself in the small dressing room, I glimpsed my torso in the mirror. I was struck by how nice that torso looked with both breasts! I looked at my face. Earlier, after I'd done self-portraits, I'd found beauty there. I'd seen strength and sweetness, traits I'd sometimes inwardly felt but never noted with a cold artistic eye. In the dressing room this morning, I saw the missing Princess coming through in my expression. The immensity of my experience hit me. Keeping my breast is such a simple, yet profound, result. Tears welled up. I looked the same, yet I am so deeply changed. This is a miracle of faith and trust manifesting in nothing changing at all. I retained my original form, my simple two-breasted-ness. Cancer has not altered my topography.

Our graphic artist friend laid out the graphic lettering, *Arken Freeth and the Adventure of the Neanderthals*, on top of the painting I'd done for Alex's young adult book. Alex will use this in the marketing to agents as an example of the genre of the book. But it looks so much like a real cover, and it does give an idea of the flavor of the story, harking back to the simple honesty of the era of *Tarzan* and the *Hardy Boys* adventures. I think it looks great and would buy it based on this cover alone! Alex read the book aloud to us at night and it is a great read. This one should make his mark.

October 29, 2003

Only three more days of radiation! Last night was the worst, as I had to stay outside in the cold evening, watching the Catlin Gable Trees crush Emma's poor soccer team. Alex and Louie are off hunting elk on a friend's ranch.

Wednesday November 12, 2003

Today must be the peak of fall color and beauty. I'm mad at myself for not taking a camera everywhere I go. Some scenes are achingly beautiful. Don't have energy to do much. The last few days of radiation were torture. I wanted to be over it so bad! The only bright spot in life getting me through it was a great series of programs on NOVA about string theory. I took notes and hope to write out what I understand of it soon. The big deal for me about string theory is that before the show, I had an insight about the unusual visual patterns plaguing my brain lately. I decided they must be "energy patterns" at the smallest level of existence.

Well, the string theory program essentially mirrored my thoughts. It seems there are non-matter patterns of vibration at the smallest level of particles in atoms. They are oval shaped and their undulating vibrations are unique to each entity. All my strings are unique to me. And the math for this idea works with both Einstein's theory of relativity and quantum physics. At a simple level, we are all nothing but God's "energy," force or vibrations.

A friend was visiting from New York and came with me to my final radiation appointment and took photos. Alex joined us and we went to breakfast. Even though I had huge plans to make special cookies and a hand-made card, I ended up simply giving boxes of pears to the valet and radiation staff. I also included one of my painting images printed on the card with a simple thank-you message.

On Wednesday, we attended the opening of Cindy Parker, who shows there is a wonderful painting life after cancer, as she is a breast cancer survivor. Her work hung alongside that of Jay Backstrand. She displays brilliant bravado and daring. A quiet shopping weekend and a long walk with friends—always a treat.

A fun fiftieth birthday party with friends at their catering business's entertainment spaces.

Re-connected with yoga and had my first shiatsu massage earlier.

January 9, 2004

The end of a week of snow, freezing rain, cabin fever and big sleeps. Every winter needs one big freeze-in. The break that comes with Christmas is all about finishing work, preparations, social activities and a great social diversion—but not a rest. Snow piled around the house so high you can't leave forces one to sleep late, stay up late, adding to more sleeping late, and dreams. All that sleeping and dreaming gets the subconscious ripe for the plans and preparations of spring. Somewhere in the cycle of life there needs to be a halt in activities, a forced slow down for internal time. Not that I only rested! The house was picked up, the Christmas decorations put away, my desk cleared, mail and correspondence caught up with, studio cleaned and paintings laid out to begin. But this cleaning coexisted with movies indulgently watched during daytime hours, long phone visits, long baths, all while the snow trapped us inside. I'm sick of it now, but it was wonderful for a short season. My final indulgence will be this year-end summation. I want to reflect, even if it's garbled together on this end, to quite a year.

January 11, 2004

Reflection on the past year. About a year ago I was taking a special class from my yoga teacher, learning about energy movement through the body. During a guided meditation I suddenly saw what I thought was a mandala. It wasn't like the mandalas I'd seen in art books, which were beautiful but static. This mandala was an active moving form, an intersection of energy, beautifully coming together and reconfiguring to go out again, like a complex freeway interchange of energy. A few days later, I found out I had breast cancer, which diverted my thoughts from this mandala image.

Throughout my treatment, however, I'd take mental breaks, wondering if it was possible for energy to move in patterns. Later in the year, I happened on a *NOVA* program about "String Theory," a theory some purists have come up with which unites Einstein's theory of relativity with quantum physics, coordinating a macro and micro view of matter. From what I could understand, the theory explains that at the smallest level of what they think matter is, matter is nothing more than energy behaving in a set, fixed pattern.

During my hours of sitting around in doctor's waiting rooms (and there was a good amount of this), my nervous hands would doodle little scribbles that had multiple patterns going on. They reminded me of symbols like variations of the cross, or the round rainbow pattern that rotates on my iMac screen when the computer is working in screensaver mode. Other times they resembled long chains of DNA, various shapes repeating on themselves and flipping from dark to light.

It was escapist to lose myself in these wonderings. Are ancient symbols simply energy movement patterns that are common throughout nature? Does the fact that the smallest bit of an atom is not anything physical mean that matter is an illusion? What laws govern energy movement? They must be important because the seeming reality of my physical surroundings sure are convincing. So what are the effects of subtle changes in these patterns and where does illness fit in?

A new, experimental treatment called cryoablation saved my breast. It was a miraculous outcome. If miracles are desired, but seemingly unavailable, what effect did my thought have on the outcome?

The world is a wonderful place, much beyond my small brain's capacity to understand it. Energy, life, matter, illusion, paints ability to create illusory images. There are so many interesting subjects to contemplate. I'm motivated to explore these elusive concepts.

Chapter 15: Dr. Littrup—A History of Cryoablation and Breast Cancer

Dr. Littrup

To understand the future of cryoablation, especially its future treating breast cancer, it is important to understand the history of cryoablation. This illustrates three main cryoablation benefits over other treatments. Various branches of medicine have been aware of these benefits for some time.

Perhaps now, with our modern imaging skills, we can understand how these three benefits come together to create a "perfect storm" of:

- treatment *visualization,*
- minimal, or at least relatively less, *pain* during and after treatment, and
- excellent *healing* after cryoablation.

For the cancer treatment world to embrace this "perfect storm," these three benefits of cryoablation need some perspective.

As unbelievable as it sounds, a Dr. James Arnott described the first cryoablation for breast cancer in 1850. He used crushed ice to cool down salt solutions to about -20 Celsius (i.e.,~-30 Fahrenheit). He used this external blend to treat patients for various *pain* conditions, chief-

259

ly cervical and breast cancers. He used icepacks to treat women with breast cancer tumors at the surface of the skin. He applied the ice packs for long periods of time.

This froze a portion of the tumor and sometimes shrank the primary tumor and even distant tumor sites. Perhaps just as important in those early days, Dr. Arnott described better tumor control and quality of life for the patient because they had less drainage and pain after treatment. However, this technique was clumsy and limited since it couldn't freeze tumors deep beneath the skin, so cryoablation languished as physicians developed more modern techniques like mastectomy. In 1947, testing proved that lumpectomy in combination with radiation was comparable to radical mastectomy. Since then, little has changed in localized breast cancer treatment.

While the use of cryoablation for breast cancer treatment languished, the science of cryogens developed. Cryogens are substances that can cause cooling, and early research focused on various ways to liquefy air, primarily oxygen and nitrogen. Then James Dewar invented the vacuum-insulated bottle. This facilitated applying liquid nitrogen to a treatment area with freezing occurring almost instantaneously.

Skin conditions were the first application for cryogens. This explains the broad use and familiarity dermatologists have with cryoablation. However, the freeze rarely extended more than a few millimeters below the skin surface.

Cooper and Lee began to use cryoablation for deeper cancer tumors by treating them with liquid nitrogen in 1961. Cooper was a brain surgeon. He began treating brain tumors by pumping liquid nitrogen down a closed tube or cryoprobe. They placed the probe directly into the tumor through a *surgical* opening.

The liquid nitrogen froze the surrounding brain tumor. The probe then doubled as a tumor retraction tool, since the tumor froze to the probe. The surgeon simply cut out the formed "tumor-icicle" while pulling it out.

The technique became known as "cryosurgery." Doctors now consider "cryoablation," a more modern comprehensive term, since cryoprobes can now extend through the skin without an incision, like a needle. Nevertheless, the Cooper apparatus and technique launched multiple applications for many medical conditions.

In the mid-1960s, better cryogen-delivery technology led to freezing of the prostate for both benign enlargement and cancer. Dr. Gonder developed instruments that applied cold through a tube placed in the urethra while measuring the temperature in the rectum for safety. Dr. Flocks also advanced the procedure by developing cryoprobes that went through the skin, allowing a more flexible access to the prostate surrounding the urethra.

A small group of cryoablation patients began reporting an amazing observation. A large percentage of patients receiving cryoablation were ones with locally advanced prostate cancer. The sheer size of these advanced tumors caused severe discomfort, and Dr. Soanes worked with Dr. Gonder to develop a technique whereby cryoablation trimmed or "debulked" the prostate cancer tumors.

An unfortunate side effect of advanced prostate cancer is that it metastasizes to bone, so many of the patients treated for debulking also had cancer in the bones.

Dr. Soanes and his research partner, Dr. Richard Ablin, noted in 1970 that a few of the prostate patients treated with cryoablation had metastases literally melt away after prostate cryoablation. This was especially true after more than one cryoablation prostate treatment.

This remission in a remote site is similar to "immunizing" a patient against his own tumor by using a tumor "vaccine" and potentially represented a huge breakthrough in cancer treatment. It is interesting that this result mirrored Dr. Arnott's observation that distant metastases regressed after placing iced saltwater bags on women's breast cancers more than 100 years earlier!

This remarkable immune effect in a small group of prostate cancer patients raised a question: why does this happen? Unfortunately, immunology was still in its infancy at the time this lightning bolt of enthusiasm swung the pendulum toward cryoablation in the urologic community. As with many "one hit wonders," the pendulum swung back hard when these "immune effects" from prostate cryoablation failed to occur every time. As a result, medicine relegated these healings to the status of "anecdotal stories" with no reliable explanation of why some people had remissions while others did not.

At this point, the use of cryoablation as a cancer treatment went down two separate roads simultaneously. On the one hand, immunotherapy research went on that continued to explore basic immunology with an effort at understanding how and why it was occurring. More on this below, but first, it is useful to explore the surgical side of cryoablation.

The other road cryoablation traveled was in perfecting the operation techniques of cryoablation. Urologists knew cryoablation could reduce the size of prostate tumors and bring relief to the patient. As well, researchers were aware that freezing could kill cancer cells. However, the prostate is a small organ located in a difficult place to operate. If a surgeon is not careful, nerves and close-by tissue can freeze, with disastrous results.

Therefore, cryosurgery for the prostate was more an art than a science. To make cryoablation a science, my old mentor, Dr. Fred Lee, and his colleague, Dr. Bahn, finally used thermocouples in surrounding tissue to measure the temperature during cryoablation. This was complemented by the use of ultrasound during cryosurgery. The ultrasound allowed the correlation of the surrounding tissue temperature with the ultrasound image of the edge of the "iceball."

Dr. Gary Onik pioneered this technique in the early 1980s. He identified the lethal zone around the leading edge of an ice ball. This zone is approximately 5 mm inside the edge of the iceball, where the temperature goes below -20 C. By determining the lethal zone and knowing where it is just with the use of ultrasound and without having to insert temperature probes, it became much easier to protect adjacent tissues that we don't want to destroy. Injecting fluid or placing balloons between the ice and the delicate organs or tissue (like bowel or nerves), allowed modern physicians to prevent freezing. Assuming we have protected tissues properly yet thoroughly destroyed the target tumor, we were finally able to make use of the healing potential of cryoablation.

The field of prostate cancer treatment has advanced so far since these early days that it is now an insurance-covered benefit, which is accepted as an alternative to surgery and radiation. Patients report satisfaction with the results of cryoablation. In many cases, when the nerves are left intact during a "male lumpectomy," they do not lose erectile function. As well, the surrounding tissue heals and continence remains. If this weren't encouraging enough, there is the hope of an immune response.

During all this time, Dr. Ablin continued to be an inspiring advocate of the use of cryosurgery to stimulate an immune effect. He had helped me slowly build a scientific foundation we can use to make a modern assessment of cryo-immunology.

One result of the recordkeeping was the discovery that the remission rate for cryoablation is the highest in some of the most lethal types of prostate cancers. This led again to the question: what is cryoablation doing in the body that leads to an immune response and cancer remission in some but not all patients?

During the time these advances in cryoablation occurred, immunotherapy research began to blossom in other cancers where spontaneous remissions occurred on an anecdotal level. Patients with advanced kidney and melanoma skin cancers sometimes had spontaneous remissions. Researchers considered these cancers a better model of remote remissions than trying to discover what triggered the isolated prostate remissions after cryoablation.

The developing field of immunology focused on how the human body sometimes achieves a spontaneous remission. A remission is a rare "eviction notice" to bad tenants such as melanoma and kidney cancer cells after they have settled throughout the house of the body.

Immunotherapy research led to the discovery of naturally occurring immune system "drugs" called cytokines. These were discovered in the body and were found to help the immune response. The powerful drugs, Interferon and interleukin-2 (IL2) were developed and became the early cytokine "stars" that helped facilitate the remission of cancer in some kidney and melanoma patients.

However, these cytokines only stimulated a remission response in approximately 15 percent of patients. This suggested that interferon and IL2 were only two dominoes in a whole string of dominoes that needed to be tripped to get the kind of response seen with prostate cancer patients who achieved remission after cryoablation.

Researchers pondered the question. What could cryoablation sometimes be doing that interferon and IL2 alone could only slightly stimulate? They soon found that information from *tumor antigens* stimulates an immunity to cancer. Tumor antigens are protein markers from a tumor, which tell the immune system the cancer is a "foreign body" needing destroying. Normally, the cancer cell is able to mask its presence in the body and the immune system ignores it, allowing it to spread, even though it is a foreign body within the patient. Immunologists discovered the information from tumor antigens needs to be "gift wrapped" and properly presented to the mother ship immune system.

The "delivery boys" that present the tumor antigen information to the immune system are dendritic cells. The connection between the cytokines (interferon and IL2) and the dendritic cells is that the dendritic cell motors run on the "fuel" of cytokines.

Earlier immunology research had already shown that tumor vaccines made of dendritic cells can be made in the lab. This is done by taking some tumor tissue (a chunk the size of the end of a pinky finger, about 2 cc) out of the human body. It is placed in a Petri dish where the tumor cells are freeze-thawed several times.

Live dendritic cells from the immune system are mixed in the Petri dish with this soup of "freeze-fractured" tumor cells. The dendritic cells behave like little archeologists and dig into the shards of tumor membrane. When they do this, they are able to recognize the tumor antigens as a protein foreign to the patient's body.

The dendritic cells are then equipped to deliver a message to the immune system that a foreign body, cancer, is invading the patient, and that it needs destroying. However, without the right mixture of cytokines priming the dendritic cells, they can't "read" the antigens in the Petri dish, and the immune response does not occur.

So, this gives us the answer to the question posed above, "Why does the immune effect sometimes happen after cryoablation?" The freezing and thawing of a tumor inside the body gives the immune system an opportunity to "read" the tumor antigens. However, an adequately prepared supply of dendritic cells is required to bore into the dead cancer cells and "read" the tumor antigens. If they are not available, freezing a tumor is like throwing a whole book of information at someone unable to read. The data of tumor antigens is there, but the body can't see the data and transmit it back to the immune system.

Therefore, to stimulate an immune response after cryoablation, we need better, more organized, cytokine "teachers." These will help dendritic cells "see" and deliver a clear and consistent message to the immune system. When this happens, the immune system tells the rest of the body's cancer cells, "You are being evicted—NOW!"

This is the current state of cryoablation. I am personally hopeful that it can lead to a new, effective treatment method for cancer. I finally received a grant from the National Cancer Institute for a clinical trial to use the above techniques in patients with lung metastases from kidney cancer. We then expanded it to include patients with lung metastases from nearly any cancer.

The pace of reoccurrence and metastasizing of the cancer can be fast in these cancers, and it is my hope that by focusing on these cancers, I will at last be able to produce a measurable immune response.

In the clinical trial, I am injecting a single cytokine, GM-CSF, into a lung tumor just before freezing it. After freezing, the patient rests for a couple of days, then inhales an aerosol of GM-CSF twice a day to continue boosting the likelihood of dendritic cells reacting against the tumor for the first week.

We then measure immune responses in the blood over the next several weeks. Dr. June Kan-Mitchell is very hopeful about the development of these blood assays to help guide future cytokine drug combinations. Similar to imaging guiding a cryoprobe to the right spot, immune monitoring blood assays are crucial to advancing this complex field. She ought to know. She helped her husband, Dr. Malcolm Mitchell, develop Melacine, a melanoma tumor vaccine.

It is interesting that only cryoablation offers the potential of exposing the tumor antigen to the immune system. Heating a tumor destroys the protein structure of the cancer, making it unavailable, or much less comprehensible, for "reading." An analogy to this would be the effect of freezing plastic wrap versus heating it, where the plastic wrap shrivels up and distorts on heating, but remains plastic wrap once thawed after freezing.

This benefit of not destroying the tumor proteins also applies to the tissue surrounding a tumor treated by cryoablation. One of the big benefits of cryoablation is that it does not denature, or destroy, the body's proteins (as heat treatments do), especially in collagen tissue.

Collagen is the "framework" that holds the body together. Cryoablation does not destroy the structure of collagen, even though freezing kills it. The body can rebuild around collagen that is left intact after freezing, much like a house can be rebuilt after it is damaged if the framing is left unharmed.

The prospect of improved cryoablation healing can again draw on the vast experience that dermatologists have had with cryoablation. Despite their liberal, broad use of liquid nitrogen, dermatologists are confident in the slight scarring and rapid healing of skin treatments.

Conversely, we have all seen unfortunate burn victims, having some unsightly scarring and distortion. This scarring has recently been found after radio-frequency heat treatments in central liver and kidney locations. This scarring leads to strictures and narrowing, which cause obstruction to bile and urine, respectively.

More convincingly, cardiologists have not seen scarring with cryoablation in the heart, compared to the scarring around pulmonary veins when radio frequency is used to stop arrhythmias or abnormal heart rhythms.

In other deep organs, cryoablation does not cause scarring, other than in the ureter (the urine tube from the kidney to bladder). Our recent series of cryoablation for benign breast tumors (fibroadenomas) as well as kidney and liver tumors, have shown approximately eighty percent volume shrinkage of the ablation zone without any significant adjacent tissue scarring, even when the ice ball has extended close to the skin surface. Radio frequency ablations in liver and kidney only show approximately thirty percent reduction in a year.

The prospects for cryoablation and breast cancer thus seem well poised for revolutionary changes from the current surgical "business as usual." Tumor shrinkage with minimal scarring should allow breast preservation for nearly all women. And with the hope of the immune effect becoming a commonplace event should the dendritic cell research prove effective, the future of breast cancer treatment with cryoablation looks very bright.

This is especially true now with the development of our single phase liquid cooling (SPLC) machine. After securing our patent and forming a company called CryoMedix LLC, my colleagues are now actively working on making it available for breast treatment.

It should be noted that certain ground rules will have to be observed to guarantee good results from cryoablation no matter what type of cancer we're treating.

We have to make sure we can see the tumor to be treated. Mammography is simply insufficient to see treatment margins. Ultrasound (US) can underestimate tumor extent while MRI may have the greatest accuracy. However, only US can easily guide treatment, so a pretreatment MRI may allow further confidence when comparing with US tumor extent during the procedure.

The well-established temperature profiles and sufficient cryoprobe placements defined by extensive prostate and liver cryoablation experience *must* be followed! Certain papers have been written stating that cryoablation results in incomplete treatment of breast cancer.

These papers have been written based on cryotherapies that used only a *single* cryoprobe. It is important to insist that breast cancer cryoablation be done with multiple cryoprobes, which have proven so effective in controlling the ice ball in prostate and liver cryoablation. But more on that later.

Ice treatment margins *must* be well visualized during treatment (preferably by expert US users) to cover all visible tumor margins. This includes conscientious selection of sufficient cryoprobe distribution to generate lethal ice to all tumor regions.

Careful imaging follow-up must occur to assure that "what you see is what you get." This is best defined by contrast enhancement by CT or MRI (depending on the organ examined), which documents that no blood flow is getting into the prior tumor area. Alternatively, an enhancing margin that increases over time can allow a "touch-up" cryoablation, usually a less-intensive re-treatment.

It is my hope that further research based on the goals outlined above, in combination with the success of the breast cryoablation case of Laura Ross-Paul, will lead to successful breast cryoablation for many other women.

Part Two: Advice to Those Considering Cryoablation for Breast Cancer

Chapter 16: Cryoablation for Today's Breast Cancer Patient

Alex

Laura and I hoped in mid-2003 that when we completed our book, patients would swamp the breast-cancer cryoablation department at Karmanos. Sadly, by 2012, this was still not true. Cryoablation has great promise, but the medical and insurance industry have been slow to embrace it as an alternative to mastectomy and lumpectomy.

As of this book's writing, Blue Cross and Medicaid offer some coverage of cryoablation for breast cancer. Despite this, it is not covered by all carriers.

In writing this book, I found there is a general fear that "cryoablation fails to kill all the cancer." When a doctor is dealing with a person's life, obviously their mandate is to do no harm. In our litigious society, this translates into "do nothing that might get you sued later." An economic corollary is "do nothing unless insurance covers it."

As long as doctors worry that cryoablation is ineffective, it will not receive enthusiastic insurance company support for treating breast cancer. Without universally easy insurance payment, cryoablation will rarely be used.

Yet, how can anyone rationalize refusing to try cryoablation for breast cancer treatment given the success it has achieved treating the prostate? The easy answer is, you can't!

When I was seeking an alternative treatment for Laura and I walked by the television set and saw an advertisement for prostate cryoablation, I thought: "If they can safely cryoablate the prostate, a difficult to reach organ tucked deep inside the body, why can't they cryoablate the breast, which is outside the body cavity and easy to get to?"

Obviously, the answer is—as proved by Laura—that cryoablation can treat breast cancer. Years of research conducted by Dr. Sable at the University of Michigan confirms this. In Dr. Sable's study, women received cryoablation and, two weeks later, a follow-up mastectomy. Researchers examined the breast tissue after removal to verify cryoablation had achieved complete tumor death. The Internet address link to Dr. Sable's paper on this research appears in the Appendix of this book for the reader's reference. The results? Yes, cryoablation killed small cancers, even with only one probe.

In doing further research, I stumbled on a reference to an intriguing paper written in 1998 by Richard J. Ablin, PhD entitled *The Use of Cryosurgery for Breast Cancer*. Ablin's article referred to an article published in 1995 in *Skin Cancer*, a Japanese journal. S. Tanaka reported using cryoablation on women with incurable breast cancer. These were women with inoperable, incurable breast cancer who had volunteered to try cryosurgery. To my amazement, this small group of patients had achieved a 44 percent non-recurrence rate at five years. Ablin's article appears in the online Archives of Surgery and is available at: http://archsurg.ama-as-sn.org/cgi/reprint/133/1/106.pdf

This non-recurrence rate appeared encouraging as we thought about cryoablation for Laura. Here were women with incurable, late-stage cancer and cryoablation had saved nearly half of them! I felt that if cryoablation could have this benefit in late-stage breast cancer, it must bode well for operable cancer found at the earliest stages of the disease.

Since this treatment seems so promising based on available literature and studies in other types of cancer, especially prostate cancer, why isn't the medical community offering it for breast cancer patients? What are the roadblocks to women receiving cryoablation for breast cancer? And how can they be removed?

There are several reasons why cryoablation is not universally available for breast cancer treatment:

- The lack of a multi-probe cryoablation machine for breast cancer treatment.
- The lack of FDA approval of the cryoablation process for treating breast cancer.
- A refusal by insurance companies to pay for cryoablation for breast cancer in the past.
- A lack of doctors trained in ultrasound cryoprobe guidance to treat breast cancer patients with cryoablation.
- Medical politics impeding cooperation between specialties. Namely, surgeons and radiation oncologists trying to block doctors with necessary image-guidance skills (diagnostic radiologists). At the same time those diagnostic radiologists were blocking doctors without an imaging "driver's license" for cryoablation.

- An incorrect belief that cryoablation is not effective in killing cancer.

Given these roadblocks, what can remove them so women can avoid a mastectomy, possibly receive the immune effect, and enjoy the same benefits men have enjoyed for over ten years treating prostate cancer using cryoablation?

The lack of FDA approval of the cryoablation process for treating breast cancer.

A cryoablation machine is considered a medical device by the FDA. In order to get FDA approval for use, one has to demonstrate that the device is safe as well as effective in the treatment of cancer. Proving that cryoablation can kill prostate cancer cells is not necessarily sufficient proof to the FDA that it can kill breast cancer. Therefore, the process can be very time consuming and expensive. Since Sanarus controls the license for their machine for breast care, it is literally up to them to get FDA approval for breast cancer treatment. Since they are a small start-up company, they have not had the revenue until recently to pay for breast cancer trials, which impacts the insurance companies, since they are reluctant to insure any treatment that is not FDA approved. And, of course, without insurance coverage it is difficult to get anyone interested in paying for their own treatment, even if the treatment is much less expensive. The only thing that could possibly help to speed up this process is funding of the Sanarus trials, either by a government entity or by individual donations. So far this has not been forthcoming. And, as a side note, even if Sanarus is able to get FDA approval, it may well be that a company which invents a different way of achieving cryoablation—for example, by using a different gas for cooling—might still need to show their machine is safe and effective, even though they can demonstrate that they can achieve the identical heating and cooling which previously worked to kill breast cancer with a Sanarus cryoablation machine.

It seems that short of government funding, crowd funding, or a change in FDA rules, the initial FDA approval for breast cancer cryoablation is going to take decades. This despite the amazing potential for breast conservation and cost savings already being demonstrated in other parts of the world.

Lack of a multi-probe cryoablation machine for breast cancer treatment

Fortunately, Dr. Littrup is a genius (though he is a humble person and won't go around bragging about himself). He may well someday receive a Nobel Prize in science if cryoablation eventually becomes a standard breast cancer treatment alternative, especially if that is combined with the cytokine therapy and results in close to 100 percent immune effect stimulation. I say this because he and Dr. Alex Babkin, a physicist who specializes in low temperature physics, invented and patented the single phase liquid cooling (SPLC) method of delivering cryoablation. Dr. Littrup hinted at this briefly in his earlier chapter. I think he did not give enough credit to this invention, so I'm taking up the baton here.

CryoMedix, LLC is the company that has developed and is commercializing this new cryoablation technology for the treatment of many different diseases, one of which is women's health applications, specifically benign and cancerous breast tumors. CryoMedix has submitted a 510K application with the FDA for the approval of this new SPLC system.

The SPLC unit measures only 10 inches wide, 10 inches deep and 25 inches high. Compare this with the five-foot-tall argon gas tank Dr. Littrup used on Laura and the fact that this machine is multi-probe, and it is easy to see that this machine will revolutionize the use of cryoablation. It will be less expensive to own and use since the liquid coolant is recycled after it is cooled, which is far less expensive than using argon.

And with the small size of the machine, low cost and ease of use, it is expected that breast cancer treatment will be performed in the physician's office instead of an outpatient surgery center or hospital operating room. One roadblock to such an advance would be the large-scale equipment needed to find the sentinel node. If there is a tumor in the node of sufficient size, current protocol requires that secondary lymph nodes be removed and examined as well, which would still require an operating room.

If mammography, MRI and biopsy—all hospital procedures—indicate a malignant breast tumor, then perhaps someday the next step in a hospital setting would be to find the sentinel node and determine whether cancer has spread to this or other nodes.

Depending on this examination, a strategy could be formulated to deal with the affected nodes. If the sentinel node analysis indicated no more nodes besides the sentinel node required removal, cryoablation could conceivably be used to destroy the sentinel node in a physician's office. Only those patients needing additional node removal would require a hospital setting.

The point of the above is that doctors will eventually treat many breast cancer cases in their own offices as outpatients. It is welcome news that some insurance companies have agreed to support this new treatment option for the potential savings by establishing a reimbursement code for breast tumor cryoablation.

Regardless of the setting, Dr. Littrup's new CryoMedix machine will someday revolutionize the ease of treatment and lower the cost of freezing a tumor. The problem is that gaining FDA approval of their device may well take ten years given the current FDA regulations surrounding medical devices. There is hope that these regulations might soon change, however, and that once a device has been proven safe, it can be used to treat patients. However this still does not get around the need for insurance companies to feel that they should pay for something that is arguably experimental. And without the complete support of insurance companies to pay for treatment, it seems likely that cryoablation for breast cancer might not be FDA-approved and insured for another five or ten years from the date of this book's publication.

Despite this gloomy outlook, Dr. Littrup's company, CryoMedix, LLC, has established a separate company called CryoFem to commercialize all cryoablation applications for women. It is expected that CryoFem will be selling its new devices, based upon CryoMedix's new cryoablation technology, to physicians for use in their offices around 2014 or 2015.

Refusal of insurance companies to pay for cryoablation for breast cancer

This is the biggest problem in making cryoablation available for breast cancer treatment. As Dr. Littrup pointed out earlier, this problem for prostate cancer treatment was in part overcome by the diligence and attention to technique perfected by Dr. Fred Lee, Sr. He set up a prostate cancer treatment clinic at Crittenton Hospital in Rochester, Michigan in 1992 and began to offer cryoablation to men with prostate cancer. Word quickly spread of an effective and safe treatment for prostate cancer, a miraculous treatment which did not usually cause incontinence.

And an added benefit was the potential of an outright cure, especially in cases of more aggressive prostate cancers. It is little wonder that prostate cancer patients "voted with their feet" when they could afford to, and went to Dr. Lee for treatment.

Understandably, urologists were concerned that they were losing patients. Sadly, Dr. Lee received a good deal of name-calling and social discourtesy for providing cryoablation to prostate cancer patients. However, his actions prompted urologists to change in the best interest of their patients and learn ultrasound guided cryoablation.

Yet, it took over seven years from 1992, when Dr. Littrup showed Dr. Lee how to perform prostate cryoablation, until the approval of cryoablation billing codes in 1999.

Without a billing code, a doctor or hospital cannot reliably expect payment for a procedure. Until then, most insurance companies try to duck any bill by stating that without such a code, they simply won't pay for "experimental" procedures.

Setting up an insurance billing code requires consistent results. Only good technology developed by skilled users who reach a consensus on standards can provide consistent results. Until cryoablation is standardized with powerful multiple probe systems, breast cancer treatment can't even get out of the starting gate.

The first rung on the ladder to a billing code is a critical mass of at least five or more papers published in peer-reviewed journals. Several articles jeopardize this milestone by stating cryoablation provides inadequate treatment of breast cancer *if* only a single probe is employed to freeze the tumor. Dr. Littrup and all others in the field agree one needs to oversee the freeze carefully while using multiple probes to direct the ice ball formation. This insures a freeze of the entire tumor.

Stating cryoablation fails while using a single probe is equal to saying a scalpel fails to cut tumors when a surgeon elects not to cut out all of a tumor. It is neither the scalpel's fault nor the fault of cryoablation; it is the fault of whoever is guiding the instrument.

Next, sufficient access to cryoablation is required in many different sites around the country. As well, sponsorship from sub-specialty organizations (e.g., American College of Radiology, American College of Surgeons, Society of Breast Surgeons, Society of Interventional Radiology) is needed in order to submit a procedure to the American Medical Association's Coding Committee.

It is ironic that medical technology progresses so rapidly, yet the medico-government bureaucracy is so slow in establishing billing codes to reimburse a proven procedure. It just gives insurance companies leverage to reject payment. This is like the age old dilemma: you can't get a job without experience, but you can't get experience without a job.

How will cryoablation be used on breast cancer at multiple facilities to create a billing code, when doctors need a billing code to get paid for performing cryoablation? Do insurance companies want doctors to work for free for years until a technique is in widespread use? Only then will they finally say, "This is no longer experimental"?

For untested, totally new technology as well as every new drug there is certainly sense in mandating safety and sufficient outcomes. Yet, this highlights a major flaw in our current evaluation process of cryoablation. The medico-government bureaucracy seems primarily designed to only evaluate drugs. This is because it is easier to perform a controlled trial of a drug since the trial has only one variable, i.e., the presence of the drug in the patient.

With something that involves an "art of application," like ablation technologies, there are many more variables introduced in a trial that must be compared. For example, adequacy of the freeze zone is critical to killing a cancer tumor, yet that is up to the surgeon's judgment. It is also dependent on the number of probes used and the correct sizing of the freeze ball to insure clean margins.

The difficulty of evaluating cryoablation's cancer killing ability had led to slow adoption for medical procedures. This despite cryoablation's long-proven ability to kill cancer in varying sites, such as the prostate, lungs, breast and liver.

It was Dr. Littrup's hope that breast cancer therapy wouldn't have to travel down the path of boutique medicine similar to that of prostate cryoablation. Given the organization and political power of the breast-cancer awareness movement, especially the Komen Race for the Cure, it may still be possible to speed up the insurance company process of accepting and coding breast cancer cryoablation.

That is one of the main motivations of all of us in writing this book. We hope to tell enough women that they can keep their breast as Laura did. We hope, in the meantime, the research of Dr. Littrup and others will finally prove that cryoablation offers a consistent "cure" for breast and other cancers by stimulating the immune system.

If enough people become aware that cryoablation offers a potential cure for breast cancer while allowing a woman to save her breast, then we believe those same people could pressure our legislators. Our representatives could then possibly require that insurance companies and Medicare/Medicaid provide coverage for this treatment if it is performed in acknowledged centers.

Short of achieving that goal soon, at a minimum, greater government funding should immediately be made available to perform trials that are currently proposed, but are going unfunded. In the end, only a large sample trial, where multiple treatment centers provide standardized cryoablation to women with appropriate tumor size and stage, will allow cryoablation a chance to prove it can heal breast cancer!

This is not an impossible goal. It seems easy when compared to going to the moon. When our country decided to go to the moon, our scientists thought it was possible, but we had to build all the hardware to get there. In the case of breast cancer cryoablation, Laura has proven we can get there already, and the hardware is available.

All we have to do is to convince the government and insurance companies to pay for this. The advances in China detailed later in this book should provide us with a humbling form of leadership that shows our country should "get with it!"

Lack of physicians trained in providing cryoablation

This is, in my mind, the second biggest problem (after insurance), which is slowing the adoption of cryoablation for breast cancer treatment. One in nine women gets breast cancer. That means of all the women alive in the US today, approximately 150,000,000, that roughly 17 million of them have already contracted breast cancer or will have it. This translates into nearly 190,000 new cases of breast cancer a year. Dr. Littrup is good, but he has to sleep and eat!

Fortunately, there is an entire legion of surgeons and radiation oncologists who are already treating breast cancer. They are treating patients day in and day out, performing mastectomies or lumpectomies combined with radiation. Surgeons, and perhaps even radiation oncologists, skilled in radioactive seed implants, can learn the imaging guidance skills needed to provide cryoablation in the same way that urologists who previously only provided prostate surgery learned to provide prostate cryoablation.

Perhaps more importantly, there is a new breed of radiologists like Dr. Littrup. These radiologists are much better with image guidance and are beginning to treat patients. In fact, a whole new radiology sub-specialty has developed in the last few years called Interventional Oncology. These radiologists treat multiple tumor regions from lung to liver, using both heat-based and cryoablation techniques that are rapidly becoming fully reimbursable procedures.

However, politics again rears it ugly head by ignoring breast cancer—nearly every other tumor type and site has become more frequently ablated than breast cancers! Whether it is surgeons who learn to use accurate image guidance or radiologists who learn clinical patient management skills, thousands of women await the unification of these specialties so that cryoablation can finally be offered for breast cancer treatment.

An important benefit of the new cryotechnology is its ability to be much more operator independent, or easier to use. Dr. Littrup actually wants to remove his expertise from the equation. His technology can accurately predict the lethal temperatures, or isotherms, of ice extending throughout and around each breast cancer tumor. This is similar to current radiation treatment where the radiation dose distribution is planned for each breast tumor. This makes it much easier to standardize, yet tailor, each breast treatment according to tumor size and extent for each woman. This also avoids the need for the awkward thermometer, or thermocouple, placements that helped standardize prostate cryoablation.

Given market forces, i.e., a desire to provide services which customers will use, it will not take long to train all these physicians in the use of ultrasound and cryoablation. Of course, they won't all learn in any given year, but gradually they will learn new skills, because all of them want what is best for their patients. It is hard to imagine any woman wanting to give up her breast if an equally safe, possibly even more effective, treatment option is available to them.

I believe the eventual adoption of breast cancer cryoablation treatment is assured. It is like water flowing downhill, it is a better way of treating breast cancer. However, the date when breast cancer cryoablation is universally adopted rests ultimately in the hands of the readers of this book. We hope that each reader explores, and then becomes politically active, if not for her own benefit then for a friend, or perhaps, for her daughter's generation.

Our website KeepingThem.com includes various links that will help facilitate your political activity in this arena if you choose to participate.

A belief that cryoablation does not kill cancer

Ten years of research has proven that cryoablation does kill cancer tumors, *if* the freeze/thaw cycle is administered properly. There is an art to doing this, just as there is an art to surgically removing tumors with safe margins during a lumpectomy.

Over time, the art of performing a lumpectomy was perfected. But in 1947, surely there were naysayers who worried that only radical mastectomy was safe, that only by removing the entire breast could one be certain of removing all the cancer from the body. However, lumpectomies and radiation proved to be equally effective in reducing mortality from breast cancer in its early stages. In the same way, cryoablation will eventually be recognized as an effective way of reducing breast cancer recurrence.

There is a key point to be made; that is, I am using the words "reducing mortality" rather than eliminating breast cancer, even if cryoablation is universally adopted.

The sad thing I learned in writing this book is that cancer is a systemic disease. That means it is in a person's entire body. So when it surfaces in the breast, or in the prostate or in the liver, it is often already out in the rest of the body.

Researchers are not completely sure how cancer spreads. There are only assumptions, because tumors are usually found in the lymph and blood system. So lymph nodes are removed as a way of slowing or eliminating the spread of cancer. But women with a mastectomy or a lumpectomy and lymph node removal can still get a recurrence of breast cancer—if not in the other breast, then somewhere else in the body. The same is true of prostate cancer. It often spreads to, or is already in, the bones when discovered late in the prostate.

So everyone looks for a whole body cure, a systemic cure, the "silver bullet" cancer cure. It is my firm belief that Dr. Littrup is on his way to finding this silver bullet. Cancer is proving to be unique, specific, and individual to each person. That means a generic vaccine against cancer may never be developed. This is because a vaccine that triggers one person's immune system to go out and kill cancer may not work in a person with a slightly different protein structure.

Like Laura's amazing dream, cancer has courted and won the unicorn of immortality; it is not a cell with a built in "destruction mechanism" like all the other tissue in our bodies. Yet, this robust disease can be killed by the body as demonstrated by the immune effect. Perhaps Dr. Littrup's research will prove that a vaccine will have to be patient specific. Perhaps only by freezing part of the tumor, and then somehow manufacturing the appropriate supply of cytokines to recruit sufficient numbers of immune cells that target each person's tumor structure, can researchers ever hope to cure cancer. The Chinese may already have perfected such a technique with a procedure they call CIC, Combined Immunotherapy for Cancer. More about this later in Chapter 21: How Fe Traveled to China and Got Her Life Back.

After studying cryoablation and all of Laura's treatment options, I began to wonder if someday patients might regret having their tumors removed rather than frozen within their body. Once this first cancer has been removed, it may be difficult to generate a vaccine-like response from the next tumor that appears. And when that next tumor appears, who knows whether the immune system at that point will be healthy enough to read the tumor antigen structure and respond to it even if cytokine therapy and freezing are done?

I was willing to bet the love of my life on this immune effect, and only time will prove me right or wrong, though as of this writing Laura has passed the ten-year cancer free mark. I also bet my own life on the added benefit of the immune effect when prostate cancer struck me in 2010.

Because my cancer was bilateral, on both sides of the prostate, I was not able to avail myself of cryoablation as it renders one impotent by freezing the nerves on both sides of the prostate. However, by 2010 a new treatment method called HIFU, High Intensity Focused Ultrasound was available outside the US, though performed by American doctors. I was able to secure treatment by Dr. Scionti, a prominent NYU Urologist and one of the pioneers in this field.

In this ultrasound procedure, the interior tissue of the prostate is destroyed by heat generated by the focusing of two ultrasound waves, which individually are hot, but not hot enough to kill tissue. Thus, like a beam of light focused by a magnifying glass, a small, controllable point where the waves combine heat the tissue up to a point high enough to kill the cells, but not so hot that they burn. Because of this, when the body reabsorbs the prostate tissue destroyed by ultrasound, the "immune affect" can also occur since the cancer protein structure is preserved to be revealed to the immune system.

After the HIFU procedure my PSA levels tested at .1 and at the one year mark they dropped to .07, a nearly undetectable level and welcome sign that the prostate cancer has likely been eliminated.

Sadly, Dr. Littrup's cytokine booster treatment is still not available. Had it been I would have availed myself of that therapy as well because cancer is an opponent to be respected. I did avail myself of the mistletoe therapy provided to Laura by Dr. Esau years ago.

I hope and pray that Dr. Littrup is able to extend his immune research. The good Lord has already saved him from death once. We need to make sure that his work is done for the good of all humanity, before he succumbs to mortality as we all must.

There are several more interesting references to cryo-surgery/cryoablation that I found on the Internet. They are located in the Appendix to this book.

One of the studies in the Appendix was published by the Journal *Radiology* and is entitled "Small (<2.0 cm) Breast Cancers: Mammographic and US Findings at US-guided Cryoablation—Initial Experience."

This article describes the results of a clinical trial where ultrasound-guided single probe freezing was performed on nine women with breast cancer. This freeze was followed up approximately two weeks later with a lumpectomy. Then the removed tissue was analyzed.

Seven of the nine women had no residual cancer, while the other two were still found to have cancer remaining. It is interesting that the failure in this trial to kill the cancer in all the women was perhaps due to the use of only one probe, rather than the multiple probes that Dr. Littrup used on Laura, which he feels is absolutely essential to get a good freeze.

Research in the United States has definitely been a slow and cautious process and this contrasts sharply with efforts by Tanaka made years ago in Japan as mentioned by Dr. Littrup.

Tanaka's 44 percent survival rate at the five-year mark after treatment is an astounding success given the fact that all these women had breast cancer considered inoperable.

I am not saying that the United States should simply accept these findings blindly, but I do feel that if cryoablation is able to heal nearly half of a group of women who could not benefit from traditional surgery then perhaps it is time to admit that cryoablation is vastly more successful in curing women with breast cancer.

If anyone could invent and patent a drug that would prevent the recurrence of breast cancer 44 percent of the time it would be a huge commercial success and none of us would begrudge the wealth bestowed on the inventors. Yet when it is a free byproduct of a low-cost treatment, it is, unbelievably, brushed under the rug!

We all either know, or know of, someone who has died of a recurrence. It is my sincere hope that this book wakes up the medical field and the public to the life saving potential cryoablation offers. Sadly, political activism will probably have to take the place of commercial incentive to make this happen.

It is our hope that soon cryoablation treatment will replace cryoablation tests, and women will keep their breasts while healing their cancer. Recent developments hold promise of a program for cryoablation for breast cancer at Karmanos Cancer Institute and other centers around the country.

Since this is a constantly changing field, clinics offering cryoablation for breast cancer treatment will hopefully spring up around the country after the writing of this book. We will do our best to list these clinics in the future at our website, KeepingThem.com, and I am sure CryoMedix will post clinic addresses as their equipment is adopted.

Chapter 17: A Cancer Patient's Bill of Rights

Alex

Cancer hits your life like a tsunami. It crashes through buildings, finds you at night, and drowns you. Cancer wrenches your life around, forcing you to pay attention to it with the constant fearful reminder: *I have cancer, my wife has cancer, my husband has cancer, someone I love has cancer.*

Whenever a happy moment comes, the cancer fear reminder dashes that happiness, for when you forget the cancer, a second later, you remember. And the remembering surprises and feels like hearing the news for the first time. A surge of fear follows, a rush of adrenaline which first energizes yet ultimately exhausts you. For what good is adrenaline against a foe you can neither fight nor flee? Cancer is within, like a guerrilla fighter opposing an occupying army. For cancer to win, all it must do is not die.

Only doctors can fight cancer and you soon realize you are a battleground, with cancer on one side and your doctor on the other. The odds of victory are uncertain and because you cannot outrun or escape your cancer, it wears down your spirit, your patience, your hope—especially when there is a recurrence.

However, with cryoablation, there is a high likelihood the cancer will go into remission and that in some cases, the resulting immune effect could possibly cure the cancer. Of course, researchers can't say this yet; it would be irresponsible to offer hope and find later they're wrong. However, the intersection of cryoablation and immunology offer great promise. Dr. Littrup's combination of the two are in one sense a crude and simple way of defeating cancer. The idea's simplicity, exposing the tumor's protein structure to the immune system, makes it elegant.

Time and research will ultimately find the cure for cancer. Perhaps it won't be cryoablation. But as I told Laura when we were trying to decide if she should go ahead with cryoablation, she did not have to cure her cancer the day of her operation. She only had to slow its progress, give it pause by surviving a few more years. Given a few years, Dr. Littrup's research into the immune effect might prove that cryoablation combined with dendritic vaccination cures cancer.

An art student of Laura's made an elaborate card after hearing Laura was battling cancer. It contained a message of love:

YOU WILL SURVIVE!

Laura made copies and mounted the card on her bulletin board, then pasted one of the copies in her journal. Her words inspired me to draft a bill of rights for the women and men going through breast cancer. This bill of rights reinforces the message, YOU WILL SURVIVE.

A Breast Cancer Patient's Bill of Rights

- You have the right to want to keep your breast, no matter what age you are.
- You have the right to ask questions, more questions, and even more questions, until you are satisfied you are making the right treatment decision.
- You have the right to expect your insurance to pay for your treatment, even if it is nontraditional.
- You have the right to be upset, angry, disappointed and plain mad that you have breast cancer.
- You have the right to expect love, support and compassion from your spouse and family, without feeling guilty.
- You have a right to want to live a healthy life to a ripe old age.
- You have a right to write to your representatives and senators expressing your viewpoint regarding treatment options, research and government funding.
- You have a right to receive God's love.

You will survive!

Chapter 18: Decision Making and Cancer Treatment

Alex

Working on this book knowing Laura's cancer treatment is behind us is truly a blessing. As I edited the book during the 2006 Winter Olympics I noticed that when athletes who won were asked to describe their joy, they almost universally said it was beyond their descriptive abilities.

I feel the same way about the miracle that was Laura's battle with breast cancer. The fear and anxiety slowly left me, though I later developed palpitations of the heart brought on, in all likelihood, by the stress I went through. I learned this is a common fate for caretakers. Palpitations respond to beta-blockers so I'm fortunate my health is still good. I think I'm right, though, in saying health-impairing stress comes from enduring inescapable situations. And I remain convinced the only way to deal with stress is to make the stress-inducing condition disappear—or somehow give up caring.

I'm glad we won the battle, because I don't know how I would ever quit caring about that cute college girl I married!

I am not a doctor nor are most readers of this book. Yet decisions are required of cancer patients and their loved ones which affect the future.

Without a medical degree, how does one evaluate alternatives? How can you feel comfortable deciding on a course from which there is no return?

I gave much thought to these matters during Laura's cancer. My industrial engineering training stressed logical, methodical, decision making. But being human, I, as much as any person, can be ruled by my emotions.

However, you cannot row your canoe in one direction without forsaking all other compass points. Decisions must be made despite our desire to avoid them. And it is often said that the sum total of our lives is the collective result of all the decisions we made. I hope that in the future, Laura and I and Dr. Littrup find that we "rowed in the right direction."

When confronted with cancer, the first decision anyone makes is whether they even want to make decisions regarding treatment. Many people are comfortable not seeking a second opinion. Some do not want to consider options because that undermines their faith in the doctor they so want to believe.

I understand and sympathize with this philosophy. I would have enjoyed not rising endlessly at 4 a.m. to research an alternative treatment on the Internet. However, in Laura's case, she wanted to avoid a mastectomy while her doctors said a lumpectomy was not an option. So Laura's desire became motivation for me to search on the Internet for a medically sound alternative.

I stumbled on a possible cancer cure. And there was an added blessing because when I began searching,

I didn't believe there was any cure for cancer, just a delaying of the inevitable.

I assume if you have read this far, you are like I was, eager to learn what the alternatives are and appreciative of advice and insight. I just want to repeat—and please keep this in mind: I trained as an engineer; I am not a doctor. I am sure many doctors would not agree with the decisions I made or the conclusions I came to about statistical studies. I am merely trying to be helpful and offer advice.

I believe my opinions are credible, however, because at least some doctors agreed with our decisions as we went through Laura's treatment.

So, to repeat, according to Dr. Henderson, head of the Karmanos Breast Cancer Institute, the gold standard of breast cancer treatment is still surgery, either a mastectomy or a lumpectomy with follow-up treatment. If you add any other treatment, you will make decisions supported by statistical probabilities of survival equal to or worse than these gold standard options.

When Laura and I were agonizing between a mastectomy and cryoablation, our daughter, fourteen at the time, offered the best perspective I have ever heard in my life regarding breast cancer. It went something like this:

"Oh, Mommy, I don't know why you're so stressed out about having your breast cut off. They just get in your way when you play soccer and you need to wear a stupid sports bra and they still hurt when you run!"

What an insight from a person recently acquiring breasts who found them an inconvenience on the athletic field!

Decision One: Diagnosis

Our first decision was based on a question. Did Laura really have breast cancer? She seemed so healthy. She exercised every day, had breast-fed our three children for nearly ten years; surely, she couldn't have breast cancer. Definitely ask for a second mammogram, or MRI, or biopsy if you doubt you have breast cancer. There are occasional false positives on mammograms. It would be like winning the lottery finding out you didn't have cancer after all.

Decision Two: Time to Explore Options

Okay, I agree with the doctors, I do have breast cancer. Now what do I do?

I don't think anyone in the medical community would argue one should ignore cancer. However, you do usually have some time if you have caught it early enough; time to explore options. The doctors assured us Laura had six weeks before the operation was mandatory, so we used that time to explore.

Since we didn't know cryoablation existed, we first researched lumpectomy hoping the doctors were wrong and a lumpectomy was possible.

The lumpectomy requires removal of the tumor plus a safe margin of surrounding tissue. The balance of the breast tissue is then radiated to kill small tumors not visible on MRI, mammogram or ultrasound.

We soon learned the size and shape of the tumors left no possibility of a lumpectomy. Her surgeon convinced us the remaining breast would not be worth keeping. A reconstructed breast would better serve Laura.

Exhausting the lumpectomy option, I continued looking for alternatives. The first alternative I found involved using microwave to heat and destroy tumors. I have to admit that I only gave microwave a cursory examination.

Microwave treatment was impractical because it would remove as much tissue as a lumpectomy. I kept researching the Internet, but I grew less optimistic with each passing day. In fact, I think by the time I noticed the PCA Cryocare ad on television, I was just getting up early and going through the motions of trying to find something, anything, to help Laura.

If you have ever been sued, you know there is a point in a lawsuit where you obsessively shuffle through the agreements for days. You highlight passages which might be stretched or interpreted in your favor in court. You eagerly point them out to your attorney. Unfortunately, he already knows about every one of them and explains why they don't apply or won't work.

My research felt similar near the end, as if I were searching with too much hope and finding impractical options. However, this early research proved useful after Laura's cryoablation because important decisions remained. After the cryoablation, Laura's immune system began to tear down and remove the frozen, dead tissue. The immune system might recognize the intact protein structure of the cancer as a foreign body. So the first decision after cryoablation related to chemotherapy and radiation disturbing the immune effect.

Decision Three: Chemotherapy

After breast cancer surgery, the next big decision for every patient concerns chemotherapy for the whole body.

I didn't understand the impact of cancer being a systemic disease when we first learned Laura had breast cancer. I thought the disease started in the breast and possibly escaped into the body. I believed if one acted fast enough, you could prevent the escape. I thought this was why they removed and biopsied the sentinel node, to see if it had gone past that point.

I learned later sentinel node biopsy determines the need for full body chemotherapy. A tumor in the sentinel node over a certain diameter indicates cancer has spread beyond the breast. If it is small enough, or if they find no tumor, then skipping chemotherapy is safe as the cancer remains in the breast.

I was surprised to learn no consensus exists about how cancer spreads from the breast. Considerable evidence shows it spreads through the bloodstream. Yet it is usually found in the lymph node closest to the tumor, hence the sentinel node biopsy. Science doesn't know if this bloodstream vs. lymph system is an "either/or" or "both" situation.

The danger in all this is that a patient can think a mastectomy, or lumpectomy and radiation, will leave her in the clear and without the need for chemotherapy. I mistakenly believed this during the early phase of Laura's treatment.

However, once we understood Laura might need chemotherapy when they discovered the tumor in Laura's sentinel node, we began researching alternatives with our neighbor, Ellie, who learned she had breast cancer about the same time as Laura. She chose a lumpectomy and radiation, and then faced chemotherapy as well. She was the one who told us about the research showing cancer was a systemic disease, and she convinced us chemotherapy was useful in getting rid of cancer through-out the body.

However, chemotherapy sounded so dangerous that I approached it with dread. I read and read and read, and became so full of statistics concerning chemotherapy outcomes that my mind rebelled. Many tests claiming positive results for chemotherapy seemed questionable because the results were short-term.

It struck me that no one knows the long-term effect of newer forms of chemotherapy, because there has not been a thirty-year trial! This is just like birth control pills. Thirty years ago, no one knew their long-term effect because the drug was new and no one had taken them for more than a few years before FDA approval. Concerns regarding blood clots, heart attacks and strokes caused a change to safer dosages in later years.

The medical community advises almost universal-ly that cancer patients should have some form of che-motherapy to improve their odds of survival. Balanced against this advice I found considerable literature which argued strongly that chemotherapy had no value and can cause other health problems. This made it difficult in helping Laura try to decide whether she should pur-sue chemotherapy.

I turned to my training as an engineer, specifically statistics. I have to admit that even with this training, I found it difficult deciding whether chemotherapy would help Laura. Our neighbor was so helpful and patient in explaining how to understand the improved odds che-motherapy provides, and in the end, our decision was to take her advice.

Oddly enough, our neighbor's advice was that Laura not take chemotherapy, because Laura's liver would probably not handle it, and it could potentially kill her. As a teenager, Laura had suffered severe abdominal pain and her parents took her to the hospital. An initial diagnosis of appendicitis was re-evaluated by the surgeon in the operating theater and he decided not to operate because he suspected her liver had swollen.

He was right in his diagnosis, her liver swelling was due to an allergic reaction to an antibiotic. This resulted in compromised liver function all her life as she suffers from a sore liver after eating fatty foods or drinking alcohol.

After our discussion with our neighbor, Laura and I visited Dr. Takahashi, Laura's Oncologist in Portland, to discuss the fragile state of Laura's liver. Dr. Takahashi recommended Laura not take chemotherapy. The risk of further liver damage was too great.

Our neighbor proceeded with chemotherapy. She knew it would be difficult but not potentially fatal. She took chemotherapy because research convinced her it would increase her odds of survival.

I am happy to report that our neighbor survived the chemotherapy with no ill effects after the treatment, though she admitted to feeling miserable some of the time during it.

Had Laura been able to endure chemotherapy, I believe she would have agreed to it, even though it would only add a few percentage points to her overall survival probability.

The odds of increasing survival chances by using chemotherapy varies based on the form of breast cancer diagnosed. In Laura's case, there was only a potential for a 3 percent improvement in Laura's survival rate beyond five years. However, with some cancers, the improvement in survival by taking chemotherapy can range as high as twenty percent.

I believe that if a person can tolerate chemotherapy, they should probably secure treatment on the chance they can lower their recurrence rate. You have to remember that when you reduce your chance of recurrence by two percent, it means two people out of a hundred will not die of cancer when they otherwise would have. It's not like you'll have chemotherapy and get a slightly milder case of cancer; it's that you might be one of those two extra survivors living to old age. For those two people, chemotherapy works 100 percent. Unfortunately, no one knows who those two people are before treatment, so it seems like a good bet to gamble that by taking chemotherapy, you might be saving your life.

In these days of genetic research, a genetically engineered cure for cancer may well be discovered in the next ten to twenty years. When Laura and I were trying to decide what she should do, I told her she was in a war that could consist of several battles. I pointed out that since a future discovery might cure her after a recurrence, all she had to do was keep winning the intermediate battles and survive until the future magic shot cancer cure arrives. In a way, science has made cancer sufferers of today like cancer itself. All they have to do to win is stay alive long enough for the miracle cure.

Scientists say that knowledge is now doubling every year. Surely in ten years when medical knowledge has increased a thousand times, a cure will exist.

In the end, knowing that cancer is a systemic disease, unless researchers show chemotherapy ruins the immune effect, I believe chemotherapy should be used.

305

It has been proven statistically to lessen the recurrence of cancer.

Decision Four: Radiation

Whether to receive radiation treatment was Laura's next big decision. Radiation is recommended after a lumpectomy to kill microscopic, undetectable tumors in the treated breast. Lymph nodes in the neck and armpit area might also have tumors and without radiation, they could spread and cause problems down the road.

All of Laura's Portland doctors were treating her as a lumpectomy patient, even though she'd had cryoablation. The only reservation we both had was the Karmanos Radiologist Dr. Tara Washington's warning that radiation could stop the body's absorption of the dead tissue.

I felt the doctors were correctly conservative in arguing for radiation as a cryoablation follow-up. But how soon after cryoablation should radiation begin?

No one could answer that question. Interference with cryoablation healing had never been a reason to delay radiation. The only fallback position was to say it was safe to wait the time a person on chemotherapy would wait before radiation. Four weeks, six weeks, two months? Who knows? Treatments vary in duration.

In the end, controversy over whether the new growth in Laura's breast was new tumor growth or new healthy tissue growth led us back to Detroit to resolve that issue as previously described.

Three months had passed by the time Laura was cleared for radiation. Up to this point, Laura's breast was healing nicely. Each day brought a reduction of the hard, dead tissue in her breast. Then she started radiation.

In a few weeks, it became obvious the body's absorption of frozen tissue had stopped. Nothing was going on in Laura's breast except a struggle by every cell to survive. Eventually, radiation ended with the hope that any small tumor sites in her breast or neck were now dead.

Did the radiation interfere with the hoped for immune effect? Only time and research will tell. Is radiation needed after cryoablation? Same answer.

One bright spot is that months after radiation, Laura's immune system went to work again. To her oncologist's surprise, the small lump of necrotic tissue gradually began getting smaller at every six-month check-up.

The only ill effect was an itchy, uncomfortable feeling in this dead tissue. As Laura says, though, it was a nice reminder she had her breast, and she didn't mind the discomfort.

Later, at the operation's three-year anniversary, Laura contracted an infection in the remaining dead tissue in her breast. During that time, this dead, or "necrotic" tissue, had slowly migrated to just below the skin's surface.

An MR of the area showed "something suspicious," worrying words we were all too familiar with. We consulted Dr. Littrup, who reassured us it was probably just inflammation and not a recurrence of cancer. He was correct, as the area was biopsied in Portland and no cancer was found.

However, soon after, a breast infection set in, right in the biopsy site. The infection did not respond to antibiotics. It resolved eventually, but only after her surgeon drained the site.

I am convinced the biopsy allowed the infection to occur and that it was unnecessary. However, we breathed a sigh of relief that it wasn't cancer after the biopsy and

Laura felt even better about her cryoablation decision. She said keeping her breast was worth the pain of a breast infection.

Unfortunately, the early "relief" at only having a breast infection turned into alarm. The breast infection returned and after a long antibiotic treatment, Laura's surgeon removed the hematoma, the last dead tissue from the freeze.

The problem disappeared for six months, and then an MR showed an inflamed area, a lymph node in one of Laura's ducts. A final minor surgery at roughly the four-year mark after her cryoablation eliminated this infection.

Who knows what caused this nagging run of infections? Was it the biopsies performed on "new healthy tissue" trying to grow and replace the hematoma that kept getting traumatized because Laura's Portland doctors thought it was a return of cancer? Or perhaps a weakness in that breast, which had suffered from several infections throughout her years of breast-feeding?

I'm sure we'll never know conclusively, but the good news is that once cryoablation has become an established procedure, alarm bells probably won't go off when doctors are able to differentiate new tissue replacing a hematoma from a return of breast cancer.

Chapter 19: Insurance

Alex

Sadly, our insurance company did not follow through on their verbal promise to cover part of Laura's treatment in Detroit, even though our Portland doctor recommended that they pay. I cannot understand their reluctance to take part in this exciting development in cancer treatment. I just hope that our experience and a growing demand for breast cancer cryoablation will finally result in breast cancer cryoablation receiving coverage like prostate cancer cryoablation.

When we began our odyssey in Detroit, Laura made a big effort to get Dr. Littrup's information to her primary Portland doctor, Dr. Brad Fancher. He originally recommended that Laura should get a mammogram, and when Laura was too busy, he took the time to write and insist she get her mammogram. His persistence saved her life, and for that, we will be forever grateful. After reviewing Dr. Littrup's information, Dr. Fancher spent a good deal of time online researching cryoablation.

Dr. Fancher eventually gave his blessing to Laura's trip to Detroit. He said that Karmanos Cancer Institute was one of the most advanced cancer treatment centers in the country, and that if they said they could safely offer cryoablation to Laura, then they would. In addition, he said he had written a letter recommending our insurer cover Laura's procedure. At this point, I felt they would cover at least part of the procedure, but to make sure, I called Dr. Fancher for clarification.

When we joined our insurance company years before Laura's cancer they required referrals from your primary doctor before paying for a specialist. However, this rule irritated so many customers that they had sent out a letter a few months before Laura's diagnosis which canceled the written referral protocol. I called Dr. Fancher to confirm we would not need a letter of referral from him. He said we didn't, and added that because this treatment was out of area—meaning outside the insurance system—coverage usually would not apply. However, since no one offered cryoablation within the coverage area of our insurance, he felt they would pay for the treatment but possibly only at half the cost.

He added that, of course, our insurance company would cover any follow-up work, such as chemotherapy or radiation, if Laura received those services in Portland.

Since Laura's "drop-dead date" for removing the tumor loomed ahead, we rushed to get back to Detroit for her assessment. I knew we no longer needed a written referral for a specialist and we had Dr. Fancher's letter requesting our insurer provide coverage. I didn't think there was anything else I needed to do.

However, looking back and after reading our policy, I now know we needed written assurance of coverage in advance. That is part of our insurer's policy agreement.

It might be a rule in your policy. Therefore, if you are considering getting cryoablation out of your coverage area, please speak with your insurance company first. You might secure coverage if you get prior approval.

I thought I had done enough and, in my defense looking back, would we have gone ahead with the cryoablation had we known the financial burden it would incur? Yes. If I had been given a choice of spending $46,000 to know absolutely that Laura would remain cancer free and have her breast eleven years later, I wouldn't have hesitated for a second.

We returned from Detroit and heard nothing from the insurance company saying not to go. Off we went to Detroit for the procedure. On the morning of the surgery, the first red flag began waving. With no formal insurance approval for Laura's treatment when she signed into the hospital, I agreed to cover it. I gave them our airline mileage card with the thought that at least we'd earn airline miles if our insurer didn't cover their half of the cost! Yet half turned out to be a false hope.

When Dr. Littrup emerged from the surgery and reported his success, he said that an odd thing had happened during the procedure. After Laura was sedated but before the operation, a hospital staff person came in and said they had contacted our insurer to verify coverage. Surprisingly, they asked Dr. Littrup to stop the surgery while Harper faxed information to Oregon so our insurance company could approve coverage. Dr. Littrup, Dr. Bouwman and the anesthesiologist met briefly. They decided it was unsafe to wake Laura and put her under later for the operation. Instead, they decided to proceed and have Harper fax information at the same time so our insurers could decide.

I am grateful to these doctors for their courageous decision. Their patient's safety and well-being came first, not some silly rules in Oregon. Dr. Littrup said he was happy to report that during the surgery the insurance person from Karmanos had returned to the operating theater. She related that our insurer stated they would cover all portions of the procedure except the cryoablation fee. They added the caveat, however, that they would cover the Karmanos work at a reduced rate, most likely fifty percent, since it was an out-of-area treatment.

I felt this was fair for us and our insurer as they were getting the equivalent of a lumpectomy from Karmanos for free, which was less than the mastectomy they would have covered in Portland, and they were getting everything else like the sentinel node at half off.

Unfortunately, while we were in Detroit, and a few days after Laura's procedure, a letter came to our Portland home from a top insurance company executive. He reversed their verbal agreement to pay half and stated they would not pay for one dime of any of Laura's treatment done out of area.

Now, keep in mind, this letter came after they told Karmanos/Harper Hospital that they would pay for everything except only half of the cryoablation part of the procedure!

When overwhelmed by work or life, I toss all our mail into a paper bag marked "To Be Sorted" with red Sharpie ink. Then I throw the bag in a corner. I came home from Detroit to a huge mail pile, usually 90 percent junk advertising, so, feeling overwhelmed, the letter landed in the bag.

It was not until Laura was well on her way to recovery from Detroit that I found the letter and realized we were facing a $46,000 medical bill.

How could I respond? The amount was so large it seemed like a joke. So one night when Laura and I were getting ready for an art opening she showed me a new dress she was planning on wearing. It showed off her cleavage and I joked that this had become "$40,000-view property."

Obviously we weren't happy about the prospect of facing this enormous medical bill, but it helped ease my sense of feeling victimized to make a joke about it. This operation was a triumph, a definite win over cancer, but I felt betrayed and lied to by our insurer.

It also angered me to think if I had prostate cancer and had learned that freezing could give me better outcomes, my procedure would receive insurance coverage! Even more amazing, Medicare would cover it!

Why aren't women's breasts considered as important as a man's prostate? Dr. Lee was smart when he established his boutique clinic offering cryoablation for prostate cancer. He knew men would pay out-of-pocket for a better chance of remaining continent and having less post-operative pain. And much more recently, with the work of Dr. Gary Onik, cryoablation now offers a good chance of avoiding erectile dysfunction.

Medicine hasn't given women the choice of paying to save their breasts. Instead, they are offered mastectomies and a rebuild with the assurance they'll look better than ever.

I won't be the judge of that. But I have to believe that once women discover they can save their breasts at boutique clinics when they finally appear, they will jump at the chance. Especially when they learn they might have an added guarantee of surviving their cancer thanks to a possible immune effect.

Since self-pay patients will probably drive demand for breast cancer cryoablation until insurance companies offer coverage, it is interesting to look at what motivated men to pay out-of-pocket.

In the beginning, Dr. Lee offered three main reasons for choosing cryoablation over radical prostatectomy (prostate removal, equivalent to mastectomy).

- Dramatically less post-operative pain and quicker recovery than surgery
- Less chance of incontinence
- A chance they may get an immune response

The following, I think, are the reasons that will drive women to pay out of pocket initially for cryoablation breast cancer treatment:

- Less post-operative pain and quicker recovery
- No tissue loss compared to lumpectomy or mastectomy
- Less worry about body image
- A chance to get an immune response

The possibility of a younger woman nursing after having breast cancer adds another positive factor.

Regarding the potential immune effect, looked at from the standpoint that lives might be saved using cryoablation, you wonder why it isn't used whenever possible if it might stimulate an immune response. Many companies have searched for chemicals which stimulate an immune response. Why not start with cryoablation, which has already proven it can trigger an immune response?

Probably because cryoablation is not a medicine they can patent. Instead of being a low-cost, highly priced pill potentially offering a reduction in cancer recurrence, it is a surgical technique costing less than current procedures. This especially sounds true when you consider that most of the expensive chemotherapy adds only a 3 percent reduction in recurrence.

Sad to say, but to my businessman's eye, it seems the lack of interest in cryoablation is because it has little potential to generate revenue. Sadly, I think the attitude is, who cares about a possible reduction in cancer's recurrence if it can't be patented?

Regardless, what followed after our insurance denial was a long series of written appeals. We even hired an attorney for a while to attend a meeting with us. At every step, our health insurance company fought us. Finally, at the last big meeting, I thought we had a chance, and I even hired a lawyer to come with us to argue our position. This meeting consisted of a panel of people from the insurance company, a nurse, a doctor and some regular people like us. And there were quite a few women.

Here was our chance, I thought. However, the senior man at the meeting and the author of our original denial letter pulled out his trump card: cryoablation was an experimental procedure.

When we had first met we understood Karmanos was planning to offer cryoablation in the future for breast cancer as a standard procedure. Dr. Littrup was developing a protocol for submission to the National Cancer Institute to get it approved and the protocol would stimulate insurer's approval in the same way they now cover prostate cryoablation.

We felt Karmanos was offering to begin its breast cancer cryoablation program with Laura because it had proven itself in the field of prostate cancer for the last ten years. Instead of being an experimental procedure, cryoablation appeared to be well along the road to recognition as being universally acceptable and desirable.

In fact, we left Detroit the first time convinced that Karmanos's attitude was that the time for experimenting was over. It was time to roll out this new procedure that worked, so I admit to being blindsided by the letter the insurance executive was quoting from, since we had never seen a copy.

Regardless, our attorney made a good point. He said our insurer bound themselves orally when their agent promised to cover everything except the cryoablation. He argued that if cryoablation was indeed experimental then, by agreement, they could decline coverage only on that portion of the treatment and pay for everything else promised over the phone.

To further bolster this argument, I pointed out that they were actually paying for all of Laura's follow-up radiation and additional hormone therapy as if she'd had a regular lumpectomy. Therefore, even if they thought the cryoablation was experimental, it was obvious our health plan's doctors were satisfied it had killed Laura's tumors, because no cancer remained in her breast and they were treating her as such.

It seemed to me our insurance company was now the one that was believing in miracle cures! They wouldn't pay for something experimental because it might not work, but they'd pay for follow-up procedures hoping it had worked. It amazed me that our non-profit insurance company would be so reluctant to cooperate with Karmanos and Dr. Littrup and ignore this inexpensive treatment option they might adopt in Oregon.

Instead of trying to be part of something new and promising and using it for their public relations and fundraising, they fought it, tooth and nail.

Still, I hoped the chance to participate in something so promising would prevail over rules and money saving.

Our attorney's gloomy attitude after the meeting surprised me. He thought we had no chance, while I hoped an oral contract was binding. It turned out the attorney was right.

We received a letter soon after confirming our insurer would not pay for anything because they had determined cryoablation was experimental. Since it had been done out of area and we didn't have previous written authorization in advance, they weren't obliged to pay for it and weren't going to.

Our attorney said our only remaining course was to sue and that we would lose. The insurance contract was too clear. He'd proceeded on our behalf with the hope that since cryoablation offered so much promise, our insurer might embrace it rather than reject it.

We gave up. Suing knowing we would lose was a waste of money. Sadly, eleven years later, our insurer still doesn't cover breast cancer cryoablation, and I'm guessing it's because of the dilemma Dr. Littrup ran into years ago with prostate cryoablation. Few surgeons are currently trained in the use of ultrasound-guided surgery. This is the province of the radiologist. And radiologists don't do surgery.

It is an unresolved turf war. Do surgeons become ultrasound readers or do radiologists become, like Dr. Littrup did, cryosurgeons?

Prostate cancer cryoablation ended up being performed primarily by urology surgeons who were losing patients to cryoablation. They responded to market demand and learned the technique. This will probably need to occur in the field of breast cancer cryoablation as well, despite the lives that might be saved and the money that certainly would be saved with immediate insurance coverage.

One factor which might hasten the acceptance of cryoablation for breast cancer is Dr. Littrup's newly invented multiple-probe cryoablation machine.

The small size and low cost of this machine compared to the large argon gas machine used in Laura's case facilitates cryoablation outside the hospital and without a general anesthetic. Dr. Littrup estimates a simple office-based breast cryoablation, separate from sentinel node biopsy, should cost around five thousand dollars.

A patient desiring breast cancer cryoablation and living in a region where it is not offered could get all the other work done at home under their current plan.

A trip to a clinic could be made for the cryoablation as a day procedure costing no more than ten thousand dollars out of pocket. This would be followed by chemotherapy and radiation treatment at home under existing insurance.

While five thousand dollars is still a great deal of money, it is a tenth of Laura's surgery. We are fortunate that we were able to afford this bill. It is our hope that this initial path toward cryoablation will be this combined "insured-not insured" process, which will make it easier for others to receive the same treatment Laura received.

And at some point, hopefully, surgeons everywhere will turn to their insurance providers and say, "We're losing our patients. We'll learn how to do breast cryoablation, so start paying for this!"

Chapter 20: Laura's Reflections Four, Seven and Twelve Years After Cryoablation

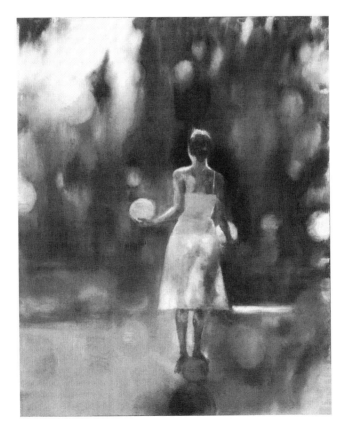

"Plug"

> *"She balances precariously, her left hand holding a breast-sized luminescent globe that acts as a beacon to light her path through the darkness."*
>
> —Laura Ross-Paul commenting on her painting *"Plug"* done towards the end of her treatment for breast cancer

Laura

Four Years Later

1/23/2007, Tuesday

It's been almost four years since first being diagnosed with breast cancer. I've had three MRI scares of something suspicious since then, but each time the triumph of the cryolumpectomy has held. The last scare resulted from an infection in the gradually diminishing hematoma of tissue killed by the freezing.

My body was still absorbing this dead tissue, but the rate of absorption had slowed ever since radiation. Unfortunately, I contracted a breast infection in this tissue. When antibiotics failed to clear it up, I returned to the surgeon I first visited when I was considering my treatment options.

Coming back into the care of this surgeon where I began my journey had the effect of helping me put my outcome into perspective. She had been so concerned for me, not wanting me to be a guinea pig for an unproven treatment. She had given me her blessing nonetheless, with a promise that she would allow me to come back into her care if the cryoablation failed to get rid of all my cancer. I felt confident returning to her care to have her resolve the infection issue.

After the surgery successfully removed the infected tissue and healed me of the infection, the biopsy showed there was no cancer in any of the removed tissue. I'm currently at the place I originally wanted to be: I still have both breasts and they are medically certified cancer free. Of course, any cancer patient will tell you that they are only as good as their next examination, but at four years out, it's looking good.

Looking back, the question that's most pertinent is: would I do it again having been through it all? When I set out on this journey, I had a very clear intention. It was to keep my breast in any way possible with doctors confirming that I was cancer free. I can now say it is as close to a miracle as it can be that we pulled that intention off.

As my thoughts go back thorough the journey of this medical miracle, one thing stands out particularly that helped with the decision making, and that is how to cope with fear. There is a lot of fear around cancer. I particularly understand this having suffered the loss of my own dear mother to breast cancer. In a way, fear can lead to a mental state of compliance. When you're afraid, it's easy to comply with the advice of your doctor. Statistics help take the emotion out of decision making so, as a result, statistical outcomes most often point the way when making a treatment decision. If the majority of cases like yours are treated in a certain way, then it's easy to think that's what you should do too. But there are decisions that require choices. For those careful choices, my experience has been that fear is not a good partner.

Intention on the other hand is a very good partner. As I've said before, my intention was to keep my breast and have it medically certified cancer free. With this in mind as I made my decisions as to how best to get rid of the cancer, and also how I wanted to live afterwards, I knew that losing a breast would offer a triumph over cancer. But I found that the medical world seemed so focused on their standard treatment method of a mastectomy that my wish to keep my breast was not given any consideration. However, I felt that a woman shouldn't have to justify her desire to keep a body part. In fact, I reasoned that, at some point, medicine went through this same process when lumpectomies were examined as a possible treatment rather than a mastectomy.

Because a lumpectomy wasn't possible in my case, but I still wanted the same outcome, I knew if I didn't at least try to find a solution that satisfied my intention, I would feel defeated. In the end, it wasn't me at all that found what I was looking for. It was my amazing husband, Alex. A television ad for prostate cryosurgery caught his eye. His brain asked the question, "Wouldn't it work for breasts?"

His terrific Internet skills and wonderful phone manners made the all-important connection to Dr. Littrup. And Dr. Littrup handed me an option, the very one I'd been seeking.

It is not surprising that my cancer treatment turned out so well, since everything else I've worked on together with my husband has prospered. Our home, our children, our business all have turned out so wonderfully.

He was willing to go down a new road with me. I would have been a fool to turn him down. I needed Alex's judgment of the Detroit doctors and their program. I needed his encouragement, his nurturing, his nursing. The outcome I wanted was only possible with a "we"—"our outcome." I could not have done this alone, but together it was very doable.

In retrospect, the hardest challenge was not the operation itself or even the decision to do it but the coordination of the hospital programs; the one where I was treated in Detroit, and the one in my hometown where the follow-up occurred. But even that challenge was met, especially as my Portland doctors' confidence in my unique cryoablation treatment increased.

I have come to have a profound appreciation for all healers, at every stage of care. I now clearly understand that complete healing takes place on four levels: physical, emotional, mental and spiritual. There are excellent healers specializing in each area. I began with a quest for a spiritual healing. Who's to say that, in the end, I didn't get it? From my vantage point now, it does seem truly miraculous.

Dr. Littrup, to me, represents the highest, most triumphant model of a medical healing innovator. In artistic vernacular, he is my Michelangelo of the healing world. He knows his science. He knows his medicine and he knows how to apply the most hopeful, helpful innovative form of healing with the biggest potential for effecting change. I think one of the best appeals of the freezing method is how it works with the immune system.

All healers are wonderful, and everyone who helped get me through my journey has been a real blessing to me. I am so grateful to all my doctors, nurses, technicians and alternative health practitioners.

Given all that's happened, it would seem logical to ask, "What would I advise a woman finding herself facing the difficult decision of what type of treatment to pursue?"

My answer is to listen to your gut. Listen to your comfort level. If hearing about cryolumpectomy makes sense to you, I would encourage you to do it if you possibly can. Support people, this goes for you, too. Until this method is easily attainable for every woman, there will need to be pioneers out there willing to make the first tries. Your friends might question you, but your reward might be very great. You might be able to keep your breast and possibly get an immune effect, just as I have.

There's been a television ad out recently that depicts a person walking up over a hill and, as the camera's perspective changes, it shows what's coming up behind: one, then several others, then more and more until a huge horde follows. That's how I envision cryolumpectomies. It's such a hopeful, fantastic solution. I know the horde is not far behind. I know my role in all of this will not become real to me until a woman out there in my future, who I have a heart connection with, tells me, "Laura, guess what—I've been diagnosed with breast cancer and I'm going to have this new method of treatment that will kill tumors by freezing them and leave practically no scar. I might even get an immune effect from it!"

When I hear that, the efforts Dr. Littrup, Alex and I have made will give a sense of satisfaction deep in my heart. I write these words to inspire others so that someday soon, cryolumpectomies will become a much sought-after treatment available to all women. Then the number of people "coming over the hill" will be a horde and not me walking alone.

It's been an epic journey, and I have grown so much in the process. The Biblical character I find inspiration from and relate to most is Jonah. Jonah didn't want the job God gave him, so he tried to run away. I didn't want to deal with breast cancer with the medical options handed to me, but I certainly didn't seek to be an innovator. I simply wanted to save my breast. As a result, I found myself in the belly of something much bigger than I could imagine. Before it set me on a sunny slope, I needed to have faith that cryoablation could treat my cancer, conserve my breast and offer a possible immunity.

I am just like Jonah, who with renewed enthusiasm, took up his post-whale task to tell the Ninevites to change their ways. I want to shout the message of change to all women everywhere and to all medical establishments, "There is a better way!"

Seven Years Later

4/19/2010

I've been getting phone calls and emails for weeks from friends letting me know that something about cryoablation as a method for treating breast cancer was in the news. So far, besides myself, there have been thirteen other women treated at Karmanos by Dr. Littrup. Two have been from Oregon. Many of those women had long phone conversations with me, which helped them make their decision. One of them just wrote to say, "This isn't new news!! For us it's old news!!!" Yes, for me it's been almost seven years. In fact, it will be exactly seven years in two days when I'm scheduled to be on an XM radio broadcast with Dr. Littrup. I couldn't be healthier! I just walked for an hour of "hill work" this morning with some of my friends. There's been many a day that "breast cancer" doesn't even enter my brain. But not lately. There have been multiple indications that the time is right to get this story out there.

When I first got back from Karmanos, there was interest by the press to cover my story as an innovative new way to treat breast cancer. The reporter working on the story finally decided to wait as she was told by experts I would have to survive for five years cancer free before I was considered "cured." My rule was to respond to questions whenever someone sought me out, but not to force my solution on anyone. We did keep a small website going. I was amazed by the number of calls I did get.

After hours of heartfelt conversations patiently listening to women agonizing over what was best for them and answering why I had done what I did, I always asked them to let me know what they decided to do. Some did. Most didn't. Some kept contact going all the way through their process. I've gotten to meet both the women from Oregon who've had their breast frozen by Dr. Littrup. Their first-hand accounts of their procedures have amazed me! Both were day procedures. The equipment has changed and only a local anesthetic is now required. The recovery time was almost immediate in terms of their energy level. One of the women, who just returned a few weeks ago, showed me her procedure site. There was literally no swelling and just the slightest hint of a bruise. By comparison what I went through was so much more. But still I'm amazingly happy with my results.

I remember my radiologist sharing a story about meeting a woman who had been among the first to be radiated. She was badly scarred compared to those going through it today, but she was very prideful of her breast. I'm with her!

My husband just sent a link to a Chinese website encouraging patients to use cryoablation for breast cancer. http://www.bgwicc.org.cn/english/2281.html

They are building a big, new breast cancer treatment center where cryoablation will be offered. It made me both happy and sad to read this. Happy that so many women were getting their breast saved. Sad that the "horde" I saw following behind me were in China and not America. One of the reasons I had confidence in Dr. Littrup is that I knew the UN had sent him to China to teach them how to use cryoablation. It's so sad the Chinese have run with this procedure but not us. What is it about our medical system that makes promising treatments so hard to get considered?

Somehow, I'm beginning to feel this is about to change. Just like Dr. Littrup once described it to me. There are other women out there who are taking responsibility for their bodies and looking for a solution that is right for them. Some are finding their way to Karmanos and Dr. Littrup—just like I did. Each day that passes builds the case that freezing a breast tumor WORKS!! It's only been a trickle so far, but I know that horde is coming.

Last summer, my college-age daughter and her friend went to Detroit to do a small internship with Dr. Littrup. While she didn't get to see a breast operated on, she did get to witness a cryo procedure. I believe she had begun to share the same frustration I've had, that this might not even be an easy-to-get procedure by the time her generation begins to see cases of breast cancer. I hope we're both wrong. I sense that women are ready to claim their right to keep their breast and still be healed from their cancer.

Twelve Years Later 3.1.14

Perhaps it's obvious from the above updates that both Alex and I thought this book would be out into the world by now. We held off releasing our story and the related information about cryoablation for breast cancer because we kept thinking a path would develop, leading to easy access for any American woman wanting to follow in my footsteps to treat her breast cancer in this breast conserving, immune-stimulating way.

So far, it hasn't happened, despite the best efforts of Dr. Littrup and the entrepreneurs supporting him and his fellow scientists. It hasn't happened here in the States, at least. It has happened in other parts of the world: Brazil, Austria and, most especially, China. As Dr. Littrup pointed out earlier, when he reflected on his trip there in the late nineties to show them his methods, the Chinese have had the opportunity to pick and choose among the best, most cutting-edge practices. Cryoablation fits rather seamlessly into their thousands-year-old medical practices based on the support of the immune system. They really got it! At a cutting-edge hospital named Fuda in Guangzhou, Southern China, they operate two cancer specialty hospitals catering to cancer sufferers from all over the world.

After Karmanos Cancer Center in Detroit quit offering their breast cancer cryoablation option, I began suggesting the Fuda program to women contacting me on our website who were looking to save their breasts.

At the end of 2012, I got an opportunity to witness Fuda first-hand when I joined a woman from Alberta Canada, Fe Zahorodniuk, to follow her treatment for an aggressive reoccurring breast cancer. While there, I attended an international conference on the subject where I was reunited with Dr. Littrup himself.

In April of 2014, my husband and I will travel to Fuda to experience for ourselves a wonderful add-on procedure that re-boots the immune system. The Fuda doctors have come up with this procedure as a continuing cancer–reoccurrence preventative. It is called Combined Immunology for Cancer (CIC). The story of my first trip to Fuda is included in this book. Since this second trip will occur after the release of our book, we will document the second trip and the CIC experience on our website, KeepingThem.com.

Back in 2003, when I experienced a very successful outcome from using my body as a guinea pig to further breast cancer treatment, I thought changing treatment options in America would be a very easy thing because the benefits of cryoablation are so obvious. After all, who wouldn't want to keep their breasts and get an immune effect? However, Alex and I were very naïve about the American medical industrial complex. Things happen slowly here! There are many hurdles to getting something new to be accepted.

This has made me even more appreciative that Dr. Littrup took on such a difficult case as mine. It has also made me even more determined to help other women get the treatment they want. I'm hopeful now, with an excellent cryoablation option offered by the Chinese, that those interested in making a change can at least take a look at a tremendously successful program to gain the confidence that it CAN and SHOULD work here in the US, the country of the pioneering efforts to first get it going. I can see it will take awhile, but perhaps that horde of energized women I saw in my vision at my three-year anniversary will have my back and help get the job done though their interest and activism. This is my fervent hope.

Cutting edge doctors like Dr. Peter Littrup and Dr. Kecheng Xu have shown us that because cancer is a disease of the whole body, personalizing treatment is a better approach, and that supporting the immune system and working with it helps cancer "exit the body at a cellular level"* (* Fuda's Dr. Kecheng Xu). As the general public catches up with this awareness, I am confident we will come closer to understanding and embracing—even demanding—the treatment option that cryoablation offers.

We live in a time when Western and Eastern approaches are meshing in all fields, even medicine. I am thankful for a modern era like this where books can be posted through Amazon and word of new ideas can be quickly spread through social networking. Perhaps, in the end, it will be the group brain known as the Internet that will allow the cream to rise to the top in all fields. I have every confidence that cryoablation to treat breast cancer will eventually emerge as the best of the treatment options!

***

Laura

Laura here again—almost twelve years after being successfully treated with cryoablation by Dr. Littrup at Karmanos Cancer Center in Detroit. I decided to fill in some back story from my life here as it may give the reader some insights to the most asked question I've gotten since taking this new path to breast conservation and cancer survival. That question is: "What gave you the courage and confidence to do cryoablation?" It's an answer that has a lot of complexity to it beyond the obvious desire to save a body part.

I believe my decision to use cryoablation started due to a death but not one from breast cancer, although that was involved too. No, it was a death due to football. I will explain further but first let me lay some background.

I was born in 1950, the second of four blue-eyed daughters. We lived in a small village called Multnomah, named after an Indian tribe from the area. Our village had been eaten up by a mid-sized city, Portland, Oregon. My ex-sailor father was a salesman of industrial equipment for the lumber industry. As a young girl, I often went on road trips with him, visiting many of the large sawmills of our state.

Since my schooling was pre-title nine, I got my physical exercise through my own devices, such as being an avid player of pick-up baseball games, which happened almost every day in my neighborhood. I even got hits off my friend's tall, athletic older brother's pitching. (My friend's brother, Wayne Twitchell, went on to be a "rookie of the year" in Major League Baseball). I was also my Camp Fire Camp's bugler, walking the length of huge Camp Namanu multiple times a day during the summer. I climbed Mt. Hood at age 15 and took every chance I could to camp in Oregon's beautiful forests.

I had a strong interest in art, which led my path academically. I found myself involved with ambitious projects, such as conceiving and executing large murals for my grade school, illustrating an award-winning yearbook for my high school and being a political cartoonist for an anti-war underground newspaper during my college years. I went on to get my Masters of Fine Art and have had a successful career as a gallery-represented artist and adjunct art professor.

My mother was a homemaker who made most of our meals, including school sack lunches, and sewed most of our clothes. I adored her. After I entered high school, she found out she had breast cancer and received a lateral mastectomy and removal of part of her ribcage. While devastating, she seemed to be in good health and recovering fully when disaster struck the first week of my senior year in high school. A drunk driver slammed into my family's car as they were returning from a family reunion at my cousin's farm. The crash killed my next youngest sister, my beloved 13-year-old Peggy. I hadn't been with them. I ended up taking care of my youngest sister Mary by myself for much of that year as my parents and older sister Kay struggled in the hospital to recover from their injuries.

Both my parents hung on to life at Good Samaritan's Intensive Care unit most of that fall. I stayed in school but had to get a job to help support Mary and myself, so time spent visiting my parents in the ICU was very precious. One evening in the late fall, I was allowed to feed my Mother her soft food supper. Just as I'd gotten started, there was a commotion in the space next to her bed as a young high school boy, around the age of the sister I had just lost, was wheeled in with a football injury.

The ICU staff flew around him, gathering equipment and inserting tubes. Suddenly time seemed to slow down dramatically. The boy raised his torso up. He twisted around looking for something or someone. His eyes found mine and locked there. Time stopped. Something very, very deep was exchanged. It felt as if our souls bonded in a state of deep peace and knowingness. Then his eyes rolled up and he collapsed limply. Buzzers went off and time started again. A nurse gave me a stern, sad look as she pulled a curtain to block my view. She later escorted me to the door saying some kind words about our time on earth and how it is shorter for some of us.

His family and a waiting room crowd full to overflowing learned of his fate by the sad, all too revealing, look in my eyes as the door opened.

But before that happened, my mother and I had the most profound conversation of my life. One that would lead and shape me, getting me through the difficult times of the next several years and affecting my decision making in life forever, especially when deciding how to treat my own future breast cancer. What was it my mother said that gave me a guidance system to make decisions by? Perhaps it will sound simple but to me it was profound.

I, of course, was trying to shelter my mom from the boy's death that had just taken place so close by. I kept to my task of offering small spoonfuls of soft food, trying to keep my emotions in check. At first she continued what we had been talking about before. But then she asked, "That boy they brought in has just died, hasn't he?"

"It's okay, Mom. Everything is okay," I answered.

"I know he just died," she said. "And I want you to know that we all will die . . . someday. For some of us, though, it's sooner than we'd like. I'm afraid I know for me it's going to be soon. I want you to know that I'll be abandoning you and I'm sorry for that. But I won't be abandoning you to be left alone in life."

"Mom, we don't have to talk about this now" was all I could get out. But she wasn't done.

"Honey, we earthly parents may not always be able to come through for you but I'm turning you over to your heavenly parents who will never let you down."

I tried to assure her I was sure she would make it.

"No, Honey. I don't think so. But I want you to promise you'll listen to me and trust your heavenly parents to take care of you. If there's ever anything you need, you just ask them. They'll take care of you. You'll see."

Our conversation was effectively over. The hospital staff next to us had quit trying to revive the football boy and the ICU team needed and wanted to clear the visitors out so the family could give his body their final good-byes as privately as possible.

The nurse I spoke of earlier came and took my arm in hers, and we slowly walked to the door.

My mom's advice helped me get through the difficult weeks, months and years that followed. I had to use her advice, as I really had nothing else. Much of my memories of those times seem to be blocked. But there are some remembrances that I'm aware of and others that have become clearer as time passed.

The first was the practical matter of getting my sister and I fed each night because we only had my meager earnings from my after-school job to pay for all our needs. Getting our evening meal happened in an unexpected way when a neighbor, the wonderful Dennis Miller, asked us over for dinner one night, and kept doing the same thing for the next eight months.

My heart's desire was to go off to Oregon State with all my friends the next fall after graduation. I had no idea how I could ever afford going to college. My mother came home from the hospital for Christmas but had to return to repair her pelvic area injured in the car accident. However, when they opened her up they discovered reoccurring cancer that was judged to be terminal. She died in the early spring.

The day my senior class did our practice for the upcoming graduation ceremony it was announced that there were quite a few unclaimed scholarships. I ran to the counseling office as soon as we finished and let my counselor know I was very interested. Subsequently, all five remaining scholarships were awarded to me, enough to attend my first year of college.

During that first term at OSU, my father remarried into a new family. I needed a family of my own. The following fall, I fell in love with a fellow war protestor who had a strong enough British heritage to insist on marriage rather than just shacking up together.

The list goes on . . . personal needs met, career needs and desires wonderfully met. If it was something I really wanted, I asked my heavenly parents, and then sat back to see how they fulfilled my request.

The only credit I can take is that I had a constantly strengthening belief that the request would be fulfilled. Some call that faith. Sometimes the request was answered in an unexpected way, but it was always fulfilled. Even seeming infertility switched into two healthy boys, and then a wonderful daughter when I wanted one but wasn't actively trying to get pregnant. So, fast forward to 2003 and a breast cancer diagnosis that looked as if a mastectomy was the only solution.

I will admit to a weak moment that came right before the one described in my journal, when, though I was alone in the room, I felt a hand around my shoulder and a strong, unafraid voice in my ear asking me why I was so sad, telling me that I would be able to keep my breast if I wanted to. Well, the thought I had right before that happened was to wonder how my heavenly parents were going to pull this one off! I still didn't know how it would be pulled off the moment that followed hearing the voice, but I had a renewed confidence and curiosity to find out. Hearing that voice's confident, unafraid tone was so powerful and affirming and it gave me so much more strength than any fear I may have had that would have led me to give in to the mastectomy.

Part Three: FUDA Hospital, Guangzhou, China

Chapter 21: How Fe Traveled to China and Got Her Life Back

Alex

I completed writing and editing our book, *They're Mine and I'm Keeping Them,* in 2006, three years after Dr. Littrup successfully treated Laura's breast cancer using his groundbreaking technique, "cryoablation." This is the freezing of malignant tumors to kill them.

However, for various reasons, cryoablation treatment for breast cancer did not become widely available in America in the years following our book's completion. While there was genuine interest from agents and publishers in bringing our book out, Laura and I decided to stop our efforts to get the book published. We didn't want to stimulate interest in a procedure that was barely available! An odd combination of patent licensing agreements, FDA approvals, hospital rules and insurance company policy limited Dr. Littrup's ability to offer the procedure and no else was offering it in the United States.

It seemed to us that telling Laura's story of saving her breast would create resentment in any woman wanting to save her breast and cure her cancer if that same person then learned that the treatment was, at best, extremely difficult to get.

As I wrote this book, Laura worked to develop a website with information regarding cryoablation, KeepingThem.com. Our goal had originally been to provide information to women seeking cryoablation treatment after reading the book.

When we decided to delay publishing until treatment was more widely available, we elected to keep the site up thinking there would be a few women searching for breast conservation alternatives to cancer treatment. We reasoned that this smaller cadre of determined patients could be treated by Dr. Littrup as part of his research budget.

Laura did the heavy lifting in talking to women who came to our site. She faithfully talked to approximately forty women interested in cryoablation for breast cancer who visited our site during the period 2006 through 2012. Approximately twelve of these women, including two from Oregon, then chose to have cryoablation performed by Dr. Littrup in Detroit. This was not an easy thing to do. Each woman was making a life-and-death decision, and there were many nights where I tried to help Laura deal with the emotion that had washed into her life while trying to help another woman—in every case a total stranger that ended up with a heart connection to Laura. I have to say, I admire my wife and the incredible energy and love she has poured into the world trying to help other women with breast cancer.

In the late 1990s, Dr. Littrup traveled to China for the UN to teach them cryoablation. The Chinese immediately and enthusiastically embraced cryoablation, primarily because their government had limited expertise and/or radiation equipment to treat cancer throughout their massive population. They were aware that treatment in the US is designed around the philosophy of early detection. However, screening programs require intense coordination and expense, primarily an investment in mammogram equipment. This equipment is not universally available in China due to the cost of providing it to such an enormous population. As a result, about 80 percent of their breast cancer cases are not discovered until a woman notices a large breast lump and invariably this becomes late stage cancer that the Chinese medical community has to treat.

Dr. Littrup's cryoablation education showed the Chinese that cryoablation offers a hope of controlling and even eliminating tumor growth in late stage cancer, so they wisely decided to put research funds into that field.

I think this phenomenon is analogous to cell phones spreading throughout the Third World because the expensive infrastructure investment of hard wire telephone connections is unnecessary with the installation of a cheap cell phone tower.

Fortunately, the Chinese soon realized that complex tumors could not be treated with a single probe machine, so they began treating breast cancer with multi-probe units. This markedly differs from the situation in America, where breast cryoablation is only used on benign cysts until such time as a manufacturer of cryoablation equipment gains FDA approval to use a multi-probe cryoablation machine on malignant breast tumors. It is interesting to note that FDA clearance has been given in the US for use of multi-probe cryoablation on prostate cancer, while it is still pending for use in breast cancer.

The use of multiple probes allowed the Chinese to treat breast cancer with as many probes as the tumor size, shape and number demanded, and their program was rewarded with early and potentially successful remissions, some of which are now almost as long as Laura's, which as of this writing is over 11 years.

In mid-2012, we learned from the Internet that FUDA Hospital was routinely treating breast cancer with cryoablation. Laura and I were considering traveling to FUDA to learn about their program when, in late 2012, Laura received an email from one of our cancer website's users. Here, in Laura's words, is the amazing story of her first trip to FUDA.

***

Laura

I received an email from the sister in-law of Fe Zahorodniuk in Alberta. Fe was diagnosed with breast cancer in 2011 and was treated by lumpectomy in early 2012. However, her Herceptin positive tumor quickly returned and, by late 2012, her outlook seemed dismal: stage 4 cancer, her body riddled with metastasized tumors. Her doctors in Canada advised a mastectomy and systemic chemotherapy, though they admitted the chances of success were very low and the possibility of mortality likely in just a few months.

However, Fe's husband, Dave, researched alternate cures and other treatment centers. His research soon led to a decision that Fe's best chance at life lay at FUDA

Hospital in Guangzhou, southern China. While Fe's husband was doing his Internet research, Fe's sister-in-law, Colleyne was helping as well and she found our website, KeepingThem.com. Once they realized that FUDA specialized in cryoablation and I had received that treatment, I was asked what I thought about it and did I think this was a good idea.

I was happy to help as best I could, letting them know I felt the potential of getting an "immune effect" carried with it the hope of having some of the metastasized sites eliminated. I told her I had been telling women about FUDA for months but she was the first one who was actually willing to go there. I asked if she'd allow us to follow her story. That is when she suggested I should come to FUDA as well to get a firsthand account. This would make my advice on our site more credible.

If Fe's treatment of fourth stage cancer could success-fully be treated in China, our book would have a happy ending, a direction to point to, and a validation of cryo-ablation's immune-stimulating effects. What a miracle that would be! What a validation of using freeze-balls to treat recurrences and secondary sites. Women coming to our site would at least have a hopeful option if they were set on keeping their breasts and possibly getting an immune effect.

It turned out Fe's case was far more difficult to treat than mine. I had primary, stage one, multiple tumors. Although I had several, they were all confined within the ducts. However, by the time Fe decided to travel to FUDA for cryoablation treatment, she had seven tumors in four different locations in her body. It was the imaging done at FUDA that found this out.

I soon learned why Fe and her husband were so interested in seeking treatment in China. It turned out that FUDA was attracting cases from all over the planet, because they were treating and reducing symptoms and extending the life of patients who were having a recurrence—patients whose primary doctors had given up treatment.

The more I learned about FUDA and the amazing record of positive treatments they were achieving, I realized that while Dr. Littrup's efforts had been ignored in the United States, they were bearing fruit in China. It seemed to me that when women contacted us in the future, we could refer them to FUDA. However, I felt compelled to travel there and verify with my own personal research that FUDA was indeed as successful as they seemed to be on the Internet.

It turned out that the custom at FUDA is for people to bring several friends or relatives to stay with them during the treatment period, which could often last longer than a month. I told Fe I would immediately start work on an Internet fundraiser to try to raise the funds to join her. That afternoon, my videographer son, Louie, helped me shoot an "ask" for a fundraiser.

Alex set up a GoFundMe.com online funding request, and he included the video and then sent it to our entire email list and Facebook websites. He then monitored the site daily as donations came in and immediately sent out individual thanks to each donor.

Alex was initially eager to travel to China, but it turned out he had a surgery scheduled at the same time Fe's treatment was scheduled, a surgery he could not delay. In addition to that conflict, he was reluctant to leave the country as he was in the final stages of helping our older son Sean advertise and distribute a documentary about *2012,* a film that Alex's company had funded and in which Alex had helped to write and edit.

At the same time, Louie was very eager to go to China because he had been thinking about doing a documentary about my cancer treatment. After I told him about the work done at FUDA, this made him more eager to travel to China in order to get more material for his documentary. Alex was happy that Louie would join me with the promise that we would later travel there, as he was eager to find out about FUDA firsthand.

Thanks to our generous friends, within three weeks, Alex's fundraising efforts had amassed enough to buy Louie's ticket while Alex and I applied our own funds for my ticket and all the other travel expenses.

Fe was already at FUDA with her sister from the Philippines, Jelly, who had joined her to share a room at the hospital and be her support system. Louie and I arrived the second week of December, just as Christmas social activities had begun in earnest back home. In China, where much of the West's Christmas decorations are manufactured, Christmas trees abounded throughout the hospital to greet us.

Our plan was to join Fe and stay for approximately 10 days and then return to Portland—just in time for Christmas. I wrote Dr. Littrup, asking if he could write an introduction to FUDA's director, Dr. Kecheng Xu, as I would need an official invitation from the hospital in order to acquire visas. The stars seemed to be aligning for us as Dr. Littrup wrote back telling me that he also had plans to be visiting FUDA, as he would be presenting a talk during an international conference going on at FUDA during the time of our stay. Not only were we going to be able to gather the story of the effects of cryoablation to treat a very difficult case thanks to Fe's generosity in sharing her story, we were to be witnesses to the world's top medical researchers and oncological professors sharing their research on using cryoablation to treat cancer.

Louie decided to look on a map of China and determine what the weather would be like. I had assumed we were going somewhere terribly cold that was near Beijing. Fortunately, Louie discovered that we were basically headed right above Hong Kong, in Guangzhou, a weather paradise in the winter!

When we heard about FUDA and the work they were doing, we decided to upgrade our website in anticipation of learning that FUDA would finally be able to fulfill the promise of cryoablation we had hoped would come from Karmanos. One feature we decided to add to the website was a blog, and with the trip looming in a few days, I learned how to blog. It would be instant journaling! I could keep my many contributors aware of the trip's progress as each day passed by. The blog of my trip follows.

Laura's China Trip Blog

Wednesday, 12.12.12

A most auspicious day to travel . . .

Louie and I are sitting in the TBIT (Tom Bradley International Terminal) at LAX, waiting for the plane to Guangzhou, China.

In nine years of keeping up a website and answering all inquiries about cryoablation to treat breast cancer, this is the first time I have known of a woman, Fe Zahorodniuk of Alberta, traveling to FUDA Hospital in

Guangzhou for cryoablation treatment. It is also the first time I have been asked to join someone in China and document her story.

When I accepted Fe's invitation, I had no idea the pioneer doctor, Dr. Peter Littrup, who had treated me in Detroit ten years earlier, had any association with FUDA. I recently learned he will be attending an international conference in FUDA when I am there. What are the odds of that? I can't help but feel events are somehow being divinely guided!

I know it's going to be emotionally tough, because Fe has Stage 4 breast cancer, which is usually untreatable. But I have a deep, strong feeling Fe is going to make it. I am a good prayer warrior, and I have been praying for Fe to be healed of cancer since we first talked. If Fe survives, telling the story of her successful treatment will bring both validation and hope.

Last night, I had a dream. I was with Louie flying on a big polished cloud high above the earth over darkened peaceful waters. We won't be flying on a cloud, but the plane will look polished and clean, I am sure!

Louie is sitting next to me in the terminal, working on his first video blog he hopes to post before we take off. We will document our trip to FUDA on video to give other women following in our footsteps an idea of what to expect at FUDA. For someone wanting to seek cryoablation for breast cancer and save her breast, FUDA is the only good option. The reality is that western women will only be comfortable when they see FUDA through a western perspective. We hope to give them that in the video and through my blog.

Friday, 12.14.12

Finally . . . I meet Fe in person!

We left Oregon on Wednesday 12.12.12 and landed in Guangzhou the morning of Friday 12.14.12. Where did Thursday go? Well, we crossed the International Date Line! It was Thursday one second and Friday the next. (Note from Alex: British sailors loved crossing the International Date Line because when sailing east to west, they got an extra day's pay for no work. The reverse was true, though, sailing west to east. I'm sure they didn't like working two days for one day's pay!)

The 16-hour direct flight from LAX to Guangzhou on Southern China Air was quite pleasant. The long, quiet parts of the flight were perfect times for me to continue to pray for Fe and also to pray that our book could get out into the world and let women know that there is an alternative to losing your breasts to cancer.

Southern China Air is very concerned about passenger comfort and well-being. In fact, the video playing on the seat-back monitors for the last half hour before we landed showed stewardesses demonstrating self-acu-pressure to help recover from the flight!

After making it through customs and finding our suitcases (thank God I had big, strong Louie with me!), we exited the airport to find a driver holding a sign with my name on it.

The driver whizzed along a freeway through this very modern, large city, arriving at FUDA hospital before 8 a.m. The driver was so kind; he walked us directly to Fe's room!

I had been so worried about what this first meeting would be like. Stage 4 cancer is so scary and things can deteriorate rapidly. I had no idea what to expect. I had also learned from David's sister that Fe had begun treatment at FUDA about two and a half weeks before my arrival. Her preliminary treatment was the implanting of twenty iodine radiation pellets around her breasts and surrounding lymph nodes and twenty around her liver. They would stay in place for fifty-nine days.

I worried that the radiation treatments might have left her in a weakened state. I was honestly shocked by her condition, but not because she had cancer; rather, because she looked so healthy!

We found Fe already up and able to walk around. She was eating normally, visiting and full of energy! I thought this was miraculous, because Fe had received her first cryoablation operation only four days before our arrival. She had six different tumor sites frozen, five in her liver and one in her breast. Following her procedure, they kept her in the ICU, Intensive Care Unit, for the next 24 hours, which is the hospital protocol.

So here she was, only three days out of the ICU. Instead of a patient on the edge of survival, I found Fe to be a spry, intelligent, bright-eyed fifty-four year-old woman of Filipino descent cheerfully visiting with her delightful sister, Jelly.

I wanted to give Fe a hug, because I was so happy—but I couldn't! She was radioactive! Even though she was wearing a protective apron of lead to protect others, hugging was too close to be safe. And I imagine she was still sensitive in her chest area from her operation.

I already felt the trip to China was worth the effort. It was obvious that FUDA is performing healing miracles! Fe told me that she had already heard of a patient who had received cryoablation for a large tumor, 11.9 cm in diameter. She said that as a comparison, MD Anderson Cancer Center in California will only treat tumors less than 2 cm in diameter.

This ability to successfully freeze larger tumors really expands the scope of patients they can treat at FUDA.

***

Note from Alex

I contacted MD Anderson's question line and they stated that they have no facilities in California at this time, that they are located primarily in Texas. However I was able to determine that there have been several clinical trials involving breast cancer and MD Anderson has participated in at least one. Fe was correct, that the maximum size of tumor being recruited for the trial is 2cm. The trial website is: http://clinicaltrials.gov/show/NCT01388777

It should be noted that while the trials are ongoing, they are not recruiting candidates at this time. Also, part of the requirement of the trial is a follow up surgery a short time after the cryoablation, so in the end, this is not a breast conserving treatment as is offered at FUDA. The trial is part of ongoing research to determine if cryo-ablation kills cancer. The staff at FUDA Hospital are confident that this question has already been answered and in fact, Laura is correct, the scope of cancers treated at FUDA is much wider than those being treated in the United States.

***

Laura

Louie and I left Fe to check into the hotel the coordinator at FUDA had arranged. She had done a great job, because the hotel was only a few blocks away from the hospital. We quickly got moved into our room and then returned to the hospital to join Fe and her sister in time for a delicious Chinese lunch of steamed fish supplied by the hospital's wonderful kitchen.

As we ate, I learned that family members could also cook meals if they wished in a communal kitchen, which was just a few floors above Fe's room. This flexibility in providing food impressed me, because FUDA is treating patients from all over the world and it is understandable that some patients would not relish Chinese cuisine.

Fe's nurses were very attentive. They were constantly coming in and out of the room, checking her temperature and IVs, weighing her and much more.

All and all, she is getting excellent care!

I mentioned to Fe that I was writing a blog, which would be seen on the website and added to our book. She wanted me to include the following statement:

Fe

"In this hospital, there's love which money can't buy. If you value your health, come to FUDA. They give you hope here. You feel it in the fiber of your flesh, in your heart and in your mind because you know you'll get better! If they can make stage five cancer patients better, they can make me better! And they don't like patients here to be sad because it will affect your immune system. They told me, we can help you, but you must help yourself! So the only thing we ask from you is to be happy."

Note from Laura

I'm not sure "stage five" is an official term but I think what Fe meant is the very ill, terminal patients she's been talking to all seem to be having a turnaround shortly after they've been treated here for a bit.

Laura

Following lunch, a whirlwind of activity began, which put the whole program together in an understandable way . . .

Mr. Li, who had picked us up from the airport and walked us to Fe's room, returned to take us to FUDA's second large new hospital, FUDA 2! It is a twenty-minute freeway drive from FUDA 1 (also referred to as Old FUDA).

FUDA 2 is a beautiful, state-of-the-art facility with the latest cutting-edge machines that form the heart of FUDA's cancer fighting arsenal. We were invited to attend an exit interview there of a patient leaving for home.

Every patient has an exit interview, which is attended by all the doctors who have worked on the departing patient. FUDA's Director and acting President, Dr. Xu, and his assistant and Vice President, Ester Law, attend all the exit meetings.

In this group meeting, the doctors present an overview of the therapies used and comment on what they felt were most effective. They also offer their opinions on future treatment and follow-ups. The patients participate, commenting on what they feel worked best and areas they are interested in pursuing (at least this is what I understood from the interpreter at my side who was filling me in).

There seems to be a very honest and objective look taken at this exit interview to record exactly what was accomplished during the patient's stay at FUDA. They determine the status of a patient's health and plan follow-up treatment if any is required.

This exit meeting concerned two patients. The first no longer had a tumor. The second was being sent home to allow the implanted chemotherapies to work for some time before returning for additional therapies such as cryoablation.

Dr. Xu explained for my benefit that this chemo treatment would kill the tumor cells but not the stem cells of the tumor, and that's why the cryoablation and immune building therapies were needed in the future.

I was asked to tell the story of my breast cancer treatment in the meeting. Vice President Ester Law translated for me. She seemed truly moved upon learning I had come to FUDA to find out what they were doing in order to spread the word to other women in the West who wanted to save their breast as I had done. There was a surreal quality to the situation because a photographer was clicking away and a videographer was filming. Such attention!

After the meeting, Louie and I were invited to Ester's office where she explained FUDA Hospital's cancer treatment philosophy. Ester explained that Dr. Xu himself had been a cancer patient and was now a survivor. The philosophy of treatment at FUDA grew from his experience. She did a beautiful job explaining how traditional treatments of surgery, radiation and chemotherapy can and do work on early stage cancer, which she estimated was about 20 percent of the patient load throughout China.

She then related that, due to China's lack of modern detection equipment, approximately 80 percent of the cases were not detected early and it was the experience in China that traditional Western treatments ultimately failed to cure most of these patients.

I don't know how these statistics hold up for American women where early detection is promoted through yearly mammogram readings, but my guess is that the push for early detection in America is exactly because they can most easily cure early stage cancer.

However, given the fact that the vast majority of cancer patients in China do not receive early detection, FUDA decided to make its mission to address the 80 percent of Chinese cases—the late detection cases where there is usually some metastasis.

To do this they have incorporated the most modern, cutting-edge technology available in the world today, while at the same time emphasizing therapies that boost the patient's immune system. (I can see why this makes sense here, as traditional Chinese medicine is a system that works by assisting and stimulating the immune system.)

Cryoablation stimulates the body to go in and replace the dead tissue with new healthy tissue. To do this, the body first sends cells that clean up and consume the dead cells. Because the cancer cells are dead, they are no longer able to mask their DNA structure from the immune system, which is how cancer survives in the body.

So after cryoablation, the immune system is able to "see" that the protein "signature" of the cancer tissue differs from that of the body. This triggers the creation of antibodies to attack the cancer, and these antibodies circulate throughout the body and are able to kill live, metastasized tumors.

This is one of the main reasons cryoablation has been so aggressively embraced here in China at FUDA; they are immune system-centric in their ancient healing arts. And to follow that model and enhance the work of the immune system, they use two more complimentary treatments at FUDA: CMI, **C**ancer **M**icrovascular **I**ntervention, and CIC, **C**ombined **I**mmunotherapy for **C**ancer.

These constitute the "Three C" Program at FUDA.

To make sure we explain these thoroughly and properly, Alex has transcribed the following material directly from a FUDA instructional bulletin that they give all new patients.

***

Alex

I have copied the text of the FUDA handout below and show it in Century Gothic font in order to make sure the reader understands this is extracted from FUDA's brochure.

The handout from FUDA is entitled, "How to Treat a Cancer Patient," and is authored by a team of doctors and scientists at Jinan University School of Medicine, FUDA Cancer Hospital, Guangzhou, China. Their motto is, "Professional, Team, Work, Sincerity, Innovation."

FUDA

Cancer is a systemic disease with tumors as a local manifestation of the disease. Once cancer occurs in a person, cancerous cells may metastasize (spread), throughout the whole body. Surgical removal of tumors in no way implies that one is cured of cancer. For example, breast cancer can relapse even if the original tumors were removed.

Like hypertension and diabetes, cancer is a chronic disease. The disease may take a few years to manifest itself—from its occurrence until the emergence of tumors. In some cases, cancer cells may exist in a stage of dormancy and never manifest themselves.

Our immune system plays an important role in controlling the development of cancer. Cancer cells may either be killed by immune cells or if they are as strong as the immune cells, nothing happens to the body. However, if the amount of immune cells decreases, leading to a decrease in their activity levels, or if cancerous cells are able to evade the detection of immune cells (a process known as immune tolerance), then the cancerous cells will spread rapidly and become life threatening.

Influenced by various factors inside and outside the body, a series of genes mutate continuously so tumors are formed. Though cancer patients may be suffering from the same cancer, their pathogenic factors and mutational genes differ. Every tumor has its specific biological features, or heterogeneity. Ignoring the heterogeneity is the main reason that cancer treatments often cannot achieve their ideal effects. It will work better if more personalized treatment is prescribed to deal with the heterogeneity.

The following principles have to be adhered to in the treatment of cancer:

1. First perform surgical removal of tumors or cryosurgical ablation, which are effective local treatment methods.

2. Conventional chemotherapy will damage immune cells. In cancer microvascular intervention, chemotherapy drugs are inserted into the tumors, thus resulting in a greater local treatment effect with minimal side effects.

3. Immunotherapy is a systemic therapy. The destruction of the last cancer cell is done through the immune cells and not by any other medicine.

Personalized therapy for cancer is a brand new therapy utilizing the molecular biological differences between cancer cells and normal cells to choose the appropriate drugs. The drugs will act on specific targeted cancer cells. This means receptors, kinases and other proteins related with cellular signal transduction to specifically kill or control cancer cells.

The Three "C's" at FUDA

CSA Cryosurgical Ablation

Using imaging-guided techniques (Ultrasound, CT or MRI), cryoprobes are inserted into tumors to lower the temperature of the targeted areas to -160 degrees

Centigrade or lower. Later the temperature is raised to 20 to 45 degrees C. This is repeated two or three times, resulting in the complete ablation of the tumor. After cancer cells have been destroyed by CSA they are left intact. Dead cancer cells will release antigens stimulating the immune system to eradicate any remaining cancer cells and reduce recurrence of cancer.

Advantages of CSA

It is applicable to both small and large tumors. It can lead to ablation of a single tumor or several tumors. It can be used on tumors near large blood vessels and the trachea without damaging those blood vessels or the trachea. It is a painless operation and it helps reduce pain caused by cancer.

CMI Cancer Micro-Vascular Intervention

One or several types of chemotherapy drugs are embedded into tiny particles or sealed within them using a special technology. Using an image–guided micro-catheter, these tiny particles containing a minimal dose of chemical drugs are inserted into tiny capillary vessels supplying blood to the tumor. The chemotherapy drugs pass through the wall of the tiny capillary vessels into the tumor. As more and more chemotherapy drugs are released into the tumor, cancerous cells are destroyed. Tiny particles cannot pass through the compact wall of normal capillaries; hence, chemotherapy drugs embedded/sealed inside tiny particles will not cause damage to other parts of the body. Furthermore, the overall side effects of CMI are reduced to the minimum.

Advantages of CMI

In applying CMI, there is a high concentration of chemotherapeutical drugs within the tumor itself with very little systemic drugs in the rest of the body. For example, a patient weighing 60 kilograms (132 pounds) with a 50-gram tumor (2 oz. or 1/8 of a pound): under conventional vascular interventional chemotherapy, 150 mg of oxaliplatin will be used. And only about .125 mg of oxaliplatin will actually reach the tumor. However, with CMI only 15 mg of oxaliplatin (a tenth of the conventional dosage) will be used and 5 mg of the drug will reach the tumor, a 40-fold increase when compared to the conventional method!

- Rapid results: a solid tumor is destroyed quickly, reducing their size and disappearance of staining of capillary blood vessels in tumors.
- Few side effects: patients can return home 3 to 4 hours after treatment with no hospitalization required.
- CMI offers an alternative treatment option. When conventional chemotherapy and interventional chemotherapy fail, CMI provides a better approach.
- It can be repeated without affecting the patient's quality of life.

CIC Combined Immunotherapy for Cancer

Conventional immune treatment project CD-CIK therapy

As the human body ages, the number of tumor killing lymphocytes gradually declines and cannot be replenished. However, these cells can be expanded in the laboratory and injected back into the body to effectively fight cancer. In the immune system, dendritic cells (DCs) are the strongest stimulator of tumor-killing lymphocytes.

***

Alex

Note of explanation by Alex: cryoablation stimulates the presence of dendritic cells, because they go into the frozen dead tissue and clean it all up. Because the freezing process does not destroy the DNA of the cancer cells, when the dendritic cells "eat up" a cancer cell, the immune system "sees" the cancer when it could not while the cancer was alive. This stimulates the immune system to make antibodies, which is the "immune effect" from cryoablation. The CIC process capitalizes on this phenomenon by boosting the immune system's response by increasing the number of tumor-killing lymphocytes that will respond to this stimulus by the dendritic cells. This is why the Chinese approach of working with the immune system and amplifying its ability to kill cancer is so effective. Laura and I traveled to China subsequent to her first trip in 2012 and had this immune system boost treatment, which I will describe in a following chapter.

***

Dendritic cells and various other lymphocyte sub-types can be isolated from the peripheral blood of patients. In the laboratory, with the help of multiple cytokines, killer cells (CIK) can be amplified by 100 to 200 times. Combined with IL-2 (interleukin 2) and polyvalent vaccine injections, the killer cells can continue to improve the anti-tumor killing effects. This therapy was approved by the FDA of the United States and the Chinese Ministry of Health and has been utilized in our hospital since 2003.

***

Alex

Note by Alex: According to Dr. Littrup, portions of FUDA's CIC process have been cleared by the FDA as well as only some of the substances used. This process is not in use in the United States primarily because lengthy trials will be needed to get full FDA approval of the entire process. In the meantime, a physician could use CIC; however, if there were any adverse reactions, the physician could be held liable for damages in applying techniques that have been cleared but not approved through trials.

Because of this, the technique is not available in the US as of the date of this writing despite the visible benefits noted in China.

***

Featured Immune Treatment Project: T Cell therapy

Another approach used in CIC is T Cell Therapy. Thanks to years of clinical treatment, experience and intensive research, the Cancer Biotherapy Center of FUDA Hospital developed T cell therapy in 2010. This therapy is specific for the treatment of advanced and metastatic tumors. Using lymphocytes that are donated by the patient's relatives, highly potent and efficient "memory" T cells are produced in the laboratory. These cells are specific for the tumor type, replacing the weak immune cells in the patient to help fight metastatic tumor cells. After two years of clinical observation, we found that the therapeutic effects of T cell therapy are strongest if it is administered in a variety of tumor immunotherapies. This therapy has been widely praised by experts both in China and abroad. The combined application of T cell and DC-CIK (Dendritic Cell and Killer T Cell) therapies shows a synergistic effect against metastatic tumor cells. This therapy has been successfully performed in over 200 cases in our hospital

Advantages of the combined therapies:

1. Very few side effects
2. Broad spectrum of anti-tumor effects
3. It provides an effective measure for the prevention of cancer relapse.

***

Laura

Wow! FUDA is possibly the most advanced and effective cancer treatment center on the planet! The three C system is wonderful.

I was astonished to learn that no one gets sick here when getting chemotherapy drugs. As explained above, during CMI those drugs are applied directly to the cancer tumor and not systemically, i.e., throughout the whole body, as is done in the West. After this treatment, the patient is given vitamins intravenously to prevent chemotherapy reactions such as losing hair and suffering from nausea.

Ester went on to explain that a lot of patients using traditional systemic chemotherapy die because the body's best disease fighter, the immune system, gets damaged from the administration of chemotherapy chemicals, which are essentially poisons. By administering a small dose only to the tumor, the body and immune system remain unharmed and able to support life.

The second technique which supports cryoablation is CIC, **C**ombined **I**mmunotherapy for **C**ancer. As explained above, tumor-killing lymphocytes in the patient's blood

363

are replicated outside the body and then returned by IV to the patient, giving her a massive immune system boost.

Dr. Xu then took time to meet with Louie and I. He spoke at length about how they had embraced cryoablation at FUDA and he gave us an amazing PowerPoint presentation that showed how cryoablation applied only at a primary tumor site resulted in the later destruction of secondary metastasized tumors in other areas of the body.

This is exactly the process I'm sure occurred in me after my cryoablation, because they found I had a small tumor in my sentinel node, indicating that at the time of my cryoablation procedure the cancer was already spreading throughout my body. But my immune system went to work (I still recall my white unicorn dream, the dream that told me that all the cancer in my body had been killed by the white unicorn . . . my white blood cells!)

Then, as if it was scripted to happen at that moment, a beautiful woman from Manila entered Dr. Xu's office to say goodbye. She was kind enough to stay and tell us her story, one that put everything I'd just learned together with a human face. Her name was Theresa and she had just finished a shopping trip with her sister before going home early to Manila after hearing she had no more cancer left to treat!

I thought that had to be the best shopping trip of her life!

We returned to our hotel after visiting the new hospital and Dr. Xu. Later that evening, FUDA's Filipino coordinator, Segundo, took us to a wonderful dinner at the beautiful Imperial Hotel. At dinner, Segundo related more of Theresa's story.

She had entered her treatment convinced she was going to die and was obviously feeling very depressed, but the staff at FUDA had given her hope and the willingness to fight for her life. Segundo told us of the remarkable transformation she had undergone at FUDA. I kept recalling her happy face after her shopping trip and how she was going home to a loving husband so grateful to have his beautiful wife back healthy and happy as well as her wonderful children who now had their mama ready to guide them fully to adulthood.

Segundo gave us a driving tour of the city after dinner. Guangzhou is magnificent! The shapes of the buildings are original, at least to my eyes. The tops of them are illuminated at night, each with its own personality. There is a space-age looking tower dominating the skyline off by itself. At night, it is lit up with a changing pattern of moving colored lights, most dazzling and beautiful.

We didn't see many westerners at dinner or out on the town, but the Chinese don't seem to pay much attention to any differences we represent. It's easy to feel at home here. In fact, there are Christmas decorations everywhere!

At dinner, the restaurant had Christmas music playing. Segundo told us that there are two Catholic churches in town that are mostly attended by Filipinos.

It's odd to have Christmas as a cultural phenomenon when disassociated from the good-will-towards-men sentiment I'm used to it representing in America. The Christmas spirit is in my heart, however. Whatever the energies or motives that brought Louie and I to China at this time, I have to believe that spirit of brother and sisterhood is part of it.

12.15.12, Saturday

(At least it's Saturday here in China)

It's only 5:30 a.m. here in China but, boy, am I awake!

Our peaceful neighborhood is waking up. Somewhere down the street, a Chinese flute is playing a wistful song.

At the risk of disturbing my roommate Louie, who seems able to sleep, I want to record some of what I've been processing. I've pulled a comfortable chair over by the window where I'm taking this opportunity to write and gather my thoughts.

The magical sounds of Guangzhou coming to life in the morning drift up through the open window as I write. My big, bedside windows offer a sky view and in the distance there are cozy-looking apartments full of decks with bikes and hanging clothes.

The sounds are so familiar in one way and so different in others. Roosters crow and there are traffic noises. Bicycle bells ring, but when someone speaks or shouts, it is all in Chinese! The scents of cooking food waft in through the window and carry a mix of spices and meats I recognize and others that I can't identify but intrigue me.

As the city wakes up, I realize there is a school nearby that bustles with loudspeakers and playful squeals of children.

Yesterday afternoon's visits with Dr. Xu and Ester brought an opportunity to learn more about what they're doing here at FUDA. FUDA is terrific with patient education and has many well-written printed materials describing their program. When we met with Fe yesterday, I found that Fe had already carefully read all the literature so she understands the therapies and why they work as she receives them.

I feel a huge part of the success at FUDA is the heart relationships that the hospital fosters. And it is a heart relationship that brought Louie and I here. It was Fe's family, calling me on her behalf, so full of fear and wanting hope from the story of my cryoablation treatment success. Fe has already taught me a lot about how family relationships work in this part of the world.

She, herself, was born in the Philippines as the baby in a family of nine children. She became a chemical engineer through the hard work of her siblings who had all worked to give each other money towards each other's education. When a good living wage became hard to come by in the Philippines, she took work as a domestic in wealthy Hong Kong, all so she could pay it forward to a younger relative's education.

I learned that when illness strikes, they also band together by sending relatives to wherever it takes to get the best treatment.

Fe is something of an ambassador. While she was getting her imaging and beginning her chemo implant treatment, she spent her first weeks at FUDA going around to visit the other patients to get their stories and encourage their progress.

She found people from her home country as well as Manila, Indonesia, Russia and the Middle East. She got stories about their cancer and found out that many were not rich people financially; rather, they were rich in heart relations with each other, which is what ultimately brought them here. They are cherished; they are valued;

and, through their loved one's assets, including companionship, they work something like the immune system itself, pulling together everything to fight through the illness of cancer back to health again.

Fe has watched miracles taking place daily while here at FUDA. Those returning home in good health have kept coming by her room to share a moment of victory over the cancer foe and to wish her well in her fight.

How utterly beautiful this was to see! This hospital that attracts cancer's worst victims is not a place of sadness and darkness. No! It's a place of hope and love and light! It's a place of NOW, minute by minute. The doctors at FUDA believe that each day the blood is different.

Each day offers a new opportunity for health. That is certainly something I will take with me back to the states.

Miracle Factory

After a short walk from our hotel to Fe's room this morning, we learned from Fe that Dr. Xu had generously arranged a guest room for Louie and I in FUDA's new hospital, which is only 20 minutes away from FUDA 1, FUDA's old hospital where Fe is staying.

Apparently, Fe had passed on the word that our fundraiser had only paid for one of our plane flights and none of our hotel expenses. This would save us a great deal of personal funds, so we eagerly accepted. Segundo and the driver, Mr. Chen, came back to the hotel to help us move.

When we checked out, the hotel desk clerk gave me my now-favorite souvenir from China: a bag to carry the new informational FUDA books and brochures. The bag was a promotional bag from a Chinese industrial stove company with a Chinese salesman in traditional Chinese garb depicted on the front of it giving a thumbs-up while gesturing towards a heavy-duty industrial stove. Even though its signage was in Chinese, the photo of the salesman certainly echoed the spirit of salesmen in the West and the uplifting image has made it my favorite shopping experience accessory. It's made of heavy materials to be used over and over for shopping, just like we are now doing in the West.

We soon arrived at New FUDA. Our room in the new hospital was a vacant wardroom on the floor that housed traditional Chinese medicine treatment rooms. Soon we could smell the sweet aromas coming from the treatments going on in those rooms.

We returned to Old FUDA after moving our luggage into New FUDA.

We visited with Fe and Jelly the rest of the morning. Jelly is Fe's older sister. She is retired now from a long career in the Philippines where she taught at a private school. She has never married but considers that to be something the right man is missing out on. I would agree, as I couldn't imagine a friendlier, more supportive companion. Fe is very lucky to have her as a roommate. They seemed to have their roles worked out as Jelly jumps up quickly whenever an opportunity to be helpful presents itself. We enjoyed listening to them tell us about their childhoods in the Philippines and their expanding knowledge of the treatments Fe is undergoing.

We were invited back to New FUDA's private dining room for lunch with Dr. Xu and Dr. Niu Lizhi, one of FUDA's main cryoablation surgeons who was also a renowned surgeon and the hospital Vice President.

Joining us were two journalists, Wilson and Sol, who were visiting from the Philippines.

They had come to learn more about FUDA and the work that goes on there. The hospital treats a large number of difficult cases from the Philippines and many grateful patients have been posting YouTube videos singing FUDA's praises. Seems the great news is spreading by word of mouth. Wilson told me a friend of his, a very respected reporter, told him to check out FUDA. Apparently, Wilson's column runs in the Philippine's most popular English language newspaper, *The Red Star.*

His column is evidently a "must-read" and covers everything from movie star activity to interesting cultural phenomenon.

Sol is the publisher of another periodical, the Philippines main business journal. He wanted to take a look at FUDA for a lifestyles column as well as investigate for some friends and relatives fighting late stage cancer.

Louie and I appreciated them switching to English when speaking to us. They seemed comfortable with China and the culture and encouraged us to try all the amazing Chinese dishes being served to us. I was impressed that Segundo, our interpreter, and Mr. Chen, our driver, were included in the lunch and everyone was treated the same.

I sat next to Dr. Xu, and he did his best to speak to me in English. His demeanor is that of a friendly, highly intelligent and respected professor, which he is. He interacts comfortably with all levels of patients, staff and guests. Watching him brought to mind the many depictions of Chinese Emperors and Head Men I'd seen in my Eastern Art History classes and textbooks.

At this private luncheon, I learned that FUDA has done more than 7,000 cryoablations. This is more than any other hospital in the world. I told Dr. Niu how I had first heard about FUDA using cryoablation for treating breast cancer. Several years ago, my husband's Internet research led to before and after pictures of a FUDA patient treated with cryoablation. This had really made an impression on Alex, because the before pictures were of a seventy-five-year-old woman whose breast cancer had burst through the skin and become gangrenous. The after cryoablation photos showed a normal-looking breast! I mentioned these pictures to Dr. Niu, and he knew exactly what I was talking about. That was his patient and he had treated her! (I bowed to him!).

He told me most cases are not such late stage and the seventy-five-year-old woman was very unusual. I asked when he thought FUDA first began using cryoablation on breast cancer. He said it was around 2003—the same year doctor Littrup treated me. He confirmed that I am truly one of the world's first and longest-surviving cryoablation breast cancer patients at almost my ten-year mark at the time of our trip.

After lunch, the journalists, Louie and I went back to Old FUDA so they could meet Fe and hear her story. I think they were just as impressed with her as I am.

She told them about her experience so far at FUDA, about her being at Stage 4 and having such a good turn around. Besides her own incredible story, she told them about all the others she's been witnessing here who were even worse.

Another patient the journalists had wanted to visit was not in her room! She had felt so healthy she had gone shopping! FUDA can really be called "The Miracle Factory."

12.16.12

Sunday Play Day!

Dr. Xu generously arranged for Louie and I to see some sights of the city today, accompanied by Segundo and driver Mr. Chen as our tour guides. At yesterday's lunch, Dr. Xu asked what I might be interested in. I told him I liked parks, nature and art so that's where we started, after first dropping Wilson and Sol off at the airport.

These two journalists were returning to the Philippines by way of Hong Kong. I told them my British Colonial in-laws were raised in Hong Kong and I always wanted to visit there after hearing their incredible stories.

However, they discouraged me from trying to travel there on this trip, as it required a time-consuming customs inspection when coming from China, even though it was part of China! We exchanged contact information, and Louie and I wished them well on their stories.

After saying goodbye to our new journalist friends, we began the tour of Guangzhou. The large city park of Guangzhou contains huge statues of the Five Goats. This is a very famous monument in Guangzhou as Guangzhou means "goats;" so, at one time it must have been famous for its goats.

In addition to the goat statue, a five-story fort and some original city walls stand at the hilltop. The fort contained a very interesting museum with art and artifacts dating from very old to the time of Mao Zedong. A gorgeous city view waited at the top balcony.

The park itself was just what I wanted to experience, because parks tell a lot about a city. This one was beautifully designed and laid out and was jammed with both locals and tourists—many from the Middle East. Some of the flora was off limits and posted as such, but much of it was designed to invite visitors in to wander among the plants.

There were a lot of older people doing Chi Gong (Qigong) exercises, something I'd only seen in television programs on China; but here it was, in the real!

Segundo is a 25-year-old Filipino whose job at FUDA is to coordinate patients coming from the Philippines. He has a huge friendly grin. He's the type of personality every guy would like for his best friend and every girl would want for a boyfriend. He and driver Mr. Chen accompanied us first to the park and, as we walked with them looking at the historical artifacts, I realized how very prideful Mr. Chen was of his culture. Indeed, everyone in the park who appeared to be native Chinese seemed happy and content.

After a couple of hours, our guides recommended a Thai restaurant in the main shopping district. After a delicious lunch, where I worked on my chopstick skills, we were off to Guangzhou's main shopping mall to shop for Christmas gifts!

Guangzhou's mall in the heart of the city is actually built over the ancient road bisecting the city. The old road sits a few yards below the new mall walkway and is exposed so people can see it. The old road is protected by railings surrounding it on either side. All along the middle of the mall's wide walkways there were crowds looking down on it. Perhaps these were shoppers pausing to take a rest, but the Chinese in general seemed to be fascinated by their own immense past, as if they couldn't believe they came from such a long, diverse, yet still intact, culture. It was if they were contemplating the scenes the old road must have witnessed.

The opposite sides of the old road couldn't have been more different! I felt like I was in New York or Los Angeles with all the top brands housed in shops featuring western advertising as fresh as the ones I'd just seen at LAX! There was an exception and I was about to appreciate it.

Segundo walked to a more custom-looking façade and said, "Here it is!" We entered what looked to be a single storefront of a trendy, local shop catering to young women. It turned out to be a long alley leading far beyond to the back of the shop. There were small, closet-sized shops on either side of a narrow alley walkway where vendors offered every kind of trendy young woman outfit and accessory imaginable.

For an American, the prices were lower than reasonable. Things designed in the West but made here were being sold at a fraction of the price! We quickly became overwhelmed. More of these venues with pocket-sized, individually run offerings followed. Vendors ensconced within offered their best English to entice us inside.

For my daughter, I chose a darling, ultra soft and fluffy white sweater covered in bright red "kiss marks."

For our two sons, I found beautifully crafted belts with stylish chrome buckles. For my husband, just what he wanted: a watch with three extra dials that show other time zones. Only later did Louie and I realize the extra dials were non-functional. Oh well! From a distance it looks great!

The press of the crowd began to tire us out. We were ready for our next major treat.

Segundo had figured out the best place in Guangzhou to get a really great, authentic Chinese massage. Down what appeared to Louie and I to look like a back alley we found our destination: "Late Night Massage." (I hadn't noticed this stop on the printed up itinerary!) Up a steep grand stairway, through a somewhat seedy bar-restaurant entrance, we entered a bamboo-decorated back room dominated by four huge lounge chairs and a flat screen TV. We were invited to sit in one of the big, squishy chairs while Segundo and Chen negotiated the financial terms of what we were about to experience.

The negotiations took at least 20 minutes with the women hostesses sounding aggressive and cajoling while our guides appeared bored and unimpressed. I imagined they were trying to get the prices down so all four of us could be treated. I had heard Dr. Xu asking Segundo if he had a way to cover the costs of our outing and Segundo replied that he did. However, I'm not sure this stop was what Dr. Xu had in mind and, for all I knew, Segundo was using his own money. (I heard later that this place had become popular with the younger male set and we certainly ended up appreciating it.)

After negotiations were settled, four young women soon entered from a back room. They were the masseus-es. They were attired in athletic polo shirts and stretch pants. They pulled back the tops of our chair footrests to reveal rectangular tubs which were first lined with thin plastic liners, then filled them with very hot water and large herb filled "tea" bags. First, our feet were soaked while our masseuses began massaging our knees and thighs and then our now softened and clean feet. So began our "three-hour massage"!

My practitioner, "#58," had the strongest fingers imaginable! They worked my acupuncture meridians and boy could she find the spots! Her technique was so accomplished I had to keep opening my eyes to see how she was doing it. That's how I discovered she was often texting on her phone as she worked my meridian lines!

I quickly melted into a pile of bones and flesh that she could push and pull however she wanted. Discovering I was flexible, she began sitting on me and pulling various appendages to their full range of motion. Before I knew it, she was totally sitting on me and working me with elbows or even feet. I looked over to Louie next to me and saw his masseuse totally walking up and down his spine! It's a good thing they gave us strong herbal tea when finished. We were so wiped out we could hardly make it back to the van. The cost for this three-hour extravaganza . . . $17 each for the full three hours!

It was a good thing we did make it to the van! A very delicious Chinese dinner awaited us at a restaurant down the street—a restaurant filled with families on a Sunday evening meal out. Our soon-to-be entrées greeted us from a wall lined with fish tanks as we entered. The Chinese seem to believe they would be cheating you were they not to include the animal's head with the meat dish you order (if it's small enough to fit on the plate). So fish and bird head, tails and feet, were included on the arriving dishes.

They also believe in mixing meats at the same meal. At this one we were treated to fish, a small duck or bird and beef—all coming with various vegetables. But first, there was a salty and delicious clear-ish soup with a big hunk of pig in it. A most scrumptious and interesting tasting herb tea accompanied our meal. The first mix of herbs and water is used to wash the small teapot with the first tea thrown out into a porcelain dish through a cover with holes in it. The tea is served in tiny cups and Mr. Chen made sure ours were always full with a fresh hot supply. It truly made the food go down easier.

The Chinese don't usually include sweets or stimulants with their meals. But a cool Chinese beer perfectly hit the spot!

During the conversation at dinner, we found out our masseuses had been discussing who we were and where we came from, because we asked Segundo what all the talking was about as they were working. There was a period Chinese movie on a flat screen going on during the massage, but they soon turned it to the American movie *Mrs. Doubtfire* starring Robin Williams and dubbed in Chinese when they heard we were from the states. The masseuses had also asked if Louie and I were a couple! Although Louie has a beard, I was over 34 when I had him! He looks just like me, to my American eyes. Couldn't they see he was obviously my son?

Cultural note if you are planning travel to China:

Most toilets in China are in the ground and need to be squatted over. The user needs to provide their own toilet paper. Most people carry small Kleenex packs with them. Ditto with napkins. A nice restaurant might provide you with a small Kleenex, but it's often required you supply your own. It's also a good idea to have hand sanitizer with you as soap is often missing in a public restroom.

Both Louie and I practically crawled into bed when we made it back to our room at the New FUDA hospital. We couldn't decide if we felt more like we'd had a strenuous workout or were just totally wiped out. Either way, it led to my first really solid night's sleep since arriving here!

12.17.13, Monday

The morning after our outing into Guangzhou with Segundo and Mr. Chen, we were promised another visit with Dr. Xu. But it turned out he was busy with a visitor, so we were offered a tour of the new FUDA Cancer Hospital where we were staying. Our tour guide was Tracy, a Chinese/English interpreter and member of the planning department, a group of very smart and socially adept young people whose office is right next to the president's and vice president's offices.

These bright, energetic assistants coordinate treatments between newly arriving patients, interpret and act as guides—basically what we in the West might consider to be PAs, or personal assistants to, well . . . everybody! It turns out this was Tracy's first such opportunity to interpret with a Westerner, and she was a little nervous, but Louie and I never would have known it. When we asked her Chinese name we were told it sounds like "Tracy" in English so that's what we called her. She had graduated from her university only a year earlier.

This was her first post-studies job. Over the next few days, Tracy was the one to help coordinate our activities and transportation. We grew very fond of her gentle, quiet intelligence, grace and charm.

Accompanying Tracy on our tour was Peng Ximei, an ex-patient who lives at the hospital. She acts as a wellness ambassador, encouraging patients by sharing her incredible story of being healed through Dr. Xu's efforts. Her story is featured in Dr. Xu's book, *Nothing but the*

Truth, which is given to all new patients upon their arrival at FUDA.

Peng Ximei's story is just one of dozens of patient stories in this book. Her story is very dramatic. She was homeless and living in the streets when she was taken in by Dr. Xu and cured from ovarian cancer. Her huge, fluid-filled abdomen first had to be drained. Then a 14-cm tumor was successfully removed by Dr. Xu's surgical team with her costs paid for by the donations of hospital personnel and fellow patients.

No one being treated at FUDA could have had it worse than Ximei, and her encouragement must surely be a tremendous uplifting experience for any new patient. More stories and healing philosophies in Dr. Xu's book set a tone that FUDA is a place where cancer can be successfully treated.

On our tour, we learned that our room at New FUDA is a typical patient room with two hospital beds, a large window letting in plenty of natural daylight and a marble-lined, modern bathroom (with a western-style sit-down toilet!).

Our room is in a wing that houses traditional Chinese medicine and our tour began by allowing us to view treatments of acupuncture and massage going on. The patients we witnessed having treatments were both nurses. Staff, family members and FUDA patients are all encouraged to use traditional Chinese medicine treatments to supplement their allopathic cures. One nurse had strained her shoulder (massage) and another had sprained her ankle (acupuncture).

As we walked down a light-filled stairway, I mentioned how beautiful and light the hospital seemed to be. The surfaces were light and reflective, the light mostly brought in by large windows at either end of the hallways and light-filled open stairways at the intersections of corridors. Besides the clean, shiny décor, there was personality aplenty.

Each ward had a large bulletin board that holds photos of healed and successfully treated patients, along with their thank-you notes. Across from each nurse's station, photos of the nursing staff were aesthetically arranged along with names and training information.

What impressed me the most were the patient information bulletin boards I noticed around the hospital. These held informational posters of how treatments used at FUDA worked to cure cancer. An English speaking nurse explained that these were changed weekly, after the patient/nurse group meeting, where a new subject is brought up to be discussed and then related to patients getting that treatment. These topics are often what the specialty of the ward might be, such as the effective treatment of liver cancer. They are led by the doctors, and all the patients and family members on the ward are invited to attend.

I was beginning to get the idea that a philosophy at FUDA is to recognize that the more a patient understands about what is going on with their healing, the better they heal. The patients at FUDA were certainly being encouraged to find out as much as they could about their treatment in order to empower them. However, it's not just medical information adorning the halls. My favorite parts of the FUDA interior landscape were the posters with sayings on them, found everywhere, that gave philosophical inspiration to the patients. My favorite was the "Philosophy of Life" poster outside Fe's room.

It read:

> "Although the world is full of suffering, it
> is also the overcoming of it."

> "Rejoicing in hope/patient in tribulation."

> "Everything can be taken from a man but
> one thing... the freedom to choose his atti-
> tude in any given set of circumstances."

> "A strong man struggles with fate."

> "A light heart lives long."

I believe, like much of China, these philosophies stem from Confucius.

There were three types of patient rooms available: a suite with a separate bedroom and bathroom for family members; a two-bedroom, designed for the patient and able to house a family member; and a four-bed ward. Each had a different price tag running from the suites for around $420 a day to the four-bed ward for around $40 a day. I was told patients had complained about the high-end price, so a committee had formed and met, and it was decided to give a price decrease the following year(!!!). At the end of the ward was a gym for anyone—patient, family member or staff—who wanted to use it. In the middle of the ward was a room containing a washer and dryer, computer and desk, chairs and a television. I was told of a larger laundry unit as well as a family kitchen for those who wanted to cook for themselves, one floor up.

Finally, we got to the end of the ward where I got my biggest surprise as to how this hospital was different. First, there was a lounge, where comfortable seating was laid out in front of a desk where an interpreter was stationed. This was a wing dedicated to Islamic patients, and I was told from 8 a.m. to midnight an interpreter was available to whoever needed their services. Across from this station was a double office offering the services of a nutrition doctor whose job was to educate patients and family members about food's important role in healing and health and to conduct educational meetings about nutrition for all on the ward.

Next to his office was a Doctor of Psychology whose job was to listen to and help any patient, family member or staff person who may have an issue. When I asked for an example, she told me about a patient who developed paranoia when hearing a knock on the door. The patient was evidently nervous about what the treatment might be that followed!

The psychologist was able to teach the patient how to train his expectation pathways to anticipate a positive experience so that he didn't dread the knock on the door.

The psychologist also told me that recently a nurse had come by to work through on-the-job fatigue caused by a recent break-up with her boyfriend. The psychologist said a lot of her job is to be a good listener, but she also has tools to help work through emotions.

In another instance, a family member was taught how to effectively give support to their relative going through treatment. Wow! I can't ever recall such easily available services when going through treatment; although, I did have a patient advocate nurse I often worked with.

My final observation came from my nose. Nothing at FUDA smelled hospital-like. When I saw a cleaning person, I asked what was being used. As best as they could describe it, I was told that it was all natural ingredients and wouldn't harm a patient but was an effective cleaner.

The final part of the trip showed us how waste was taken care of at the hospital. We started at the garbage area and I had my first of what would turn out to be three déjà vu experiences. Surrounding the garbage can area was the most beautiful rock wall full of ferns I had ever seen! (What I was sure I had already experienced somewhere in a recent dream back home, before I even knew I was coming to China!) When I remarked about the small number of garbage cans for such a big hospital I was told about a vigorous recycling program. (I then remembered seeing a big recycling facility across from FUDA 1 that took up an entire city block!)

After lunch with Tracy in the hospital cafeteria, we were shown how to arrange a ride back to Old FUDA and Fe. This turned out to be easy, as minivans and cars with drivers were constantly moving patients, family members and staff back and forth between the two hospitals.

The Transportation Department was housed in the Lobby of our new home, New FUDA. We quickly connected with a ride and found Fe resting and groggy in her room.

It actually had worked out well. We had taken the day before (Sunday) off to see the city as poor Fe had been hit with some very high fevers and was only now recovering. It was unclear what had caused the fevers, perhaps a reaction to the medication or an overstimulation of her immune system, which was by now working overtime. I strongly suspected the latter as it echoed my experience with cryoablation and is, I was later told, an indication the "immune effect" is working.

One of the brilliant treatments the Chinese have added to assist the immune system is called CIC, as explained earlier.

Fe had undergone several blood draws before her operation for this purpose. A high fever is often the body's way of affecting a cure and perhaps this is what was going on as the immune system started to kick into high gear. Or perhaps it simply was a reaction to one of Fe's medications.

Whatever the cause, the nurses were all over, making Fe comfortable and bringing down the fever. She had been washed and changed during the night and the IV bags were being particularly watched. Fe couldn't say enough about the kindness and attention given her by the staff.

Fe's tired eyes looking at us so soulfully made Louie and I both want to keep this visit short so she could rest. After catching up on Fe's newest developments, we used her phone to arrange a ride back to New FUDA. We wished her well and left her to rest.

Louie and I were now on our own to find dinner in Guangzhou. The foot traffic was surprisingly busy around the hospital. Perhaps it was because it was the evening meal hour and family and friends were meeting up to dine together. Perhaps it was just because there are a lot of Chinese! We joined the crowds on the sidewalks and walked until we found something that looked inviting where we might be able to handle getting a meal on our own. A well-lit place with a picture of a bowl of noodles on the window that was full of customers hunched over their bowls seemed inviting. We walked in and found a table and were handed a pad printed in Chinese to mark off our choices. A young man sitting at the table next to us seemed to be enjoying the noodles dangling out of his mouth, so I showed my ordering pad.

He gave me a thumbs-up and pointed to #86, so #86 it was. The waitress came by and asked us some additional details to which we had to throw our hands up in a gesture of incomprehension. She walked away muttering but brought us some warm scented water soon after. (During our entire trip we were always served warm water before a meal.) So far so good. Our bowls came and whatever we had ordered was delicious.

A chicken-based broth with noodles seems to be a staple in China. This may come with a variety of different meats (in Guangzhou it's often seafood) and vegetables. This one did the trick and neither of us could finish. Louie paid in our paper Yuan's and calculated that we spent about $1.50 each!!

When we got back to our room, an email from Dr. Littrup was waiting. He told me that it didn't appear that he'd be arriving in time for dinner the next day, so I shouldn't look for him before the conference Wednesday. Not knowing what the conference would entail, I was a bit disappointed thinking I wouldn't be getting to spend some alone time with him to find out why the program at Karmanos had stopped or if there was a plan to get anything like what they were doing in China going at Karmanos—or anywhere in the US for that matter.

I went to sleep convinced that Fe was getting the best treatment possible for a woman in her condition but still unclear if this was a realistic option for a woman from the West with a new diagnosis who might be facing a mastectomy like I had been back in 2003.

The thought crossed my mind that if Dr. Littrup hadn't treated me successfully, would the Chinese still be doing what they're doing? Had his pioneering efforts to use cryoablation for breast cancer come first, and then were copied by the Chinese or had new, parallel treatments been worked out in both the East and the West around the same time as so often happens in science and medicine?

12.18.12, Tuesday

Louie and I learned that if we got up after the 7 to 8 a.m. serving time of the cafeteria's Chinese breakfast, we could still buy a delicious Islamic breakfast from the Islamic volunteers who man a Middle Eastern meal option in the cafeteria. For some reason, they kept their breakfast hours running longer, which was good for us, because while I seemed to be able to wake up early, Louie was struggling and it often took him longer to get out of bed, no matter how many hot teas I put together for him from our room's handy hot water dispenser and the saved tea bags I managed to gather.

So it was Islamic boiled eggs, flat bread, hummus and tea that we were dining on when Tracy found us to tell us that today we could have some time to talk with FUDA's director, Dr. Xu.

As we walked down the hall of the ward housing us, we could look into rooms where acupuncture and other Chinese treatments were going on. Tracy introduced us to the traditional medicine doctor who ran the ward. He asked us if we'd like to try some treatments. We assured him we were interested but didn't have anything particularly wrong with us. Tracy checked her phone. Dr. Xu wasn't quite ready for us, so now was as good a time as ever to try it out!

Dr. Yong Chen is the most confident and knowledgeable proponent of traditional Chinese medicine imaginable. He told me he believes he could cure himself of cancer if he were ever to get it, but assured me he probably never will because of his health practices. He told Louie he would be able to take his extra weight off through acupuncture alone. He gave me a brief description of the five elements feeding off each other (wood fuels fire, fire fuels metal and so on).

Apparently, our bodies contain energetic pathways where the free flow of energy can get stuck or blocked. Freeing the blocks and stimulating the free-flow of energy is the essence of acupuncture. For at least half an hour during the beginning of treatment, a warm, sweet smelling herb called moxibustion was burned over a meridian point on my low back, followed by burning over my stomach.

The effect of that treatment was felt for days. While not being able to quite pinpoint its affect, I know I lost a craving for sweets or salty foods and just had a general feeling of, well, "wellness."

Dr. Xu greeted us warmly in his well-appointed large office. He had a large flat screen television on the wall, which was hooked up to his computer to show guests many of the hospital's wonderful success stories. He took great pleasure in showing videos of some of the impressive treatments that have taken place at FUDA under his care.

He began with Ming Zai, a boy with a huge facial tumor, and Weifeng, a young girl with another big facial tumor completely covering her right eye. The before and after photos were incredible. Both children were returned to near normal conditions. But the most impressive was

Ximei, the young woman I had met on the tour earlier with Tracy. The photo showed her as she was before treatment, a homeless woman with a huge extended stomach.

Dr. Xu had seen her one day, scavenging from the hospital garbage. He had invited her in to be examined. She had an advanced case of ovarian cancer and had been kicked out by her boyfriend when fellow villagers began rumors that she was pregnant. Her condition made it impossible for her to work and support herself, so she was literally living on the streets by the hospital.

With the support and permission of her family from the village, the doctors at FUDA were able to successfully treat her, first draining the equivalent of "100 bottles of beer" of fluid volume from her stomach. Dr. Xu led both her treatment and the hospital campaign to cover her cost, which was contributed to by staff and patients alike.

Since she had no desire to go back to her village, she now lives at the hospital and acts as an ambassador of healing, encouraging patients everyday that they can find a successful healing at FUDA as well.

Obviously, making money was not motivating these treatments. I learned that it is often news reporters that go out to the villages to write about really difficult cases and challenge the healers and hospitals of China to come up with a successful treatment. FUDA is on record for removing the largest facial tumor ever recorded.

Chuncai, nicknamed "Big Skull," was successfully treated for a 30-kg tumor that hung from his face so low he had to use his arm to support it. Watching Dr. Xu's videos I also saw that he was so loved by his family and village that they sent a brother and nephew to stay with him at the hospital to keep his spirits up during treatment. The whole village celebrated his return and he was able to use donated funds to open a small dry goods shop to support himself.

These stories were heartwarming and I learned a lot about the Chinese culture by hearing them. The villagers obviously are closely connected to each other and those in the urban centers. Even now, months later, I often hear from one of the young FUDA personnel I keep in touch with that they are spending a weekend or a week-long break going to a village to see parents or relatives.

There seems to be much pride in the heroic missions to save those in dire need, which FUDA hospital takes on. It gives confidence to the personnel and allows them to hone their skills. Indeed, an entire hospital that specializes in late stage, or fourth stage cancer, seems to be unusual for anywhere in the world. It has certainly given FUDA understanding regarding treatments that are most effective.

But my mission was to help women who were having an early detected, primary diagnosis where mastectomy was the only viable treatment option offered by Western medicine. My mission was to find out if a viable option was available at FUDA, which could allow these women to keep their breasts and get an immune effect, just like Dr. Littrup and Karmanos had done for me ten years ago.

Now that my option was no longer being offered by Karmanos, would FUDA be a place I could recommend to women contacting me through my website?

I was very grateful when the enthusiastic Dr. Xu sat down with Tracy, Louie and I to find out what my specific questions were.

Tracy really concentrated on interpreting my questions correctly. Her eyes would give a small squint when she didn't seem to understand, indicating to me that I should speak more slowly or rephrase my question. Dr. Xu wore a white dress shirt with a light blue tie covered by a soft yellow sweater. He sat in a comfortable chair next to me and, after listening to Tracy translate my questions, took off his glasses to wipe them clean.

At last, he spoke in a low but clear tone. I was worried he might be saying FUDA was not the best option, but Tracy said, "If a woman is having a diagnosis of a primary tumor and her doctor is recommending a mastectomy, if she chooses to come to FUDA to have her breast frozen instead, it should not cost her more than $10,000."

I was amazed!! He understood what I was implying, that a woman choosing cryoablation for a primary tumor treatment was already bucking the system and coming all the way to China might be too much. Would it be worth it? This answer was incredible! $10,000 was a small enough amount to put on some women's credit card or, better yet, small enough to launch an Internet funding campaign as I had done for this fact-finding trip.

This means that a woman could do as I had done, pay out of pocket for their cryoablation at FUDA to avoid a mastectomy and then return home for treatment as if they had a lumpectomy, with radiation and chemotherapy all paid for by their own insurance. One point, which I did not clarify with Dr. Xu, was the issue of receiving sentinel node diagnosis at FUDA; however, it would certainly be possible for a woman to do this in America before traveling to China if for some reason it was not available at FUDA.

Between this information, and the incredible healing I was witnessing watching Fe, my trip suddenly felt VERY worthwhile. While I was warned that every case had to be assessed on its own merits, this baseline of healing potential was very, very positive. My mind went back to the happy woman's face I'd seen posted on YouTube. A reporter from the Philippines who had researched FUDA had placed it there.

In the video, a woman with a primary diagnosis of Stage 1 breast cancer was being asked what she thought of her treatment at FUDA. With the biggest, most engaging smile imaginable, she said that she didn't want to offend her home country's medical practice, but that if a woman got the same diagnosis she had, then that woman should "Come to FUDA first! They will save your breast and you will have an immunity to your cancer!"

This video makes me cry every time I even think about it. I had always thought that if I ever met another woman who I never knew before and she told me she was going to be having (or already had) her breast cancer treated through a new method called cryoablation, I would finally feel that my efforts—as the first volunteer for Dr. Littrup to try out his cure and my subsequent advocacy work—were finally vindicated!

Even though this woman lives half way around the world and probably received cryoablation without the Chinese knowing about my particular success story, I knew in my heart she was the proof that I was looking for . . . that this method WAS starting to take off . . . big time!! And FUDA was the place championing it! FUDA was doing what I had always hoped Karmanos would do. It might not be happening in the West, but it WAS happening in the world!

Even if it takes a stream of women going east from the US to embrace cryoablation in China, it will ultimately bring attention to the possibilities the great Western pioneer, Dr. Peter Littrup, had developed. He had done all this: traveling to China in the late 90s and teaching cryoablation to a country desperate for a way to economically cure people with advanced cancer.

Even if the West is where the cryoablation machines are manufactured, it is these Eastern doctors who are using them to heal while Western doctors are ignoring them.

It is happening. People are being healed of cancer by cryoablation, just as I was. And now Dr. Xu was sitting here confirming what I had hoped was possible . . . that Western women could still get the cryoablation treatment and save their breast if they desired it! And what a beautiful possibility FUDA was turning out to be. Yes, it might be an extra effort to get all the way to China, but the facility and personnel and outcomes were all so wonderful! I was thrilled.

I knew I had been right in thinking I needed to check FUDA out for myself if I was going to have any credibility telling women they were going to be treated properly if they traveled to China.

I told an African-American woman about cryoablation before coming to China. She startled me by saying no African-American woman would be interested unless there was an African-American face telling her they had tried it and it was a good option. I used that experience to take to heart the idea that a Western woman would only want another Western woman telling her it had been checked out and was worthy and possible.

My intuition told me it would be worth going to China to be the eye witness/reporter who could pass on with true knowledge and conviction the fact that getting treatment at FUDA was both viable and smart. I was coming to the conclusion that my intuition was proving to be right!

I couldn't wait to get over to Fe's room to tell her what I had just found out.

Fe was feeling better and was happy to hear all about me hearing the exit interviews and success stories. It gave us a template to compare the treatments she was receiving.

One thing was becoming obvious: FUDA's success seems to be based on the skillful application and close coordination of many healing modalities, both Eastern and Western, whose effects are carefully monitored, evaluated and adjusted. Besides working with a "bigger bag of tricks" (to use slang to describe a wide swath of respected healing modalities), it seems to be the coordination between practitioners that felt new to me. The coordination happened easily here, because it's all part of the same hospital system. The system is set up to coordinate!

I recalled how hard it had been for me to get my doctors to talk to each other, especially when I had gone out of my home system for my initial treatment of cryoablation. So much of my energy had been spent coordinating and it was exhausting. I was able to fully appreciate all of the seamlessly choreographed comings and goings happening at Fe's bedside. They were providing Fe an orchestrated, focused healing dance.

Since we had been given a grand tour of New FUDA, Fe's sister and roommate helper, Jelly, offered to give us a tour of Old FUDA. We began at the top floor, an open, garden patio designed to give patients and their families a pleasant, quiet place to "hang out." Here there were cooking facilities provided, if family members wanted to cook for themselves. (Shelf space with pots and woks were provided for each patient). A simple exercise facility with a few exercise bikes was also available.

The main feature, however, was a garden patio, partially covered in latticework with vines growing on it. There was outdoor furniture, a wonderful city view, and even a water feature amid both potted and bedded plants and flowers. It was a bit old and weathered but pleasant and refreshing nonetheless.

Floors below housed specialty features such as a lab, operating and treatment rooms and the ICU. There is a feature unique to China, a mandate that every hospital, no matter what its specialty, must provide immediate care facilities for children.

Therefore, both the old and new FUDA hospitals had areas where parents and grandparents were gathered with their young ones doing various activities. Some children were breathing into corrugated plastic tubes with hot, steamy air coming out to ease congestion. Others were in a pharmacy specializing in pediatric medicine. Many treatment rooms had murals with smiling animal faces. Obviously, children are central to China's medical concerns.

When we returned to the peaceful quiet of Fe's room we decided to compare notes with all we'd learned about what's available at FUDA with what Fe herself had already done, using her weekly bill printouts that kept her abreast of expenses. Some of the prices were shockingly inexpensive compared to Western medical services.

Fe's treatment began with state of the art imaging, MRI and PET scans, which gave an accurate update of exactly where metastases had occurred.

Fe's treatment was then laid out. Blood was taken several times to culture her tumor-killing lymphocytes so the full effects of their immune-stimulating cryoablation could be realized by injecting the additional lymphocytes via CIC, or Combined Immunotherapy for Cancer. To reduce the largest tumors before freezing them, a catheter was placed directly into those tumors and cancer-killing drugs were injected into the tumors. This is the CMI, or Cancer Microvascular Intervention.

The tumors in her breast and liver were later frozen using multiple probes guided by ultrasound and CT. (This is called CSA, or Cryosurgical Ablation.) During the Cryosurgical Ablation operation, small iodine radioactive pellets were placed around her surgical sites (radiation therapy).

Her post-operation procedure included all types of medicine and vitamin IVs as well as traditional Chinese medicine procedures to alleviate symptoms. Just like I had experienced, pain was not a big concern as freezing is amazingly non-morbid.

While going over these treatment summations, both Fe and I became aware that there were small spots showing up in her bones and that these were tumors, which had not been frozen. My conclusion was that, just like Dr. Xu had shown me in the video success stories, these should be able to be removed by Fe's own immune system as all those newly cultured lymphocytes went into action. Fe made a note to specifically ask about it.

Louie and I reminded Fe and Jelly that the International Conference would be starting first thing in the morning, so we weren't exactly sure when we'd see her next, but I gave her my assurance that we would bring Dr. Littrup for a visit as soon as it was possible. While I didn't verbalize it, I knew I'd be more relaxed about Fe's treatment getting his expert approval. He would know what questions to ask and how to access the answers.

Our driver knocked on the door, so we fondly said our goodbyes and caught a ride back to New FUDA for a cafeteria dinner with Segundo. He was quite nervous about his job of coordinating the arrivals of the 15 cancer specialist-researcher-professor doctors flying in the next morning from all over the world for the start of the conference. We assured him he was more than capable if our experience with him was any indicator. We said our goodnights and headed for an early evening turn-in ourselves.

All these treatments and the general Chinese approach were given an amazing metaphorical summation by Louie when we got back to our room to process. He likened FUDA's form of attacking cancer to the fighting techniques of his favorite childhood cartoon anime, "Voltron."

In the cartoon there were five main fighters who each had an armor that made them into flying, fighting machines. As trouble commenced, the appropriate fighter to take on the job did the fighting. But when big trouble happened, as it always did, the five fighters joined together and created one big fighting machine to take it on. The point of the anime, it seemed to Louie and I, was that the combined efforts of specialists resulted in winning results. Quite similar to the combined specialized treatments going on at FUDA!

As I watched the sky grow dark from my third story window, my mind tried to process the amazing experience this trip to Guangzhou was bringing me. Tomorrow, I would finally be re-united with my doctor, the amazing Dr. Peter Littrup, who had saved my breast and healed me of cancer in 2003—the same doctor who was partially responsible for helping his technique take off in other parts of the world, especially here in China.

This would be a very different type of meeting, happening on the other side of the world. I wondered if he was in awe as much as I was at the odds our paths would cross in such a way.

12.19.12 Wednesday

The next morning was the beginning of the FUDA International Symposium on Cancer, so we were finally up early enough to experience eating with the hospital's kitchen crew, all decked out in their red and yellow uniforms.

There was some kind of doughy, lightly fried pastry with a sweetish paste inside a "bow" that seemed in come in several versions. But the most memorable, delicious new taste came from a dark bean mush that tasted slightly sweet. (I learned later it was made of mung beans.)

"Heaven!" It was very satiating and I crave it still. Whatever the "bows" were made of, they didn't make us feel sick but, instead, satisfied!

If only I'd known how delicious and satisfying the breakfast at the New FUDA cafeteria was! I would have been rallying Louie out of bed earlier!

Whoever said the best tea comes from China wasn't kidding. I would add that the best tea I have ever had was in China. If I had tea as good as this in the States, coffee would never be a morning temptation!

At breakfast, we sat amongst regular hospital staff. All I had to do was point to something on someone's tray and they would gladly use their chopsticks to pick it up and offer it to us. It soon became apparent that these workers were accustomed to sitting at the same tables Louie and I had chosen to use. We were in their space, but they didn't seem to be territorial. Rather, they were happy to pose when I indicated I wanted to take photos. They seemed curious and polite.

No one from the youthful "planning committee" came looking for us this morning. After breakfast, we found most of them in the hospital's 4th floor lecture hall. A festive and organized scene awaited us. Young women in dark blue blazers and skirts handed us Attendee Badges to wear around our necks and we were given a large bag full of books and brochures, including Dr. Xu's *Nothing but the Truth* and even the new medical textbook *Modern Cryosurgery for Cancer,* co-written by doctors Niklai N. Korpan (from Austria) and Kecheng Xu and Lizhi Niu (from China).

I recognized many of the hospital's nurses in the audience chairs, most wearing a smart, stylish wool coat appropriate for the winter season. Since they weren't in uniform, I assumed they were going to the conference on their day off from work. It was impressive that they had such passion for their work.

Louie and I found some seats about six rows back from a stage that was beautifully put together with a large printed backdrop of turquoise blue with bright red and yellow-Asian looking decorative marks framing the letters announcing the Symposium, "FUDA International

Symposium on Cancer (Cryo Immunology-Stem Cells) And 2nd FUDA Technology Consultative Committee Conference."

On either side of the stage, mounted above head level, were large flat screen television monitors. On the floor, in front of the stage, a large, technical-looking dark orb of molded plastic sat on a pedestal. The sides of the room were slightly curved from top to bottom and covered by grids of flat screen monitors showing various aspects of the hospital services.

Wow! Everything looked so futuristic, high-tech and inviting, yet imposing, at the same time.

As soon as we sat down Segundo came up to us rather breathless and said he'd been looking all over for us. He wanted to know if we'd like to say hello to "Dr. Peter," as Dr. Littrup is known in China. We went with him to a smaller, wood-paneled room behind the stage where all the presenting doctors/professors had gathered and were wearing flowered lapel corsages.

From behind, I immediately recognized Dr. Peter as he turned to greet me with a warm handshake that turned into a hug. Louie was introduced, and Dr. Peter then said, "Wow! Pretty interesting we're meeting again here, on the other side of the world!" We didn't have long for a conversation, but he assured me he'd find a time we could meet in private, later that evening.

We took our places in the audience and the conference began with warm greetings by Dr. Xu's right-hand assistant, Ester Law, who spoke beautiful English, being from the Philippines. She also gave opening remarks in Chinese. After opening remarks from a Communist Party Member, the first presenting professors were introduced.

Dr. Nikolai Korpan, a rosy, robust-looking professor with a big smile and merry eyes was the President of the International Institute for Cryosurgery from Hospital Rudolfinerhaus in Vienna Austria. He began with a presentation entitled "Cancer Cryoimmunology-Theory, Experimental and Clinical Experience since 1982." It was an interesting overview and I learned that Prof. Korpan had used cryoablation to treat over 700 Austrian women with breast cancer.

That made me sit up and pay attention! At least somewhere in the world besides China a very active breast cancer cryoablation program was functioning!

The next presenter was from the States, Dr. Michael Sabel. He is also a teaching professor from Michigan, like Dr. Littrup. Dr. Sable works at a different research university. I was aware of his work as he was conducting a study on women during the time I was looking for treatment.

He was freezing women's breasts to make sure the freezing worked to kill the cancer. However, Dr. Sabel was following his freezes up with a mastectomy. I looked into his program but was not interested in the follow-up treatment, although I always wondered if any of the women refused the later mastectomy.

Prof. Sabel's talk was on "Cryoablation and the Modulation of Tumor Microenviroment." He spoke so fast and used so many medical terms and references I realized most of it was over my head. He seemed to be explaining how to translate his clinical experiences into usable data. One thing I heard for the first time was that over-freezing can shut down the immune system instead of stimulating it.

This is called "Cryo Shock." Apparently this over-stimulation can release dangerous cells. He referenced pre-treating tumors before freezing with chemotherapy injected directly into the tumors, like they do at FUDA, to give the most systemic control and greatest benefit in treating primary tumors.

He also mentioned the importance of having multiple probes for a "fast flow freeze," which seems to work best.

Uh oh! It was beginning to dawn on me how medicine works. Despite the fact that Prof. Sabel gave statistics about cryoablation's use since the early 80s, these top professors were still trying to figure out exactly how to use it best! There may be many great success stories like mine along the way but getting the nuance of it was proving to look like a long and complicated process.

The next presentation was quite spellbinding. The tall, lean, bespectacled and most elegant Prof. Lizhi Niu, FUDA's Vice President and head of the surgical program, spoke on "Cryotherapy for Pancreatic Cancer."

This did not appear to me to be an easily impressed crowd, especially the fellow professors, but you could hear an audible breath suck when his statistics were presented. Many patients were quite long-lived after treatment, up to five years so far. Apparently, pancreatic cancer is very tricky to operate on because there are so many valves and openings in the pancreas. Excited, even aggressive, questioning followed Prof. Niu's presentation and the questions seemed to center around how the delicate infrastructure connections within the pancreas were protected during a freeze.

Prof. Niu definitely became a new hero to me by totally maintaining his quiet composure during this onslaught! He used his beautiful, long, delicate fingers to assist the explanation, which seemed to center around protective gels and certain skills he'd developed. He didn't voice the skill needed, but the way he answered, he made it obvious it could be done successfully—if you knew what you were doing!

Wow! Now I'm figuring out that skill is certainly a big factor, as it must be in all operations. How can this be trained? From a patient's point of view, how can this be assessed?

Two more presentations followed, but they were by Chinese professors speaking in Chinese. Even though translations followed, the information was related to stem cells and not cryoablation, so I didn't take any notes.

The cafeteria was understandably more crowded than usual at lunch. The professors were being hosted in FUDA's private dining room with Dr. Xu.

Louie and I picked out our chosen food items and found our favorite table. An attractive woman named "Linda" soon joined us. (Like Tracy, this is probably the name that sounds closest to what her name is in Chinese). Linda's card told me that she was "Domestic Medical Foreign Affairs Dept. Director." She had quite a few staff members with her. She explained that she had just come back from the Middle East and would be returning there after the conference.

It was beginning to make sense that the high number of patients from the Middle East would need a liaison and staff to facilitate their coming to FUDA. Obviously, the Chinese were putting a lot of effort into servicing patients in populations that are politically close to their country. Linda seemed both wise and compassionate and very professional. The outreach operation coordinating with the treatment operation, to work as a whole, was impressive to me.

Dr. Littrup surprised me after lunch when he asked if I would mind if he introduced me during his upcoming presentation. We both marveled that I was almost a ten-year survivor. His was the first presentation after lunch, and it was entitled, "Cryoablation of Metastases & Cost Effective Improved Survival: An Immunotherapy Effect."

The photo visual behind his statistical information was very interesting. It seemed to be a photograph of his feet in professional attire (suit-pants and dress shoes) dangling over a landscape many hundreds of feet below, as if jumping in business clothes from an airplane. I got the idea this may have been used before for a medical presentation where his work might be considered radical or risky.

The brief run-down of his involvement with cryoablation was anything but risky sounding, with impressive statistics on survival rates involving liver, lung and soft tissue cases, which is his specialty. He stated he has done over 1000 operations to date, certainly one of the world's highest records. He explained it was his experience that cryoablation appears less morbid with less pain and better absorption than heat or laser treatments.

He spoke of his years of experience working with Dr. Fred Lee, pioneering techniques of using cryoablation for prostate cancer where he found the best technique is to have one probe per centimeter of tumor size (so a 5-cm tumor would require five probes) in order to get a fast freeze for the best effect. His experience was that the absorption rate of the frozen tissue should be such that the area of frozen but as yet unabsorbed tissue should be smaller than the original tumor by six months after the procedure, noting that local recurrences were very low and location specific.

Then his talk moved to cost comparisons through traditional treatments that involve chemotherapy, noting that chemo can run as high as $50,000 to $100,000. By comparison, cryoablation, even with follow-up MRIs to track progress, was considerably less expensive and cost-effective.

He summed up his experience with the notation that the faster you can freeze, the faster it stimulates necrosis, the body's healing response, and boosts the immune system. He concluded that "freezing hard and fast = greatest survival."

He wanted to mention the importance of bringing about an outcome a patient desired as a way for explaining why he tried cryoablation for other types of cancers that didn't yet have a protocol (like breast cancer) where organ conservation (like the breast) was a factor. It was then that I was asked to stand as an example of a survivor of almost 10 years for breast cancer.

I was shocked at the loud, audible breath-suck as all the heads in the room quickly turned towards me as I rose from my seat. This seemed to be a great surprise, having one of Dr. Peter's own long-lived patients amongst this esteemed crowd—an immediate example of the success of an un-protocoled experiment.

I was quickly given a clapping ovation. I smiled widely and gave a little wave as I quickly sat down, noting and appreciating Dr. Xu's huge, contagious smile from across the room. I guess I had put a human face on what all these statistics meant. Such an appreciative clapping gesture validated these doctor's human concern as they met to move forward a new, promising technique at the highest professional level.

My heart was moved. I now had yet another reason I was glad to have come!

The conference continued with presentations on immunotherapy, integrative and personalized medicine as well as cell therapy, among other subjects that were related. Louie decided to go back and take a nap (this was an early morning for him!). But I stayed to listen, even though most of it was technically over my head. One thing being in China was teaching me was that the heart can pick up a lot of information that the head cannot, and I was fascinated by what drew this group to these new, promising innovations.

One of the most fascinating presentations to me involved the addition of immunotherapy to the protocol of cryoablation, something I had only been recently introduced to by hearing about Fe's treatment. Her blood had been taken, incubated for 14 days, and then given back to her to stimulate the immune system's killer T cells. This procedure takes advantage of cryoablation's immune stimulating effects so that the newly released cytokines coming from the dendritic cells can go back to the lymph nodes and tell the killer T cells what to look for and destroy. (This is an "artist's version" of the effect. It probably comes from watching so many cowboy movies in my youth where the Calvary scouts find the bad guys first, and then go tell the troops!).

The culturing of the blood provides this hugely important army of cancer destroyers, the killer T's. The concluding statistics showed that using the Combined Immunotherapy with Cryoablation significantly prolongs survival more than using cryoablation only or chemotherapy plus cryoablation. Impressive! Oh how I wished this technique was available in the states!

At a certain point I left the conference to go back to my room. It was my only opportunity to get packed for the trip home the next day and I wanted to change clothes for the evening's activities (and to rally Louie!). We made it back for the final thank you's and the group photo. The Chinese are the best photo documenters I have ever seen! I was surprised when Dr. Xu gestured for me to be a part of the photo.

As I approached the stage, I was pulled to the very center of the group! In the resulting photo, I saw that both Dr. Peter's and Dr. Xu's hands were on my shoulders. This gesture made me feel that both men truly had a patient's needs at the heart of their motivation.

An air of relief and relaxation came over the group, especially the Chinese hosts, as Ester rounded us all up for the bus trip to the restaurant where the post-presentation banquet was to be held. Again, I was amazed that they included Louie and I at this important event halfway around the world—especially when our decision to come had been so recent and without any knowledge of an impending important conference such as this.

What if I had ignored Fe's offer to have me join her? What if my friends had not been so generous and quick in their response to our funding request that helped pay for Louie's ticket? So many decisions had seemed to hang by a thread. But the reality of the heart connections I was quickly making was not lost on me. I was connecting with a community of people from across the globe with very like minds when it comes to the best way to treat cancer. It's a way that takes time but ultimately is so less morbid and certainly highly successful.

I settled in to enjoy the view as the modern, comfortable bus drove us through the very beautiful city of Guangzhou to our banquet destination, a fabulous large restaurant overlooking the glittering river.

Our second floor banquet hall offered the most breathtaking view. We were all immediately drawn to the balcony where much picture taking ensued. The visiting doctors/professors were shutterbugs like me, including "Dr. Peter" (as I found out all the Chinese like to call Dr. Littrup).

As various groups formed for photo taking, Dr. Peter began to reminisce how much had changed in China, especially Guangzhou. "None of this was here the first time I visited back in 1996," he told me as he leaned over the balcony to look at the reflective river and the brightly lit buildings beyond. "In fact, I was let out on something of a dirt road when I wanted to do some exploring of my own!" I knew he had been asked by the UN to travel widely, including here, to share his work on cryoablation.

The change from dirt roads to brand-new buildings and freeways of this very modern city echoed the Chinese medical community's quick embrace of Dr. Peter's pioneering ideas about treating cancer through working with the body's own immune system. Here, unlike the West, his ideas had been planted in fertile soil.

As we were called inside, I experienced what was to become my biggest eye-opener into Chinese culture: how to party!

The doctors/professors continued picture taking with their colleagues seated inside at the front of the room. Louie and I were invited to take a seat anywhere to our liking. However, before settling, one of the Chinese doctors from FUDA approached me. In accented but good

English he told me that he had heard I was interested in the immune blood therapy that Fe had been treated with (I was. It seemed to be unique to FUDA).

He asked if I would be interested in visiting his lab at top floor of the hospital the following morning. It would have to be early as he had a commitment mid-morning. I accepted, of course, and thanked him very much. He was both rather quiet and shy and I wondered about his offer. I suspected that he was more interested in Dr. Peter's inclusion but was perhaps too shy to ask him directly.

I couldn't believe I really could be appearing as a conduit for such important information getting out to potential Western patients. No, I think he saw me as a link to a hero. I was thrilled by this offer, however. As far as I was aware, nothing like this amazing treatment existed in the West, and I was very anxious to get Dr. Peter's take on it.

Suddenly, a classic Chinese movie appeared on a big screen at the front of the room. Ester was dancing around with a microphone, encouraging others to take it to sing along. So this was the Chinese version of Karaoke: singing to old, classic movies! Soon, an older, gentlemanly professor took the offer and started belting out the words in perfect pitch.

He knew the song! His hand gestured towards the screen then to his heart as he gave it his all. This was received by wild, happy clapping and when he finished, another elder statesman took up the mike. My mind quickly started connecting the dots from my observations during this trip.

The room where we slept was close to a school and we often heard music coming from what must have been a rooftop playground during much of the day. Could it be that these songs were familiar to these older gentlemen from their youth through the educational system? (Judging by their age that would mean the movie and songs must have come out of the Cultural Revolution era. I became aware of my Western cynicism, as I couldn't really tell if the passionate delivery was "camp" or reverence).

Ester was dancing around, gesturing for others to join her. What had been a formal gathering was quickly changing into a happy party! The transition was remarkable; I noticed at least one other Westerner looking on in amazement. The spirit was contagious, and soon the disk jockey was searching for anything from the West so Louie could have a go. All that they could find was the Eagles's "Hotel California." Not the best karaoke song ever, but he gave it his all, and I joined in to give my support. This went on while food was being brought out with pauses for toasts.

Once the toasts started, they were continuous, with the doctors/professors leading the toasts by going from table to table, lauding in most high regard their friends and colleagues. (So the Chinese way to get a banquet going? The more the toasts, the more alcohol is consumed!) There was delicious food at the table, but so much was going on that it was mostly being ignored. It was hard to get a conversation going with tablemates!

Soon, a bit of a hush came over the room. I looked over to see Dr. Peter had taken the microphone and was getting ready for his turn at karaoke. What would his song be? Ahh . . . Elvis . . . at his most infectious: "Jail House Rock"! Dr. Peter just nailed it, complete with the twisting, gyrating body moves of the King himself! Now everybody was dancing! This definitely was a bonding experience!

While I marveled at this scene—unlike any I ever expected to see—a pang of sorrow came over me that this was my last night. I could see this closely bonding mass of mostly suits and ties truly was a group capable of changing the way cancer gets treated for the better. Bravo attendees of the FUDA International Symposium on Cancer!

With so much unwinding behind us, tables began to fill and food began to get eaten. But soon, a very unexpected surprise came. I had noticed Dr. Xu going from table to table, warmly engaging with each participant. But he eventually made his way to a large table at the back of the room that quickly caught my interest.

On it was a long white piece of rice paper from a large roll. Next to it, hung from a beautiful antique-looking holder, were a variety of calligraphy brushes. Suddenly, it flashed through my mind what I'd seen throughout the lobby and halls leading to this room. Something with echoes back home in all the best Chinese restaurants . . . beautifully framed, large, horizontal calligraphy.

Since Asian Art had been my favorite art history subject in school (I'd taken two years of it), I was familiar with this tradition. But what was new to me here was the very idea that the learned and brilliant Dr. Xu, former army officer, hospital administrator and international foundation president, could also be a calligraphy master!

I was one of the first to move closer to see what he was up to. He confidently took a brush and started making Chinese characters . . . beautifully! I noticed that the table had ink drippings on it. The old heavy table must be a permanent fixture in this room. Perhaps this is a tradition I was totally unaware of. Perhaps it explained the beautiful framing and displays of such works I'd seen in the West. Much more than a lovely piece of writing was going on. A special event was being celebrated. A guest was being honored. A commemorative souvenir was being made.

I'm sure there was a protocol at work. As he finished the first set of characters, Dr. Xu gestured towards Prof. Nikolai Korpan of Vienna, the first presenter and the man with whom Dr. Xu shares a co-presidency of International Society of Cryosurgery.

The young members of the planning committee quickly mounted the work on the padded board behind the table and the two presidents shook hands vigorously as lights flashed from dozens of cameras and cell phones. A beautiful image to cap a magical evening! Next to be so honored was Dr. Peter, who received a most hearty applause. And so it went as all the visitors were given a precious souvenir of this important event.

There was one non-professor attendee to also get a calligraphy trophy. As I was fiddling with my smart phone camera I heard, "Madam Laura, Madam Laura!" "It's your turn!" Not only did Dr. Xu honor me with my own scroll, but he also handed the brush over to me. I had seen him give attention and responsibility to young members of his staff. Perhaps this was something of a test as well as an honor . . . I absolutely didn't want to let this magnificent leader down. I took a large brush and began to write . . . "A great man" . . . (the room became hushed and questioning, soft Chinese voices could be heard). Not even I knew what would come next, but then it did come, the only phase that seemed to match what I'd come to feel about Dr. Xu . . . "Lives by his Heart!"

I finished with a dedication to him personally: "with great affection and appreciation to Dr. Xu, from (my formal, professional name) Laura Ross-Paul, December 18th, 2012."

After the subsequent photo-taking and applause, I was very happy to have sweet, gentle Tracy by my side, assuring me I had done well and that my scroll gift from Dr. Xu would be folded and packed, ready for travel, in the morning.

The evening unwound, and Dr. Peter asked if Louie and I wanted to join him at his hotel for a drink, which we gladly took him up on.

On the bus to the hotel both Louie and I noted to each other one of the traditional herbals we'd seen available in the restaurant's lobby: made from elk testicles, we wondered what it was for. Being from a family where my husband has hunted elk most of his adult life and he taught our sons to hunt as well, it had caught both our eyes.

Finally, we had a moment alone with Dr. Peter! We found a quiet spot on some facing couches by the bar, under the huge hotel staircase. Dr. Xu, Ester, Dr. Korpan, and some others must have had the same idea as they took seats at another couch grouping nearby.

After figuring out a fruit drink we could combine with some gin (the Chinese bartender hadn't a clue about making a gin and tonic), we settled into a catching up session about our lives since we had first made some history with my long-ago revolutionary breast cancer treatment.

I explained the deep emotions instilled in me though wanting so desperately to help other women looking to follow my footsteps and have their breasts treated with cryoablation and how that had eventually led me to China after I became aware this option was no longer available at Karmanos where I had been treated.

Dr. Peter revealed he had his own health problems to contend with and lamented that they had certainly interfered with where he had hoped to be at this point. We both lauded the Chinese for what they were doing and affirmed hopes for getting it going in the US.

Soon, Dr. Xu's group had broken up, and Louie and I were offered a ride back to our room at the hospital. By this time, the fatigue and spirits had gotten the better of our judgment and we assured them we would get a cab. They asked if we knew what to tell the driver. I found a card in my pocket with the hospital address, so they left us to our own devices.

They had been right to worry, however; we soon learned, according to Louie's GPS, that the cab the hotel door man had called for us began heading towards to the distant Old FUDA, (where Fe was) and not the much closer New FUDA! Thank God for Louie's smart phone skills. To save face, he instructed me to remain in the cab as he briefly entered the lobby of the wrong hospital, pretending he was picking something up, and then we gave the driver instructions to where we really needed to go. (Thankfully, we had enough Yuan to cover the cost of the un-needed extra miles!!).

The two white elephant carvings in front of New FUDA were so welcoming when we reached our home away from home that we decided to take our photo in front of them!

12.19.13—Last day!

As I lay on my hospital bed the morning of our last day, I tried to savor the moment and all the things

I would miss about FUDA, Guangzhou and China. Certainly my big, bedside sky view with all the cozy-looking apartments in the distance, full of decks with bikes and hanging clothes. I would also miss the enthusiastic loudspeaker voices and playful squeals coming from the school nearby.

I will very much miss Fe and her sister Jelly, who now felt like family members: Fe for her bravery and strong belief in the rightness of her treatment and Jelly for her sweet cheerfulness and gentle manner.

I definitely had made heart connections with Segundo and Tracy and Madam Ester and Dr. Xu. Experiencing their focused dedication and enthusiasm for dealing so directly with what many feel is one of life's worst afflictions, late stage cancer, and doing it with such compassion and grace, bringing levity to every opportunity that would allow it. It all had made a huge impression on me. I don't know what I was expecting, but this somehow had the feel of a large, extended family of which I had become a part. I knew I would be forever changed by my experience.

Segundo already had collected Dr. Littrup from his hotel when we bumped into him looking for us on the way to our 4th floor appointment with Dr. Chen at the Immunotherapy Lab. Dr. Chen greeted us outside his lab and asked us to use shoe covers to enter.

The top floor lab had a shiny, spotless hallway with glass and chrome walls on either side allowing us to look into labs with neatly arranged medical equipment. On the walls were some visually effective posters in English that depicted the reactions that happen when culturing a patient's blood to grow Killer T cells. Besides the cellular depictions of the process, robust figures of a man and a woman were depicted successfully traversing a steep hill. It was visually very easy to understand the process by looking at the posters.

Soon, we were invited into Dr. Chen's small but organized office. He had some studies ready to show Dr. Littrup, so the two of them soon got into a scientific discussion that appeared to be a challenge for Tracy's interpretive skills and Dr. Chen's English. One thing I picked up on that I hadn't known before is that the immune stimulating effects come through three differ-ent types of cytokine stimulation: one that lasts for three days after cryoablation, one that lasts for approximately three months after ablation, and one that lasts a lifetime.

This relates back to what Dr. Xu had told me about the benefit of getting CIC at any time after one's initial treatment. He explained that there is always a cell die off as we age, but having a CIC boost benefits the effec-tiveness of creating more of these lifetime Killer T's that have the knowledge of exactly the type of cancer that had been originally cryoablated. (No wonder 10 years ago Dr. Littrup had told me to put off radiation for at least three months! It gave my immune system a chance to fully develop its response).

I made a mental note that I would certainly return sometime in the future to have this done with my hus-band, Alex, who had had ablation to treat his prostate cancer in 2010. We would both benefit and he would get a chance to see China in the process!

Not surprisingly, Dr. Peter was very interested in the additional healing effects of the culturing of the blood (CIC) the Chinese used at FUDA. When he finally ran out of questions, it appeared Dr. Chen had something he wanted to say. "Dr. Peter, I have read all of your papers and books. Everything. You are like a God to me." There was a long pause when both doctors looked each other in the eye. I could only imagine what was going through their minds. Dr. Peter's mouth had slightly dropped open and, when I referenced the comment later, he acknowledged he had gotten this before in China.

He said it with a slight lament that I imagined was because, so far, his wonderful, pioneering efforts in this field were still widely unknown in the States.

Soon, it was time for Dr. Chen to go to his meeting. We walked him down the stairs and were met by Ester and Dr. Xu who had been looking for Dr. Peter to attend the same meeting. Louie and I were asked to join. It was held in the conference room and the only seat I could find was next to what appeared to be reporters crammed against the wall behind all the doctors/professors sitting at a large conference table.

Louie soon left to finish packing but I stayed awhile, feeling this might be a chance to be a fly on the wall of something important and historic.

The doctors/professors were presenting statistical evidence from their practices and research. It was mostly in English, but many presenters were obviously more comfortable speaking in Chinese, and Ester Law was asked to interpret from time to time. After each brief PowerPoint presentation, questions were rather aggressively asked and debated.

The Chinese presented statistics on pancreatic cancer that included a man, now in his 80s, who had survived post-cancer treatment for 127 months (over ten years!). There were lots of questions about techniques. The treatment used in these cases did not seem so different than what I'd understood was effective with

Fe: carefully doing lots of imaging to map out the situation; using iodine seed implants and inserted chemotherapy (CMI) to reduce tumor size; using immunotherapy (CIC) to build an effective response to cryoablation; and variations on all the above per a patient's needs.

The American, Dr. Michael Sabel, suggested creating an International Registry, with standardized forms to collect data that would stand up to peer review form (I wasn't sure if that meant these statistics coming from China were different than how they are done in the West, but I appreciated the idea of coordination. What the Chinese were accomplishing was obviously highly respected).

I listened more to the presentations and questions but became a little discouraged that even these top researchers were still debating the best way to do things. I realized this was a necessary process for any new medical procedure, but I had already waited ten long years for cryoablation to be readily available to all women, everywhere, to both save breasts and save lives.

Perhaps this type of medical comparing of notes is a constant for all types of treatment, which leads to advancement even as treatment is being offered. But in the West, we haven't even gotten to square one with regards to cryoablation.

Breast cancer treatment has not significantly changed in almost forty years, although I'm sure refinement of existing procedures has happened.

While I admired all the learned doctors debating so passionately, I had to leave the room to breathe the fresh air of hope. I wanted to spend my last afternoon with Fe.

Louie and I finished our packing (thank goodness he'd chosen a new backpack for his Christmas present when we had shopped in the mall; we needed the room to pack all the books and brochures we'd been given along with the Christmas gifts).

We put on the clothes we would be wearing on the long plane ride home. Our plan was to collect Dr. Peter who was most interested in visiting Fe with us. But when we returned to the meeting site, all the doctors were quickly being ushered into the elevators for an excursion to a Chinese restaurant for lunch. Ester's big smile and encouragement to join them forced us into a split-second decision. On the elevator ride, both Segundo and Tracy assured us we'd still have plenty of time for our visit with Fe. They assured us they'd make all the driving arrangements to get us to the airport in plenty of time for our flight.

Our buses soon pulled into a modern shopping mall center with an ample, large parking lot, similar to what might be found in almost every city in the states. We were told that this was one of Guangzhou's most famous seafood restaurants and, being close to the South China Sea, we knew seafood was the city's specialty. The restaurant's entrance was inside a modern hotel lobby with high ceilings and ultra-modern design features. Being close to Christmas, there were decorations everywhere. I was fascinated by a life-sized metal sculpture of a horse in the lobby and stopped to have my photo taken with it. I almost missed the group being quickly ushered into several private dining rooms and was glad that a tall, beautiful Chinese woman who was with our group had waited for me.

She spoke soft, elegant English to show me where to go. The doctors/professors had been taken to their own private dining room, but we were invited to join the table of a room full of new faces, also guests for the luncheon. Luckily, my new companion, Shenshan Chen, sat down next to me.

One of my friends from Oregon is also a very tall, handsome Chinese. Shizen, my acupuncturist and "bone setter," is from the far north of China and I asked Shenshan if that might be where she was from. She said it was. I was entranced and fascinated by her quiet, dignified manner, so poised and elegant.

She reminded me of my tall, quietly elegant British mother-in-law who had been raised in Hong Kong. Shenshan explained that she had been trained and worked as a doctor but soon transitioned into working as a sales representative for medical equipment. Her hair was pulled back in a ponytail and her beautiful dark eyes contrasted with her pale, glowing skin. I told her I thought she could be a movie star, to which she gave a small, polite smile.

Almost as soon as we sat down serving dishes of food began to be brought and put on the turning circle in the middle of the table. As the conversations around us were mostly in Chinese, I got a chance to look around the room. A very elegant, tasteful sculpture in three parts occupied much of the far wall. I couldn't tell what the sculpture was made from but it had a slight iridescence and resembled forms from the sea.

It was beautiful, like no decoration I had ever seen. (It would be the second of three strong déjà vus I had while in China.) The walls were paneled wood with carved moldings, both ancient and modern somehow. Large windows let in plenty of sunlight.

A distinguished older gentleman sat to Louie's left and used English to make sure Louie and I were getting enough to eat. He wanted to know if we had tried all of the various dishes. When I looked down at my plate, a bowl of the special seafood and chicken soup Guangzhou is famous for had appeared. Floating on top were what looked like a Chinese version of our Northwest banana slug, complete with stripes! Suddenly, my appetite went away.

I asked the question, "What is this creature called?"

"It's a sea slug" came the answer. After a long pause where I noticed all eyes were on me, Shenshan asked, "Don't you like your Chinese food?" I took up the flat spoon next to my bowl and took a full slurp, sea slug and all!

"Delicious!" I said, and it was, although something like a gummy worm in texture.

I felt it was time to introduce ourselves to the other distinguished looking gentlemen around the table and I started by asking the one to Louie's left what his association with the group was. This brought hilarious laughter. Another gentleman let me know that we were sitting by the distinguished president of the medical school FUDA is associated with, Jinan University School of Medicine.

I gave him a slight bow and apologetic smile. Oh my! What had Louie and I gotten ourselves into?

Our luncheon ended with a visit from Dr. Xu who was obviously old, dear friends with this group. Shenshan quietly interpreted their conversation as having something to do with a research program involving all the top medical specialists of China that Dr. Xu was hoping to get going in the future.

I looked at him admiringly. At an age when many administrators would be thinking of retiring, he was laying out big plans for the future. I wondered at the ample heart he must have to fuel such passionate dreams.

We returned to New FUDA to fetch our luggage. Louie and I were so happy to find Segundo and our driver Mr. Chen playfully making funny faces at each other on either side of a glass wall while they waited for us in the lobby. They were there to take us directly to Old FUDA and Fe. We gathered our bags and brought them to the lobby where we had to wait for Dr. Peter. A professional photographer was taking his photo with the rest of the group.

Ester saw our bags and asked if we were leaving, telling us that we were invited to a river cruise dinner. It sounded lovely, but we told her we'd be on our plane by then. Dr. Xu himself seemed to pick up on the goodbyes being said. Soon, he, Ester, Tracy and Segundo were all escorting Dr. Peter, Louie and I to our car.

To be sent off from this great adventure in the hospital's driveway by such top brass brought a tear to my eye. Had I not come, I never would have known about such wonderful people and such great work going on here on the other side of the planet!

Fe was ready and waiting for our impending visit. She looked radiant, though slightly nervous sitting upright on her bed as we entered her bright, light-filled room. As if to commemorate the importance of the visit, Jelly picked up her iPad and began recording the visit.

Dr. Peter took Fe's hand and warmly let her know how happy he was they were finally getting to meet. Fe began her response by singing the praises of the staff, who started gathering for introductions beside her bed. Fe's doctor, Dr. Quincy Lihua, answered some of Dr. Littrup's questions but soon had to return to her duties.

We all sat down for a visit. As Dr. Peter asked questions of Fe, I would sometimes steer her towards things she had told me about her treatments or anecdotal things she had heard from other patients.

Soon, Fe was showing Dr. Peter the long spreadsheet of her hospital costs as they were accruing. Kept by her bedside, it was an excellent list of the treatments she had received. It quickly surfaced that Fe and I were both concerned that some of the spots in her bones had not been frozen. Did Dr. Peter think this was because they were being used as indicators of the immune system's ability to kill small, secondary sites on its own? Did her doctors expect them to diminish and disappear soon? Dr. Xu had shown me this often happens in the PowerPoint presentation I'd seen in his office earlier.

Dr. Peter wasn't sure but expected that was the case and assured Fe they were not her greatest concern right now. He looked at me and seemed to be sorting out in his head the differences with the protocols he was familiar with. Certainly, the addition of the CIC was the main treatment that was missing in the West.

"It seems to be unique to what's going on here. I can't think of anything like it. It's too bad, but I'm sure it would take a long time to get through trials in the states," he said.

Something rang a bell in my brain, and I meant to ask Dr. Littrup if he was aware of the fact that, according to the FUDA brochure, no trials were needed; the FDA had already approved CIC! I resolved to communicate with him later, though, because the main focus was now Dr. Peter's visit with Fe. (Sadly, I've learned since that the problem with CIC here in the states is that portions of it have been cleared by the FDA but not approved through the use of trials, so the potential liability of damage from using CIC here, even though it would be allowed, prevents its use.)

Dr. Peter asked Fe's doctor if he could be given certain records, so he could make up a case file on her treatment. Fe readily gave her permission, so her doctor quickly left to put together a package for him.

I was proud of Fe's bravery in coming to China and wanted her to hear Dr. Peter's opinion as to whether he thought this was her best chance at survival. He told her he thought it was but also had some ideas about medical trials going on in his own city of Detroit, which he thought Fe might qualify for if things didn't work out.

I voiced the fact that I felt Fe and her husband were spending their entire life savings on these treatments to which he replied that the doctor, Dr. Pat Lorusso, running the trials in Detroit, was very good about getting drug companies to cover costs since it was drug-based therapy.

I wrote down the information to send to Fe's husband David, but in my heart, I said a prayer that the FUDA therapies would be enough. I had both seen and heard of miracles here. I knew the determination these brilliant Chinese doctors had to not let a foe like cancer win, to not give up until they were victorious.

Fe had come a long way and had already endured so much. I knew she had a fighting spirit even bigger than my own. She was determined too! Fe comes in a small but solid package. I knew it would eventually be just as important to get her story out as it was to share mine. When the strong wills of medicine and mind come together, miracles can happen. China had taught me this; or rather, it had reaffirmed this belief in me.

Soon a driver had come to take Dr. Peter to observe a cryoablation procedure going on back at the New FUDA hospital, which would be followed by the scheduled river cruise. Dr. Peter expressed regrets I would be missing it. I assured him it would be a trip highlight for him. Both the river and the city are so beautiful.

We all posed for one last group picture—Fe with her blue radiation prevention apron on—and then he left.

I could tell Fe was exhausted. Her head leaned back on her pillow and her soft brown eyes locked with mine. She had one last favor to ask me. She had not been able to get her doctor to print out instructions of what would be needed for her heparin port cleansing once she got back home. David also had written me of this concern.

Since Canada has a national medical program, appointments had to be set up in advance, but orders had to come from FUDA. I wasn't sure if I could pull it off, but I went out to the hall to find Fe's doctor. I told her I wanted to leave with a copy of the order that I could send to Fe's husband, so he had a physical copy at the ready. And would she please also send him an electronic version immediately?

I told her I only had a half an hour left before I had to leave, and I asked if she could get to it immediately. She smiled and turned around and then went into her office and began working at her computer. Whew!

The ride to the airport was slightly surreal. For miles and miles we passed beautiful landscaping on either side of the freeway with all the plants looking like a well-groomed Chinese garden. Louie pointed out a playful grouping of a family of molded plastic goats, cheerfully waving goodbye as we left the city.

On the city outskirts, we passed what looked like a whole city of unfinished, unused high-rise apartment buildings. Was this a miscalculation of expected growth or buildings waiting for projected occupants?

A woman begging for our leftover coins greeted us at the door of the beautiful, modern airport. This continued inside with different beggars while we waited to get our boarding passes. We passed a large pile of brightly striped luggage owned by a group from Africa waiting nearby. (My third and final déjà vu).

We took advantage of the last of our paper money to buy some gifts and snack items for home: incense in beautiful carved boxes; playing cards with groupings of generals depicted on them; delicious pastel biscuits, all individually wrapped. (Checking in our luggage had freed our hands to carry these additional packages as carry-on luggage!)

Going through customs we stood behind the only other Westerner we saw in line. The woman, about my age, said she had been visiting an orphanage run by her daughter. She told us that just the night before, an adorable baby girl had been left in a basket on the orphanage's doorstep, all carefully dressed in clean, soft clothing with a note giving her name. The woman speculated the parents perhaps couldn't afford to keep her as additional children are taxed.

Louie did not look like his passport photo, so he made the officer smile when he covered his beard with his hands and pulled back his long bangs. A line waiting for early boarding in first class had already gathered when we arrived at the terminal.

Among those standing in it, I was actually sorry to witness a pouty woman dressed in a very short skirt and extra tall heels asking her husband for money. This was so different than anything I'd seen before this moment in China.

Luckily, an English-speaking Chinese college student with an American accent, got behind us in the coach line. We had a wonderful visit in our own language before the line moved, and we found our seats all the way at the back of the plane. Soon, I would be drifting in and out of sleep as I began the first of four movies, some Chinese, some American. Louie had given me the window seat and the extra ledge allowed a spot for my tired head.

Epilogue

Within days of arriving home, Dr. Peter sent me an album of photos from the river cruise and sightseeing trips the doctors/professors were treated to during the last two days of their conference. They were beautiful and showed old temples, markets and monuments.

Both Fe and David continue to correspond with me. After two more trips to China, Fe's tumors are finally all gone! She will be having imaging in Canada after the date of this writing to check for any reoccurrence but she is back by David's side, working full-time, helping to run their cleaning business.

I will let her words, sent via various emails, finish the story of this incredible adventure.

Bless you, Fe. Bless your bravery and belief in a system so vey foreign and far away. Bless you, good people of FUDA, for reaching out to offer your miracle practices and give hope to all who have been given up on by traditional cancer treatment practices. Bless you, Dr. Peter Littrup for your pioneering efforts in bringing the technique of cryoablation to America and for continuing to be its biggest advocate here.

Thank you and bless you, Louie Paul, my talented second son, for your quick, enthusiastic decision to join me to document this adventure. I hope your resulting video and film give attention to this story and help effect change.

And thank you, my loving husband, Alex, for supporting my quest to save my breast and cure my cancer years ago. You found Dr. Peter Littrup after endless hours of Internet searching and then helped me convince the staff at Karmanos that I was a good candidate for experimental cryoablation. Then you took on the financial burden of my treatment when insurance refused to pay, as well as funding most of the cost of our trip to China.

Without your belief in me and my desire to keep my breast years ago, I would certainly have undergone a mastectomy, and who knows? I might have died of a recurrence within a few years of my mastectomy, just like my mother did, since my liver could not have tolerated chemotherapy, and I would not have had a chance at receiving a full systemic killing of any residual cancer.

I firmly believe I got the protection of the immune effect from my cryoablation, and am convinced that saved me all these years from a recurrence. There is no way to prove I am right or wrong, but in the end, I have acted with faith in God and he has given me his blessed protection and guidance every step of the way.

And as of this writing I have lived cancer free for an astonishing ten years, an accomplishment of healing celebrated when Dr. Xu and Dr. Littrup placed their hands on my shoulders in the group photograph. I am living proof that their treatments work . . . they can give a full life back to a cancer patient.

***

Alex

Alex here. I would like to take this opportunity to thank Laura for making her trip to China and for the excellent writing she contributed above. I so admire her courage and determination to get the message out to women in America, a message that assures women here that they have a real chance to save their breast and cure their cancer.

This message tells women they do not have to have their breasts removed to cure their cancer. In fact, by having a mastectomy, they may sadly be missing an opportunity to cure that cancer through the immune effect induced by cryoablation.

This is an odd thing to say: a mastectomy may not save your life, as conventional wisdom maintains in the United States, but it is the truth that Laura learned in China. It needs to be spread now throughout America and the Western world.

Honestly, the Chinese have taken the best of our technology and applied it to the desperate conditions of their huge country in which 80 percent of cancers are not discovered until they are a late stage, systemic condition. Necessity is the mother of invention; in China's case, it seems that necessity is the mother of invention and technical adoption, for they have perfected and gone beyond the pioneering, inventive work of

Dr. Littrup by combining their new CIC and CMI therapies with cryoablation.

Choosing cryoablation to save her breast and then working to get this message out and traveling to China took great courage on Laura's part, but I know that she has been divinely led in this quest that I have had the opportunity to help her with. I am convinced that her guardian angel told her to trust Dr. Littrup and his experimental procedure years ago.

Remember that at the time, her Portland doctor was telling her that if she had cryoablation she would get a recurrence and die of cancer.

Instead, Laura stood up to this fear and embraced this strange new treatment of freezing, and she has lived cancer free since 2003.

I don't think it is often that a person can be married to their biggest hero. In my case, I consider myself so fortunate to be married to such a wonderful woman who is also my hero, and to have had the chance to help her achieve the goal she declared so long ago when her mother died of cancer and she prayed that she would find a cure for breast cancer.

One could argue that she failed miserably, because she is an artist and not a cancer researcher; but to my way of thinking, she chose cryoablation and stayed alive, then went to China and . . . found a cure for breast cancer!

When I read about Laura doing the calligraphy poster for Dr. Xu, it struck me that the following saying applies to my amazing wife:

"A great woman . . . lives by her heart."

May the telling of this story inspire a change in the way we in the West view and treat breast cancer. As

Dr. Peter, Dr. Xu, Fe and Laura have all experienced: it IS possible to KEEP your breast AND get immunity to your cancer.

***

Additional thoughts about the 2012 FUDA Trip from Laura:

Laura

It took a while for me to digest and process the trip to FUDA and its implications for cancer treatment here in America. Writing now months after the trip, I think I've finally realized why the Chinese health treatment system, at least the part I visited in FUDA, does so well.

A significant reason their method works so successfully might be related to the Chinese culture itself.

Chinese medicine has embraced the concept of supporting the immune system for thousands of years. Their whole philosophy of acupuncture and herb-based medications is built around this immune system cooperation model.

With Western medicine, cancer is seen as an enemy of the body, requiring complete elimination by extreme methods to insure total victory. The goal at FUDA seems to be slightly different. Instead of seeing cancer as a foreign enemy, the disease seems to be treated as a system out of whack with the body taking extreme measures, because its normal processes are not doing the job. Treatments are chosen for their ability to assist the body back into its normal healthy function. Affected organs are protected as much as possible. The body has a system to attack foreign bodies; i.e. the immune system, where dendritic cells emitting cytokines (acting like little janitors) locate foreign cells and report them to the lymph's killer T cells, which go on to attach and eliminate them. Rather than harming the immune system just when it's needed most, as is done in the West, at FUDA the immune system is supported through both cryoablation and Combined Immunotherapy for Cancer (CIC).

The second difference that stands out to me is FUDA's individualized approach. In the West, breast cancer patients are offered "protocols" for treatment based on statistical evidence. The protocols feel like a one size fits all system, with the most extreme treatments being encouraged, (mastectomy) to garner the best results.

Treatments at FUDA favor keeping body parts and the tailoring of treatment to suit the individual situation, with adjustments being made as responses are analyzed.

I believe this is a cultural difference, because the Western protocols act as a protection in our litigious society. At FUDA, the hospital's reputation as a successful place of healing is a motivator. A fear factor of being sued does not seem to be part of the equation.

Before:

"If this was pioneered here and the machines are made here, why have I never heard about it? *

During:

"If this was pioneered in the states and the machines that do it are made and come from the States, why isn't it being done there?" **

After:

"If we pioneered it here, and the machines that do it come from here, why aren't we doing it here?" ***

* Most often asked question before going to China.

** Most often asked question while in Guangzhou.

*** Most often asked question after my trip to China.

If you have finished reading this story and are just as incensed as I am that there isn't (yet) a good answer to these questions, I hope you will tell others about these possibilities.

Sharing the word at a grassroots level is a start toward effecting change. If you know, or are, in a position to influence a closer look through a Western medical system, I hope you will check out our website, KeepingThem. com, as well as the FUDA website, FUDAHospital.com.

My husband Alex and I thank you from the bottom of our hearts.

Chapter 22: Fe's Recurrence

Alex

Laura and I were upset to learn from Fe in late 2013 that her doctors in Canada had conducted a PET Scan and detected five small tumors in her lymph system. These tumors had appeared since the earlier analysis that she was cancer free after her trip to FUDA in 2012. This was a severe blow to Fe, but also confirmation that cancer is a systemic disease and that once it has metastasized and gained a foothold in the body, it is difficult to contain and completely eliminate.

In response to this recurrence, Fe scheduled a return trip to FUDA for more treatment in early April 2014. This coincided with a trip Laura and I had already planned to make to FUDA and China as well. We were excited on the one hand to see Fe in China but sad that the reason she was there was to treat a recurrence. On the bright side, it was miraculous that FUDA could still offer Fe treatment options! She had not lost her war with cancer; she was just going to have to endure another battle.

Prior to learning about Fe's situation, Laura and I had already decided to travel to FUDA for their CIC treatment. After learning about CIC, we became convinced that CIC offered an opportunity to both of us to give ourselves a lifelong immunity to our respective cancers.

Dr. Littrup used cryoablation in 2003 to treat Laura's breast cancer and cryoablation is a proven method of stimulating an immune response to cancer in the body.

I was diagnosed with early stage prostate cancer in 2010. Through a fortunate series of occurrences, I discovered Dr. Scionti of NYU's Urology Department who used High Intensity Focused Ultrasound (HIFU) to treat my prostate cancer in June of 2010. The HIFU procedure uses overlapping ultrasound beams to heat tissue to a temperature high enough to kill a tumor but not so high that it alters the protein structure of the tumor (which happens, for example, using laser treatment).

HIFU thus has the potential of creating dead cancer cells with their protein structure intact, just like cryoablation does. There is a controversy among researchers as to whether HIFU can stimulate the immune effect, where the immune system recognizes the cancer as a foreign body with a different DNA structure and develops an immunity to the cancer.

For this reason, we understood that the CIC treatment at FUDA could boost Laura's immune system response but might not be effective for me. I decided to pursue the treatment in the hope that the researchers who say HIFU stimulates the immune effect are correct.

Laura and I contacted Segundo in the Patient Consultation Services Department of FUDA and coordinated our visit. In the CIC process, a person's blood is drawn and cytokines are isolated from the blood. Those cytokines are then used to induce the growth of CIK's,

Cytokine Induced Killer Cells. These cultured CIKC's are then infused into the patient's body by IV drip over a four-day period. This infusion, combined with other injections, complete the CIC process and stimulate an immune response in the patient that can fight a future cancer recurrence.

It turned out that the culturing of the CIK's takes about a week, and that the cells can be stored by freezing them until a patient is able to have them infused.

Like many viewers of Public Television, we have seen a million ads for Viking River Cruises, so we decided to take a 12-day trip around China with Viking while our CIK's were being cultured. We then returned to FUDA after the journey to have the CIK's infused into us. And since we would be at the hospital the same time as Fe, we would also be able to follow her treatment progress.

We left for China on April 2, 2014. Unless you have taken a flight of over thirteen hours duration, you can probably not be sympathetic with my complaints of discomfort. It is like someone complaining about their first world problems such as having to charge their iPhone at a random electrical outlet because the battery runs down so quickly. On the one hand, it's frustrating an iPhone's battery seems to die soon after you charge it; on the other hand, it's hard to complain about owning an iPhone because they are so handy!

Just trust me that when I tell you that if you are six-foot-two, old and have bad knees from too much skiing (I still ski), plus basketball late into your adult years, a thirteen-hour-plus flight is not fun. Sure, I watched four two-hour movies, had some great Cathay Pacific meals and some wine, but that still left me trying to sleep—impossible with sore knees—for another five and a half hours! I have always wondered how airlines sell those business class bed seats at a cost of $5,000 each seat round trip, but now I understand why they were full after flying to China and back. If you have the money . . . the nice, fold-back-into-a-private-bed seats are priceless!

Regardless, we arrived in Guangzhou, and after a confusing welcoming by an airport agent with a wheelchair for me—I told him I'd been skiing the weekend before and absolutely didn't need a wheelchair . . . he said the hospital had told him to greet me with it—we were driven to FUDA in a hospital van.

We checked in and paid for our planned treatment, and then we were shown to our room. Laura had unfortunately booked a very small room. I suffer from claustrophobia, a remnant from an awful experience in my youth, so I was not doing well in the tiny room.

In addition, it turned out that after checking into the hospital and trying to pay for our treatment with our debit card, our debit card was blocked, even though I had specifically notified the bank about our visit there and planned use of the card. This meant that we could not buy any food either from the hospital (they only took cash for food for some reason) or from street vendors, the only other source of food near the hospital.

I tried calling our bank but was not able to get through on either of our cell phones. I began to panic, because I was claustrophobic, horribly fatigued from the flight and very hungry with very little money left to buy food! I told Lori that we needed to use the last of our cash to get a cab to a hotel that worked with Westerners so that we could use our visa cards to buy food.

She asked that we hang on for a bit, because she was going to call Segundo. I was not encouraged when we learned that he was out of town on holiday! He did call back, however, and promised to help us out.

We settled into our room, and then Fe and Jelly came to greet us! It was so wonderful meeting them. Despite her new bout of cancer, Fe was positive and energetic.

Here is Laura's description of our meeting.

Laura

We were only in our room a short time when Fe and her sister Jelly knocked on our door. Fe immediately started crying. We gave each other a big hug, and I could feel her heart energy in my chest. So sweet. She actually looked great! I knew she had been on a special diet heavy on the vegetables and greens, mostly raw, with some meat protein. She just glowed! She had brought us a big bag of fresh fruit from the street market and some pressed fruit rolls brought from Canada. Looking at Fe's glowing skin, I gave some serious thought to adopting her diet! She told us she only cooks a few days a week and puts it all up in containers for convenience since she has gone back to working full time, assisting her husband David run their cleaning business.

We had a great visit catching up and comparing notes about our flights. Apparently, her connection in Tokyo had been tight. She made her plane by running but her bag didn't make it. When she finally got it a few days later, her personal notebook with everyone's contact information was missing from the front pocket.

I gave her an advanced copy of our book and she was so sad that she hadn't stayed cancer free as we had hoped for our ending. I had to assure her that she really looked great and that it wasn't over yet. Whatever was showing up in her lymph nodes I felt might be her body's way of fighting what she had. At any rate, she had returned to the place where she knew she could get the help she needed. Unfortunately, the PET scans from Canada had to be redone, so she wasn't really sure exactly what the treatments were that she might be getting. After agreeing we both were in good hands with these doctors, we all decided to get some dinner in the hospital's cafeteria.

Alex continues the story about both Fe and us.

Alex

Fe is small, barely four-foot-six or so and very lean. She has a huge abundance of energy despite her cancer and she had an abundance of amazing stories from her life in the Philippines.

Jelly is taller and quieter. When you see Fe with her sister Jelly, you would not think they are sisters. And Jelly is so patient and kind-hearted! She offered to cook some Filipino food for us even though she had already been cooking for both of them for a week (they preferred their own food to the hospital food and the hospital provides a kitchen). Jelly is also a very positive influence for Fe, because I soon noticed that whenever Fe would give voice to her fears about treatment or her cancer, Jelly would cheerfully chime in that everything was going to be just fine. And she was right!

At FUDA, Fe was having imaging for new cancer sites. Her Canadian doctors had found some irregularities in her lymph nodes of the neck region, which had brought her back to FUDA for more in-depth imaging and treatment.

For some reason my jet lag hit me after I had eaten some food and I collapsed in sleep. Laura still had energy, so she joined Fe and Jelly in their room for a long talk. Apparently, the imaging done in Canada hadn't been sent to the Chinese so had to be repeated, which upset Fe since she would have to pay for it again. She was also upset that much of the staff was away on an important Chinese holiday that involves travel back to hometowns where dead relatives are prayed for. She tried to come at a non-holiday time to avoid delays in treatment, but the slow-down happened anyway. Since this was a weekend, Laura assured her things would get rolling in the morning and she most likely would have time to get all the necessary treatment done before her return ticket date.

The next day began a big turnaround for our stay at FUDA. Segundo called and said he had organized a new, larger room for us. We immediately went to see the room. It had a computer connected to the Internet as well as three times the space and a large desk for me to write. While we still hadn't solved the cash/debit card problem and our inability to buy food, I was at least not as concerned because I wasn't starving, thanks to Fe and Jelly, and the energy of a good night's sleep gave me optimism.

Packing our stuff to transfer to our new room, we received a surprise visit from Dr. Xu and Dr. Niu. It was wonderful to meet these amazing men. They both exuded a calm and professionalism that inspired confidence. After visiting and having some pictures together,

Dr. Xu offered to have his driver and his assistant Coco take us to see some sights of the city and then have dinner as his treat that night. The universe was solving our food problem even if my bank wasn't! And later in the day, I was able to use Skype to stay on hold long enough to contact my bank and finally get through to them to resolve the lock on my debit card. Now we could get cash and buy food in China! (Note to travelers: You must give banks your full itinerary of ALL the cities you will be traveling to in China!).

During the course of our first, four-day stay in Guangzhou for withdrawing our blood for the CIC process, I was able to get to know the wonderful people Laura had met in her previous trip. Among them were the visionary Dr. Xu, who is the head of the hospital, Dr. Niu, the senior cryoablation surgeon, and Dr. Lee, another surgeon. I also met Madame Ester, the marketing liaison for the hospital.

I met the younger support staff who work with international patients. Segundo is a Filipino in his late twenties who originally trained as a nurse. He joined FUDA in 2010, specifically to work with the many Filipino patients who come to FUDA.

I also had an opportunity to meet Coco, Tracy and Katie. In China, schoolchildren pick an "English/American" style name to have a Western persona in school as they learn English. This name sticks with them the rest of their lives. These names represent an interest of the person at the time they picked the name; for example, Coco picked "Coco" because of her interest in Coco Chanel as a young girl.

The Chinese are an amazing and delightful people! As I had already learned in my life from my days of

competing with them in the Oregon State University
Engineering program, they are extremely smart—some
of the smartest people in the world. They are also hardworking and disciplined. However, it was not until this
trip that I realized they are also extremely playful, fun-
loving, and gracious hosts to visitors of their beloved
country.

Coco instantly charmed us when she passed a
wedding shop that evening while giving us a tour of
Guangzhou. She had Laura take a picture of her posing
as if she were wearing a dress displayed in the shop's
window. After taking the picture, Laura inquired as to
her boyfriend status. Coco admitted that she still needed the boy in order to have the wedding!

So for the rest of our visit, I assured her that if she
invited us to the wedding, we would come to China and
attend. However, I teased her and told her that since
she was such a wonderful catch, we might be able to
attend the wedding prior to our leaving China. We soon
began referring to her as our Chinese adopted daughter
when we posted our Instagram photos. Our real daughter, Emma, after seeing Coco's pictures on Instagram,
commented that she was glad we had found her long-
lost Chinese sister.

While in Guangzhou, we saw ancient archeological
displays of early life under the Emperors in 3,500 BCE.
We visited a meeting hall once used by Sun Yat Sen,
the Father of the Republic of China. Sun Yat Sen led
the people's revolt against the Qing Dynasty, the last
emperor of China.

The meeting hall of his party, the Kuomintang, is
preserved in Guangzhou for public visits. Dr. Sun Yat
Sen is still revered as one of the greatest leaders of

modern China, despite the fact that his intended plan of government, a democratic monarchy like England, never gained traction and was swept aside in the turmoil of warlords fighting each other; and later, the Japanese invasion; and finally the triumph of Mao over Chiang Kai Shek. Dr. Sun's main contribution to China's history is that he emboldened the people to put their needs first and overthrow the Emperor system of government that had ruled for thousands of years.

During the following days, we had blood drawn and various other tests completed to get our CIC treatment going. It only took a few days and, at last, we were ready for our Viking Cruise of "The Imperial Jewels of China" due to begin in Beijing. On our last night before starting our Viking River Cruise, Dr. Xu hosted a dinner for us at a delightful seafood restaurant. As Laura related previously, the Chinese display the seafood live in tanks and you have to pick out what you will be eating so that it can be prepared fresh. We wandered around the tanks and I noticed one tank full of three-foot long sea snakes that swam around their tank with their head raised aggressively. They looked to me like they would bite one's finger if offered to close to the tank.

A young mother with three little girls around the age of eight or nine must have thought the same thing, because she held her finger about four feet above the tank's surface and gradually lowered her pointed finger towards the water. The little girls were standing on the woman's left side, their eyes barely above the edge of the glass tank and wide with horror as the woman's finger descended towards the snake-filled water. I had stepped to within just a few feet of the mother's right side to see what would happen.

The mother pulled her hand back quickly and the girls smiled and heaved a sigh of relief. But as they did, I extended my hand to the point where the mother's had been and continued to lower it closer to the water with my finger pointed. The little girls' eyes, and now the mother's, focused on my hand, convinced that this crazy old Western tourist would take up the dare where the mother had left it and indeed get bitten by a poisonous snake.

Suddenly, my right hand darted out towards my left hand, my fingers shaped like the jaws of a snake. My right hand "snake" bit my left pointer finger. The mother and three little girls jumped back in terror then began to laugh as they realized I had played a joke on them. I smiled and said, "Nee How" meaning "Hello,"— my one Chinese phrase—and they smiled. Further proof of the delightfully playful personality of the Chinese.

Dinner was very interesting. It was held in a lavish private dining room with Laura and me, Drs. Xu, Niu and Lee and another gentleman, Dr. Liyang, and Dr. Xu's driver all dining together. During the dinner, we learned that all of the doctors dining with us had grown up in the countryside and after passing numerous rigorous tests, had been sent to medical school by the communist party in their youth and had then all gone to work for the army as doctors.

I related that I had grown up in very small towns in Oregon and had worked in the fields since the age of ten and later in a cannery until graduating from college and beginning my engineering career. We also told them that Laura had been a field worker as a young child, and I think this established a bond between us, as I don't think many Westerners that travel to China give off the impression that they once labored in the fields harvesting crops.

Dr. Xu expressed interest in translating the last third of our book into Chinese and publishing it in China to which we instantly agreed. We were so delighted that our efforts to spread information about FUDA and cryoablation for breast cancer would be coming to fruition.

Dr. Niu shared with us that his son Mike would be traveling to England next year for graduate study and asked that we visit with him and Mike on our return to Guangzhou and offer advice to him regarding education and career.

Dr. Liyang astounded us by describing his research work. Previously a professor at Duke University in the US, he had transferred to work in China at another hospital, because his research would be better supported by the National Health Program. And his work was stunning! He showed that he could extract stem cells from human urine and somehow generate new cells that could cure liver disease in mice.

We asked if we could spend time with him upon our return to Guangzhou and he agreed.

We were also so impressed by Dr. Lee. It turns out that although he has a residence not far from Guangzhou, he stays at the hospital overnight during the week in order to better treat his patients. He looked as if he were about fifty years old, and I was amazed to learn he was sixty-five, my age, and still working long hours when most men retire. The medical team at FUDA is definitely dedicated and hardworking.

After having our blood drawn and making arrangements for our return, we flew to Beijing on the 8th of April to begin our Viking cruise.

I'm sure that most people in America who watch public television have seen the sumptuous Viking ads and wondered if the actual cruise was as good as the scenes advertised. I am delighted to report that the ads fall short of how wonderful this Viking cruise was!

There were about 240 people on the cruise. Our first six days of the trip were based in hotels, and we were taken sightseeing each day on nice 40-passenger busses. We were assigned an English-speaking Chinese tour guide who stayed with our 40-person group during the entire trip. Mathew was our guide's "English" name and he kept us entertained on the bus rides, providing us with history and anecdotes of life in China.

We were given radio receivers with earphones so that once we arrived at a tour site, he could lead us around on the tour and also tell us the highlights of what we were seeing. Other tours utilized megaphones for the guides, and we were soon glad of the earphones so that we weren't blamed for being loud Americans!

Our tour began in Beijing. I hadn't really thought about the size of Beijing until we were driving around the city and listening to our guide.

The population of Beijing is a staggering 21 million people and they live primarily in a fifty-mile diameter circle inside the 6th Ring Road. I realized that to compare Beijing to Oregon's cities, you would have to take the urban density of relatively small, downtown Portland and duplicate that density and size of buildings until they occupied the space north to south from Portland to Salem. From the west, that city would run from the foothills of the Coast Range to the base of the Cascade Mountains on the east.

While populated, the majority of this fifty-mile diameter circle of land in Oregon now holds, at the most, 1.1 million people. It absolutely staggered me to realize that to duplicate Beijing in Oregon you would need to increase the population in the same space in Oregon by a factor of twenty!

It is easy to see how the pollution in Beijing is sometimes so bad that children are ordered to stay home because the air is dangerous to inhale. This, despite the fact that they estimate about a third of the pollution of Beijing actually originates in the surrounding cities and not in Beijing itself!

While we were in China in the big cities, I am guessing that the average visibility due to smog was about a mile. The sun was always a pale disc in the sky and you could comfortably stare straight at it for a long time. The only city that was not this badly polluted was Shanghai, which is right on the coast.

Even out in the country, when we were on the ship going down the Yangtze River, we often encountered pollution. Rarely was the sun blindingly bright as it is in America.

Though I enjoyed seeing China on our tour, I have to admit that the country scared me. The people are so industrious, hardworking and wanting to succeed that they either have forgotten or are ignoring the fact that pollution is unforgiving and can destroy a country and eventually even a planet.

For example, while we were there, a study was released by the government that claimed 20 percent of China's farmland is badly contaminated with cadmium,

mercury, lead and other dangerous metals and com-
pounds to the point where the food grown in this soil is
bad for people's health. The study recommended that
six inches of topsoil be removed from this massive acre-
age of farmland.

Having seen what China has done in the construction of such gigantic projects as the Three Gorges Dam,
I am sure that they are more than capable of removing
this titanic amount of contaminated soil. I am confident
that they will do so, because I sincerely believe that the
will of the people of China is to have the best country in
the world, and nothing can hold them back.

In fact, after the first day of touring Guangzhou,
I was so stunned by the amount of construction and
modern buildings that I told Lori the skyline reminded
me of the spaceport in the 2009 Star Trek movie, and
that the Chinese are so industrious and hardworking,
I predicted they would be the first country to travel to
Mars.

Despite my concern about China's population and
pollution, I have to say it is the most interesting Asian
country I have ever visited. I have traveled extensively
in India and, by comparison, China is more interesting,
because it looms so large in the future fate of humanity.
When Napoleon traveled to China, he observed: "That
is a sleeping dragon. Let him sleep! If he wakes, he will
shake the world."

Moreover, it seemed to me that everything I saw in
China confirmed that the country has a history of doing
things in a big way and, translated into the modern
era, that means that China is indeed going to shake the
world! On our first day's tour, I could not believe how
large Tiananmen Square was, to be followed by disbelief

447

that the Forbidden City was vastly larger! Then, when we exited the Forbidden City, we crossed a moat, and I learned that the dirt from digging the moat was stacked up next to the Forbidden City!

This mound of earth is called Prospect Hill. It is a two-hundred-foot-high mountain about three hundred yards to the north of the Forbidden City. It is literally a man-made mountain built six hundred years ago using nothing but shovels and buckets. It staggered me to imagine any group of people having the willpower and stamina to achieve such building feats.

We spent our afternoon touring the Summer Palace, a second palace located by a man-made lake. There we saw temples, the world's longest (about 700 yards) covered walkway, a full-sized sculptured marble "boat" and numerous temples stretching up the hill by the lake. This summer palace is connected to a twenty-mile-long canal running across Beijing to the Forbidden City.

The Summer Palace was the summer residence of the Royal Court, and they traveled there by barge in the canal. It must have been a grand spectacle and a huge event when the Emperor traveled on his royal barge through the city for all to see.

On the second day in Beijing, we traveled to the Great Wall, which sits to the north of the city. We drove for over an hour and not until the last ten miles did we lose the high-rise buildings and get into a suburban, industrial, occasional farming setting.

Laura and I climbed from the tourist center at the Great Wall to a guard tower high atop a mountain. It was a difficult climb up huge, steep stairs and often across blocks of stone set at such a steep angle that my shoes sometimes slid across the surface. The end of our

448

climb rewarded us with endless vistas, for here, the air was clearer. We could see guard towers where the wall marched to the horizon in both directions. When we were done taking pictures, Laura started down a steep set of stairs. I asked her where she was going, and she said back to the bus.

The guardhouse had turned her around, and she was actually walking to Northeast China. I told her if she went that way, we would see the rest of China on foot, which is almost literally true, the Great Wall of China is so large, it is the only human structure visible from outer space.

This says so much about the Chinese. The works they do are the largest and most significant ever achieved by humanity. For example, they invented paper-making, the compass, gunpowder and print-ing, to name just a few of their amazing, life-changing inventions—a tradition they are definitely following now in the field of medicine!

We flew from Beijing to Xian and saw the Terra Cotta warriors. Again, the size of this display astounded me with the gargantuan canvas that the Chinese paint on in their public works. When you see photographs of a few of the warriors and more lined up behind, you get no sense how many of them there are. An architect on the tour with us calculated with me that the build-ing, a massive open-arch metal structure housing the Terra Cotta warriors' open pit, was approximately 250 yards long by 75 yards wide and contained an astound-ing 6,000 larger-than-life warrior statues! There are three other smaller pits at the site that contain cavalry, archers and generals. It literally is a statue army that was built by an estimated 700,000 workers.

This statue army lies close to a pyramid of dirt, which holds the tomb of Emperor Qin. The army's purpose was to guard the Emperor from his enemies in the afterlife. The tomb itself has not yet been excavated pending development of techniques that will allow archeologists to penetrate the interior with remote cameras that will not disturb the atmosphere inside and possibly degrade the contents. This has sadly happened to the terra cotta warriors. Brightly colored when unearthed, the color fades in hours after contact with the atmosphere.

We flew to Chongqing and boarded our ship to cruise down the Yangtze. The ship was even better than I imagined, and we were so lucky to have our old college friends Lonnie and Tammy just across the hall from us.

Lonnie and Tammy were such fun companions! Despite the fact that we were assigned to different tour groups, we spent time with them shopping for pearls in Beijing and exploring the Temple of Heaven. Once on board, Tammy and Laura did Tai Chi early each morning. Lonnie and I somehow missed this activity in an effort at improving our health through extra sleeping.

The meals on board the Viking ship were sumptuous and so well prepared that just getting to eat like this for a five-day cruise made the whole trip incredibly luxurious.

Our first stop along the river was to see the Shibaozhai Pagoda. This 12-story pavilion was built on a massive vertical face of rock in 1650 AD. We climbed the 99 steps to "heaven" to see the Buddhist Temple at the top.

We then sailed down to the Qutang Gorge and transferred to a smaller sightseeing vessel that took us up the Daning River in the Lesser Three Gorges. Incredible vistas of clouds, mountains and waterfalls surrounded us. Laura snapped hundreds of pictures and has already begun a "Waterfall" art series, which I can't wait to see.

We were able to see one of the ancient coffins laid to rest in a niche in a high vertical cliff. Wild monkeys were also spotted darting around the trees near shore.

We then passed through the enormous five stage locks of the Three Gorges Dam at night, which dropped us to the lower river level. A tour of the Dam site followed, which, took my breath away. This is the largest hydroelectric project on the planet; once again, the Chinese tradition of doing something incredibly large and important was apparent.

We cruised down the Yangtze, stopping at a local school sponsored by Viking Cruise Line donations. There we were entertained by the schoolchildren singing Jingle Bells with us. This was my first glimpse of the reality of the Chinese countryside, the "real China" as our friends at the hospital spoke of it, the place where 800 million Chinese live while engaged primarily in subsistence farming. A nice little boy escorted me to his desk and chair, and when I sat back I received a nasty poke in the back.

The chair had no back, just the remains of the two vertical posts, which once held the back supports and now just held a protruding nail, which I had bumped into. That nail told me so much about the conditions in the "real China." This was a different world from the five-star hotels we were growing accustomed to.

The river tour ended when we disembarked at Wu Han. The river continues to Shanghai, but the land is flat cropland, so Viking flies its clients to Shanghai to spend more time there.

We had a full day of sightseeing Shanghai, though I found it to be most beautiful at night. The old section of town along the riverbank was an interesting contrast of buildings from the 1880s and high-rise towers covered by pulsing colored lights. Tour boats with blazing colored lights filled the river and added to the spectacular vista of large buildings, buzzing humanity and a display of electric power that put any Christmas decorations in America to shame. And these buildings shimmer in alternating colored lights every night of the year!

After a final breakfast at the wonderful Shang-ri La Hotel and a goodbye to our college friends and the friends we had made on the cruise, we were on our way to the airport. What had seemed to be a long, 12-day trip at the outset was suddenly over too soon!

It was nice to return to FUDA and settle into one place where we could get some rest. The Viking tour had been so full of activities and long hikes like the Great Wall that we were pretty tired! We settled into our room and spent a long afternoon sleeping peacefully. At one point, we were told that Dr. Niu wanted to host us for a meal that night.

We were treated to a wonderful Chinese dinner prepared especially by the hospital staff and served in a private dining room off the main cafeteria eating area. Dr. Niu was there, as well as Coco, Segundo and Dr. Niu's son, Mike.

Mike had received an undergraduate degree and was planning to travel to England in the fall of 2014 to do post-graduate work. He was not sure what he wanted to go into. When we were first told weeks before that we would be meeting with Mike, I had an intuition that he would become a businessman and possibly get an MBA in England.

But in talking to him, he was expressing an interest in getting a teaching degree in English or becoming a journalist.

Then I mentioned the fact that Laura was an accomplished palm reader and that she should read his palm. Mike instantly accepted her offer. However, she needed her glasses, so while she went to the room to fetch them, I explained to the others that Laura had learned palm reading from an amazing Cuban psychic who had come to our college and stayed at my fraternity.

They seemed skeptical, being scientifically trained, so I thought I would tell them a story about the psychic that might give credibility to the fact that Laura had been taught by a master of palm reading, and she was really good at it.

The Cuban psychic was in his late 20s and was traveling around the United States visiting college campuses during the late 60s. I related that not only could he do palm readings, he also was able to find hidden objects within seconds after returning to a room. In addition, before he left us, he predicted that one of us would die within a year. We all thought one of our members who was in ROTC would die in Vietnam. However, his prediction sadly came true when one of our members died in an auto accident within a year of the psychic's prediction.

Our dinner hosts were amazed to hear this story and as I finished, Laura came in and proceeded with her palm reading session. She immediately identified Dr. Niu's son Mike as being adept at business and

encouraged him to pursue that as a career! Then she
read Dr. Niu's palm and told him that the remainder
of his life would be happy and long. He said he was
very glad to hear this because treating cancer patients
constantly made him worry that he could grow ill and
die young.

The others in the room all had their turn getting a
palm reading, and it was fun to see how Laura literally
became "Madame Laura, Palm Reader" and how her
observations agreed with people's thoughts and experiences.

After dinner, we went to Fe's room, our first visit
with her since our return from the Viking cruise. She
was in good spirits. In our absence, she had received
the CMI Cancer Micro-Vascular Intervention.

Small particles with chemotherapy drugs inside
had been embedded by Fe's doctor close to the small
tumors, which had sprouted up since Fe's previous
treatment in 2013. The doctors used an image–guided
micro-catheter to insert these tiny particles into tiny
capillary vessels supplying blood to the tumors.

Over the period of a week, the chemotherapy drugs
pass through the wall of the tiny capillary vessels into
the tumor. As more and more chemotherapy drugs are
released into the tumor, cancerous cells are destroyed.
The tiny particles developed by FUDA cannot pass
through the compact wall of normal capillaries; hence,
chemotherapy drugs embedded/sealed inside tiny
particles will not cause damage to other parts of the
body. Because of this, the overall side effects of CMI are
reduced to a minimum.

It was impressive to see Fe looking so healthy and
think that she was getting the benefit of chemotherapy

without losing her hair or being exhausted. This is because the concentration of the chemotherapy drugs delivered to each tumor was very high while the concentration of chemotherapy drugs in the rest of Fe's body was very small.

Fe said that the only problem she would have in the future from this CMI treatment was the fact that the pellets would show up on airline security cameras so she would have to go through the manual inspection each time. This is obviously a small price to pay for beating cancer and avoiding the typical side effects of chemotherapy.

Fe said she had started the CIC treatment as well and that she was having some fevers and chills on this, her third day, but that because she'd had the procedure previously, it wasn't affecting her as badly this second time.

The next morning, Dr. Lucky came to our room and again reviewed our treatment plan with us. She was very knowledgeable and spoke excellent English, so we felt confident that we were in good hands. At 11 a.m., two nurses arrived. They were very skillful in finding veins on the back of our hands and inserting IV drips.

Soon, we were receiving about half a pint of a clear liquid that contained the dendritic cells and various other lymphocyte subtypes that had been isolated from our blood and then amplified in quantity approximately 200 times using cytokines, or proteins. The result was an infusion of a huge amount of killer cells into our blood, killer cells that could kill not only cancer but also a variety of other diseases we had been exposed to in the past such as chicken pox or mumps.

They then gave us IL-2 (interleukin 2) and polyvalent vaccine injections, which improved the killer cells ability to kill tumors if they were in our body.

It's interesting to note that while this therapy was developed in the USA and has been partially approved by the FDA, bureaucratic rules in America (as explained earlier) prevent its use. Yet, it is used safely and with good results in China!

Laura and I felt a little dizzy and tired after our first round of infusion, as Dr. Lucky had warned us. Despite the fact that we had slept for quite a bit of this first day of treatment, we went to bed feeling groggy and exhausted around 8 p.m.

It had turned very warm in Guangzhou with almost 100 percent humidity. Despite this, we soon found that the air conditioning made us too cold when we started having fevers, so we opened our window. It was a long night for both of us.

We would feel cold and pile on our blankets despite the warm, humid room. Then, the fever would break and we would wake up exhausted, soaked in sweat and needing to change our pajamas (which the hospital had fortunately supplied in ample numbers).

It reminded me of when I was an eleven-year-old boy and we were planning travel to Europe in 1959. Typhoid fever was still a risk in post-war Europe, so I had to have a series of immunizations for the disease. These injections induced fevers of 104 to 105 degrees Fahrenheit in me as well as hallucinations. Fortunately for us, the CIC fevers were not as high as that.

However, with our windows open, the domestic sounds from the apartment block next to the hospital would drift into our fourth story room until about three in the morning. The heat, humidity and sing-song Chinese conversations mixed with the sounds of the street and combined with my fevers to make me feel at times as if I were in the night-time village scenes from the movie, *Apocalypse Now.*

I don't know if our DNA has such a thing as a memory, but I started feeling somehow as if I were a prisoner in China and that I would never be allowed to leave. If our DNA does have a memory, then I'm convinced that I was somehow experiencing the memories of my British grandparents and aunts who had been placed into a Japanese slave labor camp in Hong Kong during World War Two. Don't ask me how, but I really think I picked up on my grandfather's slow descent into death by starvation as he gave most of his food to his children.

The heat, humidity and this fever-induced sense of imprisonment left me feeling depressed. I was all right during the daytime when I could look around and visit with the wonderful hospital staff and, of course, Laura. It was the nights I dreaded.

And to make matters worse, Laura's liver became swollen and tender. I wrote an email to Segundo and asked if it was safe for Laura to continue, because she had suffered liver damage as a teenager due to an allergic reaction to an antibiotic. At that time, her liver became very swollen and her doctor thought she had appendicitis. However, the surgeon refused to operate, insisting that she did not have appendicitis symptoms and that he suspected a liver problem. That diagnosis was correct and fortunate, because the operation might have killed her!

Nevertheless, her liver has been compromised since then, and something about the CIC process had triggered a liver reaction, so they scheduled her for an ultrasound exam of the liver during the third day of our treatments.

Fortunately, after the second night our reactions to the CIC lessened as did my nightmares. Despite this, I was very anxious to get home and found myself unable to sleep in the middle of the night. Sometimes I would watch videos I had made on my phone of my dogs chasing balls or of fishing and skiing trips I had been on.

On the third day of our treatment, a nurse came by in the morning and told me to get ready for a visit by a local government official in fifteen minutes. She asked where Laura was, and I said she'd gone to acupuncture on the hospital's second floor so the nurse rushed off to get her while telling me to shower and clean up!

It turned out that the Province Vice Governor was in town and had heard that we were at FUDA being treated. He'd also learned we had written a book about Laura's cancer treatment, which included a description of the work going on at FUDA.

He had decided to pay us a visit! Laura was not in acupuncture as it turned out but was having ultrasound done. Luckily, instead of going to acupuncture, she decided to go back to the room. It was at the top of the stairs, still dressed in her hospital garb, she bumped into Dr. Xu and about 8 to 10 reporters and camera personal escorting the Vice Governor, Mr. Lin Shaochun, to our room. The lights came on, and Laura was introduced to the Vice Governor, right then and there. Once Dr. Xu explained who this esteemed visitor was, her eyes widened and she apologized for being dressed in her pajamas, which received a hearty laugh from the crowd. She invited the Vice Governor to our room . . . just as I finished dressing.

One second the room was peaceful and quiet, the next it was Laura, crews, lights—and I found myself shaking the Vice Governor's hand. He spoke and an interpreter explained to us that he was welcoming us to China and was grateful that we had chosen FUDA Hospital for further treatment of our cancer.

I replied that we were fortunate to be getting treatment at FUDA, because it was one of the most advanced cancer treatment hospitals in the world.

Then, they filmed Laura and me speaking with Dr. Xu and shaking hands. Then they brought Fe in. Her treatment was finished and she was leaving the next day. What a transition from when I first met her almost two weeks earlier!

She was so much healthier and robust-looking. She is very small and slim, and she actually did a little dance for the TV cameras to show that she was beating her cancer and felt better!

After the film crew left, we were told that we would be featured in a news story and that the reporters wanted to return the next day for some follow-up footage.

As if all this excitement weren't enough, we were now late for a luncheon with Madame Esther Law. Laura had made friends with Esther on her previous trip, and it turned out this was the only day we could get together before Esther left for an international travel commitment.

Esther represents the hospital at various conferences and also in the media all over the world. Her job is to spread the word about FUDA and attract

customers in need of the FUDA services since this is
a private hospital without government support. FUDA
thrives on its ability to successfully treat patients from
around the world who have found themselves without
any viable treatment options.

And what a dynamo Esther is. I can see why she is
so perfect for her job. She has a presence of focused
energy about her and nothing seems to slip past her in
a conversation. She has met dignitaries, researchers,
scientists, government officials and royalty in her travels. The hospital has blossomed with happy patients as
a result of her work. Her support staff is fluent in many
languages, and they handle all the coordination of a
patient's visit.

Segundo, who had helped us, is a member of
Esther's staff, and he is fluent in English, Chinese and
Filipino.

Esther hosted us for lunch along with Fe and her
sister Jelly. It was a lovely luncheon in a private suite
of a traditional Chinese food restaurant. We had a
lively discussion about many topics, from the FUDA
hospital outreach program that has attracted Asians,
Iranians, Iraqis, Australians, Canadians, Brits and New
Zealanders to the success motivation classes of Tony
Robinson and others that Esther admires.

It turned out that Esther is from Malaysia and has
a husband and child there. She maintains a residence
and office in Guangzhou as well as a home in Malaysia.
She returns home every few weeks to spend time with
her family. What a dynamic and accomplished person!

We returned to Fe's room and spent much of the
evening with her. Her prognosis was excellent. The latest PET scan showed her tumors were now gone.

The tumors were Herceptin receptor positive, and FUDA had already administered Herceptin to her. In some cases, this can cause cardiac problems, but Fe had no issues tolerating the drug.

Her FUDA doctors dispatched her back to Canada with instructions for her to continue Herceptin therapy, which can be used for many years to keep her cancer at bay.

What a change from her first trip to FUDA when her Canadian doctors had told her she was in Stage 4 of progressive breast cancer and the likelihood of living out the year was very low. Now, two years later, she had done a dance on Chinese national television with her newfound healthy body! Her tumors in her lymph system were gone, and now she had the hope of long-term survival with the application of Herceptin therapy in Canada.

Fe and Jelly said goodbye that night, as they had an early flight the next morning.

And that same morning, after being made woozy and weak from our CIC infusion, we learned that the CNCC film crew indeed had returned and definitely wanted to film Laura having an ultrasound! She was told to enter a closed door and enter the room. Once inside, the TV cameras were set up to film. The radiologist for the hospital could see that Laura was not comfortable with exposing herself to literally millions of Chinese. This was a moment when understanding the language would have helped. His large opened eyes somehow signaled a discomfort matching her own. Then he gave her a confident look and proceeded to lay his ultrasound tool on her midriff with a blanket covering all but a sliver of skin. Whew!

Then the film crew staged me coming down the hall and fetching Laura from the room, us shaking hands with the doctor and then walking back down the hall. Of course, no one spoke much English and the corridor was very, very long, so as we walked down the hall, we had no idea when they wanted us to stop.

The camera lights followed us and they continued filming for what seemed like minutes until we mercifully turned the corner at the long corridor's end and disappeared from view! Even if we had stayed in China long enough to see ourselves on CNCC TV, we would have no idea what exactly the story said, as we do not speak Chinese! I hope that it would make clear, as was the case, that Laura had no liver damage at all from the CIC treatment and, indeed, her liver was functioning normally.

That evening, our next to the last in China, our newly adopted daughter through a heart connection, Coco, and her friend, the wonderful Katie, took us out to dinner on their own time and expense. They wanted to treat us at a Thai restaurant they enjoyed. Getting to it allowed us to get a chance to see Guangzhou's crowded streets and sidewalks at rush hour. Never again will we ever think of our beloved city of Portland, Oregon as crowded! Sitting in the restaurant with two lovely bright girls, surrounded by the Chinese clientele, made us feel almost at home. The twenty-something's of China certainly represent China's bright future and our hearts were heavy as we realized how much we soon would be missing our new friends.

Later that evening, we were delighted to have a visit from Dr. Liyang. He had brought along a laptop with a PowerPoint presentation. He had worked at Duke in the

United States but had grown frustrated with the slow pace of his research due to FDA restrictions. Despite raising $58 million for research into his patents, he had turned his back on America and its stifling regulation of all things medical and returned to his birthplace.

And the work he has done stunned us! He can collect stem cells from a person's urine. He then takes a human egg and removes the nucleus, replacing it with the nucleus of the stem cell. This creates a human ovum clone in a Petrie dish with genetically young telomeres (as opposed to a clone transferring from a non-stem cell donor nucleus, which as a newborn is already as old as the clone source). Moreover, this process is ethical, because he is not taking a living ovum destined to become a human being. Instead, he has created one from a non-living egg and a donor stem cell.

This created ovum grows in a Petrie dish and the cells start to differentiate. We could see a small heart beating in Dr. Liyang's video! While we watched, he told us to remember what we were seeing. He had only accomplished growing a beating heart in a Petrie dish two weeks before, and he estimated we were the first Caucasian eyes to view it.

When Laura teased that he was going to get a Nobel prize for his work, he shocked us by replying he'd been on the list twice before, but his research was motivated by the high number of Chinese who get liver disease every year—at least 400,000—with very few donor livers to treat them.

After the cells in the Petrie dish differentiate sufficiently, Dr. Liyang extracts the origin cells for the liver. These cells are then ready to be inserted into a diseased liver.

To conduct tests on mice before proceeding to human testing, Dr. Liyang had to develop a mouse that would not reject human tissue. He was able to create such a line of experimental animals. He was then able to induce liver disease into the mouse. To treat the now slowly dying mouse, Dr. Liyang then found that if he injected the liver cells from the ovum into the spleen of the mouse, the mouse would distribute these new cells where needed. He said that within a period of two weeks, the diseased mouse liver had been replaced by human liver tissue that retained the size and shape of the original mouse liver.

The first mouse has now been alive for more than a year and Dr. Liyang is proceeding to work on primates. Once he has shown it is safe in primates, he will move forward with experimenting on humans.

The impact of Dr. Liyang's work will be astounding as liver disease kills millions of people each year around the planet. The only "cure" so far is not a cure at all. It's the donation of a liver, which saves only a fraction of those with liver disease each year, since we only have one liver and to have a donor, someone has to die, be healthy and be an organ donor.

Dr. Liyang estimates that the process of giving someone a new, healthy liver will take about a month and cost about $120,000—a small price to extend one's life for decades.

Dr. Xu, the hospital director, also treated us to a PowerPoint presentation in his office the next day regarding his research into insulin production. He amazed us by showing a patient that had suffered from pancreatic cancer—the same type that had killed Steve Jobs.

Yet, Dr. Xu had not only saved his patient's life by using cryoablation and CIC, he had gone on to be able to produce insulin in a manner that is less costly than the current technique of making insulin. We were glad when we got to the fourth morning and had our last infusion and injection. After one last session of fevers, we were on the road back to normal!

We were now finishing up our treatment and preparing to go back to the states. While CIC was not a pleasant experience, it was tolerable. I feel the fevers and chills were worth it given the possibility that our immune systems had at least an 80 percent chance of preventing a cancer recurrence. In addition, I was confident the process would improve our ability to ward off any other diseases we have been exposed to, such as the flu or shingles, or diseases we'd been immunized against such as typhoid fever or smallpox.

Suddenly, with the end of CIC, our trip was over. The seemingly endless horizon of being in China for a month shortened to a night where I could barely sleep for fear of missing our 6 a.m. alarm! And then with the dawn, we were wheeling our carry-on luggage down the now-familiar hospital hallway and riding in the hospital bus to the airport.

The ever-present smog and pollution of Guangzhou had worsened and reduced visibility to less than a mile, as we rode to the airport. Despite the pollution, the early hour and the fact that it was a Saturday, all of Guangzhou seemed hard at work: delivering, building, carrying, researching, treating, recycling, talking . . . in short, working.

We passed truck after truck with labor teams of thirty or forty men crowded in the back, eyes squinted against the wind, on their way to perform manual labor somewhere. Other trucks loaded to bursting with barrels or crates tied on with weak-looking rope raced down the road along with us, their drivers a picture of purpose and concentration.

I am convinced that the Chinese are absolutely the hardest-working people I have ever seen in my life. I always thought the Germans were the hardest working, but the Chinese put the Germans to utter shame in comparison.

This work ethic has allowed the Chinese to advance the progress of humanity through a series of inventions and developments that have written large on human history. At FUDA Hospital they are following this tradition by creating treatments that can defeat advanced cancer cases.

Napoleon was right, that China would shake the world if awakened. But that is not necessarily a bad thing for the world, because when it comes to treating cancer, FUDA is leading the world to a cure.

Chapter 23: Conclusion

Alex

While writing the conclusion to this book, I remembered the happiness the Sonja Henie movie gave me when it reminded me of Laura in Sun Valley. I was suddenly struck with curiosity, wondering if Sonja was still alive and what kind of career she had after the Sun Valley film. I looked for her name on the Internet and read that the beautiful and talented Sonja had died at the age of fifty-seven after a long battle with leukemia, or cancer of the white blood cells.

It hit me like a hammer blow. I had seen so much of Laura in Sonja and so much of Sonja in Laura in that film: the sense of humor, the joy for life, the passion for accomplishment that made Sonja a great athlete and movie star and Laura a great painter, mother, outdoor person, partner and activist. In Sonja's fate, I saw Laura's potential fate: a long struggle with cancer followed by death before reaching sixty.

If it hadn't been for the pioneering work of Dr. Littrup, the possibility that the immune effect has actually cured Laura, or perhaps a combination of the hormone suppression, radiation, the naturopaths and acupuncture, in the end, who knows—Laura might not have survived her bout with cancer.

I sincerely hope that someday there is a cure for all types of cancer, so that the world will not be robbed of someone like Sonja Henie far before her time, and which occurred with the passing of Elizabeth Edwards, who was treated in the traditional way for breast cancer shortly after Laura.

After writing this book, I have to say that I'm overwhelmed by three words: love, faith and courage.

As a person gets older, they begin to experience very important events in their lives. Tragedies, triumphs . . . They are part of life and so are the sayings that accompany them, such as "a sigh of relief."

I didn't really know what a sigh of relief was until Laura was pronounced cancer free by the doctors in Detroit who were using the advanced gas chromatograph scanning machine. There was no more cancer anywhere in Laura's body! When I heard that, I heaved a sigh of relief and slept like a log for weeks afterwards. This was confirmed later when the site of Laura's breast infection near the cryoablation site showed no cancer at the three-year mark!

That sigh of relief was the result of those three words: love, faith and courage.

Laura showed tremendous courage throughout her ordeal. She wanted to keep her breast, and she wanted to cure her cancer. Despite many of the doctors in her hometown arguing against it, Laura had the courage to proceed down the path of cryoablation.

At the same time, she had faith in my ability to help her sort out her options and, indeed, to even find those options somewhere else out in the world. I had faith that somehow, somewhere, I could find a way for her to keep her breast and cure her cancer. My deep love for her motivated me to look so hard, and it was her love for her mother and the prayers she said as a teenager that someday she could help to find a cure for breast cancer that gave her the motivation to pursue cryoablation.

At the time she offered up those prayers as a young girl, she imagined herself as a medical researcher. However, every lab needs its guinea pig, and she realized that if that was the role she needed to play to try and find a cure for cancer, she would do it gladly.

Then we both had to have faith in the advice of all the doctors in Detroit at Karmanos, and especially in Dr. Littrup, and that they in turn had to have faith in us, that we would be fair and open-minded in the event the cancer returned.

Finally, we all had to have faith that the science was right, that cryoablation can kill cancer. And realizing that was the ultimate issue, we can't help but feel a deep and abiding love for all those brave women who for more than ten years submitted to cryoablation first and then allowed a mastectomy to occur two weeks later so that their tissue could be analyzed to confirm that cryoablation does kill cancer cells.

It is to all those brave, pioneering women that we dedicate this book and tell them, with all our hearts, "Thank you."

Thoughts from patient Fe

Fe wanted to share her thoughts with the readers so I have compiled her emails and comments here without editing to allow her own voice to come through.

Fe was first treated in December of 2012, and then she returned to Canada. In March of 2013 she returned for follow-up treatment. Her words are from her various emails to Laura.

Hi Laura,

I have been here (FUDA) since March 6th and will be leaving April 3rd 2013.

My treatment has been very hectic since I arrived. My PET scan result was very progressive. No cancer was seen in my primary breast or liver. My bone tumors have all disappeared. The only remaining cancer is a little spot in a lymph node in my left shoulder. I am wishing I was cancer free without the little spot that is left! Sigh!

I am now on my 8th day of full IVs in bed. I am bored already and having intense cabin fever. They are bombarding me with full blast treatment.

My first day I had a PET scan. Then the next day a transarterial. The following day they implanted 10 new iodine pellets around the lymph node tumor in my left shoulder. That's why I'm in bed this long; it has been a wearing treatment.

My surgeon said after this stay I will just be back for follow-up treatments, but they can't say when, because they want to make sure the anti-cancer IVs that are being administered will work properly in my system.

I am up early this morning to do some paper work and soon I will be having my Herceptin and other follow-up IVs.

My Dr. said I could have my Herceptin in Canada, because I told them we can't afford the rest of the follow-up treatments. My PICC they have inserted here in my left arm will stay until my Herceptin is administered back in Canada.

Once again, I should be cancer free without that little small spot in my shoulder.

God the healer was so good to me. All the consultants, surgeons and doctors came to congratulate my progress and give me hugs until it became a very hilarious scene in my room. All of them felt my ecstatic cry of joy was an achievement on their part.

I think I have truly touched these Chinese medical experts' hearts in one way or another.

I have seen the head nurse and my doctor in tears of joy at the success of my treatment.

My husband, David, was so happy as, just like me, he wanted me to be cancer free.

The nurses and doctors here are my heroes. I'll keep you posted regarding my treatment and progress once I've returned to Canada.

Love and prayers,
Fe Juan Zahorodniuk

Notes on March 15, 2013

Hi Laura,

My room was swarming with doctors, four surgeons yesterday. One of them is my surgeon, so I asked him about my one small lymph node with the 10 iodine seed implants.

He said the tumor will take time to dissolve but he reassured me, it will be gone for sure. I asked him twice if it will really be gone and he said "YES" very surely and strongly.

Since I am not yet totally cancer free, I want to tell you that I believe I soon will be based on what my doctor told me at FUDA. He said that my standing right now is not even considered stage 1 cancer, so I've progressed from stage 4 to "less than stage 1."

God's healing miracles have made this possible. Thanks for your prayers as well and for joining me at FUDA!

Love & prayers
Fe Juan Zahorodniuk

From March 21, 2013

Hi Laura,

I wanted to give you a list of people I realize I owe my life to.

Without them I wouldn't have made it.

Dr. Li Haibo, vice president of the Old FUDA hospital, my surgeon for iodine seed implants and cryoablation.

Dr. Zhou, my Transarterial Chemo Embolization (TACE) doctor.

Dr. Shi Juan Juan and Dr. Zhou Jangfen, Physicians.

Dr. Park Piao from New FUDA hospital who did my fourth transarterial. He is the Director of Micro vessel Intervention Therapy.

Wei Changqun, head nurse for Periphery Inserted Central Catheter (PICC).

Thanks for letting me thank them in your book.

Fe

And then in May of 2014 after Fe's return to Guangzhou for further treatment, Fe wrote:

March 22, 2013

My heartfelt thanks to my husband David, my hero, willingly committed to extend my life to our last penny.

Shelly, Eleanor and Brian, whose generosity of heart cannot be fathomed.

My sister Jelly, my guardian angel who is always on my side at FUDA fighting for my life.

Erin, my sister-in-law who accompanied me on my first treatment.

Collyne & Wes who burned their midnight oil for researches.

Lastly, to Laura & Alex who know the content of my soul & being.

Status of Fe's 5th treatment

I have been dealing with recurrence of breast cancer since late 2013 when multiple lymph nodes—not organs—were found to have cancer.

Regrettably, we blame ourselves for the cancer recurrence. We had run short of funds from previous treatments by naturopaths, herbalists and, of course, Fuda. In October 2013, I was supposed to return to

FUDA for Immunotheraphy to keep the cancer cells at a level that's non-detectable and stable. However, we could not afford that return trip and, as a result, tumors returned in my lymph system.

This meant that I had to travel to FUDA in the spring of 2014 for more aggressive treatment of the lymph nodes. After that treatment, I am now on a regimen of Herceptin, which should prevent a further recurrence as long as I stay on that drug.

This brings me to our next subject of funding and suggestions to people reading this on how you may fund a trip to Fuda. It is strongly recommended that if you are relying on in-country funding or reimbursement from your home country that you contact the Health Services branch of your government before you go on your trip to see if any treatments may be covered. Our experience in Alberta, Canada was that Alberta Health Services declined to reimburse us for the following treatments in China: Herceptin, Iodine seeds and cryo-surgery.

Fundraisers among friends and family can often be very helpful to lessen the financial burden. The odds are very good that a lot of people care about you enough to help save your life and help you receive less punishing treatments than conventional treatments.

Sources

Unlike a scholarly paper, if I made reference to a publication in the text I simply quoted it there along with the reference information rather than numbering and footnoting the reference. Therefore, the number system below is just a way of organizing each reference, some of which have already been described and others that I think might be of interest to the more technically oriented reader.

In some cases below, I have taken the liberty of copying part of the article text that I found most interesting and placing it directly below the reference information.

My biggest disappointment in writing this book has been my inability to procure a copy of the work done by Tanaka and published in *Skin Cancer*. I think this will prove to be a very important study, but it was beyond my resources to locate a copy of this work at the time of writing as it was published years earlier in Japan and has never been translated to English to my knowledge.

In the end, the important part of his study is the result: 42 percent of women who were treated with cryoablation had no recurrence of cancer at five years. Before cryoablation in America can claim this kind of success rate, many studies will have to be done. Tana-ka's results should be a clarion call of promise that cryo-ablation may well hold the key to curing cancer.

Now it is up to all of us to ensure that cryoablation is given a chance to prove itself.

1. "Tumor protector identified. Study finds VEGF in-hibits cancer-fighting dendritic cells." http://www.mc.vanderbilt.edu/reporter/?ID=95 (10/28/05 17:59:10).

"In an article appearing in the journal *Nature Medicine*, investigators show that vascular endo-thelial growth factor (VEGF) serves as a crucial ac-complice in cancer cells' ability to escape the human body's natural impulse to defend itself."

2. "Scancell - Science - ImmunoBody™ Vaccines." http://www.scancell.co.uk/pages/science/immuno-body_vaccines.htm (10/28/05 18:09:43).

"Cancer vaccines represent a highly attractive ap-proach to cancer therapy. In contrast to current treatments such as chemotherapy and radiotherapy, small non-toxic doses of a vaccine may be adminis-tered to a patient to stimulate an immune response. It is generally accepted that to be effective against cancer, a vaccine needs to target dendritic cells to stimulate both parts of the cellular immune system; the helper cell system (known as the CD4-mediat-ed response), which stimulates inflammation at the tumour site; and the cytotoxic T-lymphocyte or CTL response (known as the CD8-mediated response) in which cells of the immune system are primed to recognise and kill specific cells."

3. "NML and SANAS represent South Africa internationally Pretoria." http://www.nml.csir.co.za/news/20010322/ 20010322articles.htm (11/02/05 19:45:12)

"Cryogenics

The study and use of materials at very low temperature. The upper limit of cryogenic temperatures has not been agreed on, but it is suggested that the term cryogenics be applied to all temperatures below –150 °C."

4. "Cryoablation probe patent." http://www.fresh-patents.com/Cryoablation-probe-dt20041028p-tan20040215294.php (11/02/05 19:48:52)

A gas-based cryoablation probe is provided with a shaft having a closed distal end adapted for insertion into a body. A supply conduit is disposed longitudinally within the shaft for flowing gas towards the distal end, and a return conduit is disposed longitudinally within the shaft for flowing gas from the distal end. The gas is maintained at a lower pressure within the return conduit than in the supply conduit. A heat exchanger is disposed within the shaft in thermal communication with the supply conduit and return conduit to exchange heat from gas in the supply conduit to gas in the return conduit. A vacuum jacket is adapted to provide thermal isolation of the heat exchanger from the shaft.

"Agent: Townsend And Townsend And Crew, LLP. San Francisco, CA, US.

"Inventors: Peter J. Littrup, Alexei V. Babkin, Robert Duncan, Pramod Kerkar, Sergey T. Boldarev. BRIEF SUMMARY OF THE INVENTION [0010] Embodiments of the invention thus provide a cryoablation probe that overcomes certain deficiencies of the prior art. In some embodiments, a gas-based cryoablation probe is provided with a shaft having a closed distal end adapted for insertion into a body. A supply conduit is disposed longitudinally within the shaft for flowing gas towards the distal end, and a return conduit is disposed longitudinally within the shaft for flowing gas from the distal end. The gas is maintained at a lower pressure within the return conduit than in the supply conduit. A heat exchanger is disposed within the shaft in thermal communication with the supply conduit and return conduit to exchange heat from gas in the supply conduit to gas in the return conduit. A vacuum jacket is adapted to provide thermal isolation of the heat exchanger from the shaft."

5. "Features." http://www.med.wayne.edu/PR/
AnnualReport/00-01/F-freezing%20the%20dead-
ly%20spread.htm (11/02/05 20:00:10)

"Last fall, Dr. Peter Littrup became the first person in the country to use Endocare's CRYOcare System to treat a lung tumor using only computed tomography guidance (CT, or "CAT scan"). With new cryoablation technology, Dr. Littrup froze a cancerous lung tumor at minus 40 degrees centigrade, a temperature cancer cells cannot survive.

"Endocare Inc. develops and manufactures cryosurgical and stent technologies for applications in oncology and urology. Its initial devices have concentrated on prostate cancer, but new technologies are in development for treating tumors in the kidney, breast, lung and liver. Sanarus Medical, Inc., specializes in the development of innovative surgical devices and technologies for the treatment of tumors in women, focusing on breast tumors and gynecological diseases.

"'We plan to continue our collaborations and, though we are still in early clinical stages, we'd like to see cryoablation emerge as a comfortable, minimally invasive adjunct—or possible alternative—to current treatments for cancer patients,' Dr. Littrup said."[5]

6. "A 'second chance' at life." http://www.advocate-health.com/immc/info/library/ham/win04/immc8.html?heart (11/02/05 20:01:20)

"A 'second chance' at life Detroit physician saved from a fatal heart condition by Illinois Masonic doctors.

"A renowned Detroit radiologist, Peter Littrup, M.D., has cared for hundreds of people. Last September, though, he experienced what it's like to be a patient. While in Chicago for a medical conference, Dr. Littrup was visiting friend Seth Kaplan, M.D., and his family in Lincoln Park when he began having chest pain. "It felt like someone was ripping my chest apart," he says.

"Realizing Dr. Littrup needed immediate attention, Dr. Kaplan, a practicing ophthalmologist also board-certified in emergency medicine, took him to Advocate Illinois Masonic Medical Center.

"According to Alvaro Montoya, M.D., a cardiothoracic surgeon at Illinois Masonic, Dr. Littrup's aorta had partially ruptured—a dangerous condition that required immediate surgery. 'A five-hour procedure repaired the dissection by replacing the aorta and aortic valve and re-implanting the coronary arteries," Dr. Montoya says. "The survival rate for someone with an aortic dissection is very low, but Dr. Littrup was awake and alert after surgery and was able to return to Detroit five days later. He's a very lucky man.'

"It's a sentiment Dr. Littrup himself shares. 'The medical staff miraculously saved me, giving me a second chance at life.'"

7. "Cryosurgical Ablation of Miscellaneous Solid Tumors Other Than Liver or Prostate Tumors." http://www.regence.com/trgmedpol/surgery/sur132.html (12/02/05 21:17:49)

"Cryosurgical ablation (hereafter "cryosurgery") involves freezing of target tissues, most often by inserting into the tumor a probe through which coolant is circulated. Cryosurgery may be performed as an open surgical technique or as a closed procedure under laparoscopic or ultrasound guidance. The hypothesized advantages of cryosurgery include improved local control and benefits common to any minimally invasive procedure (e.g., preserving normal organ tissue, decreasing morbidity, decreasing length of hospitalization). Potential complications of cryosurgery include those caused by hypothermic damage to normal tissue adjacent to the tumor, structural damage along the probe track and secondary tumors, if cancerous cells are seeded during probe removal.

"Breast Cancer

"Three studies described the outcome of cryosurgery for advanced primary or recurrent breast cancer in

72 patients. (3-5) Cryosurgery was performed percutaneously with ultrasound guidance (n=15) or during an open surgical procedure (n=57). Patients were
treated for advanced primary disease (44 percent) or
recurrent tumors (56 percent). Tanaka reported the
largest retrospective series: 9 patients with advanced
primary tumors and 40 with recurrent disease. (3)
The author reported 44 percent survival of primary
breast cancer patients (n=9) at 3 and 5 years, but
did not report survival duration or other outcomes
for those with recurrent or metastatic disease. The
report also did not adequately describe selection cri-
teria for those enrolled in the study, details of the
procedure and procedure-related adverse events. The
other studies were smaller series of patients and also
were inadequate with respect to study design, analysis and reporting of results. (4-6) Furthermore, the
study by Pfleiderer and colleagues was a pilot trial
to evaluate technical limitations of the procedure.
(4) Tumors were excised and evaluated by pathology
days to weeks after cryosurgery, and the authors reported incomplete necrosis in tumors greater than
23 mm in diameter.

"One case series by Sabel and colleagues explored
the role of cryoablation as an alternative to surgical
excision as a primary treatment of early stage breast
cancer. (7) This phase 1 study included 29 patients
who underwent cryoablation of primary breast cancers measuring less than 2 cm in diameter, followed

1 to 4 weeks later by standard surgical excision. Cryoablation was successful in patients with invasive ductal carcinoma less than 1.5 cm in diameter and with less than 25 percent ductal carcinoma in situ identified in a prior biopsy specimen."

8. "Arch Surg—The Use of Cryosurgery for Breast Cancer, January 1998, Ablin 133 (1): 106." http://arch-surg.ama-assn.org/cgi/content/extract/133/1/106 (12/02/05 21:22:58)

"In their report regarding the use of cryosurgery for breast cancer, Staren et al[1] bring to bear the latest technology permitting the precise placement of cryoprobes and monitoring of the cryolesion. However, it is important to communicate that cryosurgery of breast cancer, for small and localized as well as advanced and unresectable disease, has been used for almost 30 years. As early as 1968 and through 1994, Tanaka[2] has treated 9 primary advanced and 40 recurrent breast cancers with cryosurgery. All cases were considered incurable: advanced, unresectable, and resistant to radiotherapy, chemotherapy and endocrine therapy. The 3- and 5-year survival rate for these primary advanced breast cancers treated cryosurgically was 44 percent.[2]

"In 1976, LePivert[3] reported the cryosurgical treatment of 7 cases of locally advanced breast cancer (5 stage III, 2 stage IV) using single and multiple cryoprobes."

9. "In Situ Ablation Of Breast Tumors. What Is The State Of The Art?" http://www.cancernews.com/category.asp?Cat=3&AID=226 (12/02/05 21:27:03)

"It is also important to bear in mind that surgery is still the 'gold standard' for the treatment of breast cancer, and for cancers detected at an early stage, the results are excellent. With lumpectomy and radiation for small tumors, recurrence rates are low and survival is high. And while there may be some cosmetic alteration, usually women are very pleased with the appearance of the breast after lumpectomy and radiation. Studies with thousands of women, followed for many years, will be necessary to show that the results with in situ ablation are just as good before it can replace surgery as first line therapy. It is too early to say which method will be the 'state of the art' for breast cancer ablation. It is most likely that different techniques may be necessary for different patients. Each of these techniques holds tremendous potential, and continued research is crucial. At this time, most of the on-going trials consist of in situ ablation followed by standard surgical resection. It is important for women to participate in these studies, for this information will hopefully allow women in the near future to have their breast cancers treated without surgical excision."

10. "Breast Cancer: Cryosurgery successfully treats some early-stage tumors, May 25, 2004." http://www.obgyn.net/newsheadlines/womens_health-

Breast_Cancer-20040525-18.asp (12/02/05 21:30:17)

"2004 MAY 25—(NewsRx.com & NewsRx.net)—Imagine being treated for breast cancer right in your doctor's office, with an incision as small as a pinprick to show for it.

"New research from seven cancer centers suggests this might be possible one day.

"In a process called cryoablation, surgeons freeze the tumors to kill the cells. The technique is already used as a non-surgical treatment for benign breast disease. Results of the new study, published in the May 2004 issue of the Annals of Surgical Oncology, found cryoablation is effective at killing cancerous cells in small tumors.

"Although still an experimental treatment for breast cancer, these findings move cryosurgery one step closer to clinical application for early stage disease.

"As mammograms and other imaging techniques become more sophisticated, doctors are able to find breast cancer earlier, when tumors are very small. Progress in detection has led to an increased interest in developing alternatives to traditional surgery for early-stage cancer.

"'This trial shows that cryoablation is a safe,

well-tolerated, office-based procedure that holds real promise for treating early-stage breast cancer,' says Michael Sabel, M.D., a surgical oncologist from the University of Michigan Comprehensive Cancer Center and lead author of the study.

"Of the 27 procedures performed in the study, cryoablation successfully destroyed all cancers less than 1.0 centimeters in diameter. The procedure was equally effective for tumors between 1.0 and 1.5 centimeters in those women with a type of cancer called invasive ductal carcinoma who did not have significant ductal carcinoma in situ, a non-invasive breast cancer, in the surrounding tissue. Cryoablation was not shown effective for tumors larger than 1.5 centimeters in diameter.

"'Right now, its application should be limited to patients with invasive ductal carcinomas no larger than 1.5 centimeters. But we're continuing to determine the boundaries of the procedure,' Sabel says.

"He notes that a follow-up study will begin soon at U-M and other centers to learn more. 'But as is the case with this study,' he cautions, 'patients enrolled in that study will be required to undergo a lumpectomy following the procedure. More data is needed before we'll be able to offer cryosurgery alone as a treatment for breast cancer.'

"Funding for the study came from Sanarus Medical Inc., who developed the cryoablation probe used in the study."

11. "Cryosurgery More Effective in Treating Some Prostate Cancer." http://www.pslgroup.com/dg/7ffa. htm (12/02/05 21:43:52)

"PITTSBURGH, April 30, 1996—A recent study conducted by urologists and researchers at Allegheny General Hospital (AGH) and published in the March issue of *Urology* confirms that prostate cryosurgery is at least twice as effective as traditional methods of treating localized prostate cancer.

"Led by Ralph Miller, M.D., and Jeffrey Cohen, M.D., AGH urologists and professors at Medical College of Pennsylvania and Hahnemann University, the study of patients who underwent prostate cryosurgery at AGH offers greater hope for men who wish to avoid radical prostatectomy and radiation therapy as treatment options.

"According to the study, cryosurgical removal of the diseased prostate tissue has a failure rate of just 35 percent compared to traditional therapies, which have failure rates as high as 85 percent.

"The study also supports that removal of the cancerous prostate tissue can be performed with fewer complications than previously encountered, involving less pain for the patient and a quicker recovery.

"Additionally, the study notes, newer cryotechnology enables surgeons to bring larger volumes of tissue to lower temperatures than previously possible, increasing the capabilities of the technique."

12. "Untitled." http://www.prostatepointers.org/ prostate/lay/apilgrim/chapter12.html (12/02/05 21:53:20)

"Results of Cryosurgery

"Dr. Gary Onik reported negative biopsies in 82.6 percent of his patients at 3 months following cryosurgery. Dr. Fred Lee found no cancer in 92 percent of his patients at 3 months. The University of California San Francisco reported that 89 percent had negative biopsies at 3 months. Dr. Jeff Cohen showed 69 percent negative biopsy at 21 or more months after the cryo.

"Dr. Fred Lee is preparing to publish 6-year data on his patients. His data appears to be better than that for radical prostatectomy.

Cryosurgery is a genuine alternative for the patient. Yet there is a need to accumulate long-term survival data.

"It was suggested by certain academic sources that a

randomized study is needed to compare surgery and cryosurgery. To do it properly, a large number of patients with similar stage disease would be randomized to either cryosurgery or radical surgery. The patient would have little to say about which treatment they were assigned. The difficulty of conducting such a study is the moral dilemma of how to select the patients for such treatment."

13. "Berkeley Engineering—Forefront." http://www. coe.berkeley.edu/forefront/fall02/cancer.html (12/02/05 21:56:32)

"In the study, researchers froze melanoma cells at about -14 degrees Celsius, a temperature at which cells on the outer rim of a frozen lesion often survive cryosurgery. The cells were then treated with trace amounts of bleomycin, which is toxic to cancer cells but can be ineffective because it has difficulty penetrating cells. What the researchers learned was that freezing helped the bleomycin enter the cells. Even tiny amounts of the toxic chemical, several magnitudes smaller than what is typically used in patients, killed most of the cancer cells.

"Rubinsky hopes that by combining the two therapies scientists can create a regimen that's more effective and less debilitating than either strategy used alone. 'When you add chemotherapy to cryosurgery you have a minimally invasive technique that has the precision of a scalpel,' he says. The next step is to find the best way to administer bleomycin or other chemotherapy agents to the cancerous cells, says Onik, Rubinsky's longtime collaborator on cryosurgery research. 'We don't know whether it's better to inject the bleomycin intravenously or to inject it directly into the cancer,' says Onik, now director of surgical imaging at Celebration Health, a treatment center in Orlando, Florida. 'Certain details still have to be worked out.'"

14. "Immunologic Response to Cryoablation of Breast Cancer—Storming Media." http://www.stormingmedia.us/55/5512/A551234.html (12/02/05 21:58:19)

"Abstract

"The objective of this project is to characterize the anti-tumor immunologic response to cryosurgery, a new minimally invasive approach to the ablation of breast cancer. The work consists of both murine and human studies, expanding upon reports that cryosurgery of primary tumors has been reported to be capable of developing specific anti-tumor immunological responses that can prevent the growth of micrometastasis. Because of conflicts with other grant support the grant was relinquished effective August 31, 2003. While the project is ongoing, several interesting findings were discovered. Murine studies, utilizing the MT-901 mammary adenocarcinoma cell line in BALB/c mice, demonstrated a Th1 cytokine response to cryoablation as compared to surgical excision. Mice treated with cryoablation had long-term tumor specific memory as demonstrated by tumor re-challenge. Immunologic studies demonstrated an early but brief antibody response, a regional T-cell response and a systemic NK cell response, although no long-lasting systemic T-cell response could be identified. A manuscript is presently in preparation. Human immunologic studies have been initiated, but the results are too early for interpretation at this time."

15. "CRYOSURGERY—Annual Review of Biomedical Engineering, 2(1):157—Abstract." http://arjournals. annualreviews.org/doi/abs/10.1146/annurev.bio-eng.2.1.157 (12/15/05 22:45:57)

"Cryosurgery is a surgical technique that employs freezing to destroy undesirable tissue. Developed first in the middle of the nineteenth century it has recently incorporated new imaging technologies and is a fast growing minimally invasive surgical technique. A historical review of the field of cryosurgery is presented, showing how technological advances have affected the development of the field. This is followed by a more in-depth survey of two important topics in cryosurgery: (a) the biochemical and biophysical mechanisms of tissue destruction during cryosurgery and (b) monitoring and imaging techniques for cryosurgery."

16. "Mistletoe." http://www.wholehealthmd.com/
    refshelf/substances_view/1,1525,10109,00.html
    (03/04/06 07:21:16)

"What Is It?

"Long before holiday revelers started a custom of
kissing under the mistletoe, traditional folk healers
used this evergreen shrub to treat various ailments.
While they recognized early on that the sticky white
berries of the mistletoe plant were poisonous, they
brewed the leathery leaves into a therapeutic tea, a
remedy that has long endured for ailments ranging
from nervous tension to skin sores.

"A liquid extract containing key medicinal compo-
nents of the mistletoe plant has also been used for
decades to treat cancer, mainly in Europe and parts
of Asia. This practice is considered quite controver-
sial in the United States, however. Recent news reports were sparked by the revelation that actress
Suzanne Somers was using mistletoe to treat her
breast cancer."

"Health Benefits

"Folk healers in Europe and particularly in Asia have
long relied on mistletoe for treating everything from
rapid heart rates and high blood pressure to epilepsy.

"But by far the most popular use of mistletoe to-

492

day—particularly in Europe—is for treating cancer. Austrian philosopher Rudolf Steiner introduced this idea in 1916 as an outgrowth of a system of thought called 'anthroposophy.' According to Steiner, tumors represent an error in the regulation of the physical or spiritual body.

"In Steiner's view, just as mistletoe is a parasite on a host tree, so is cancer a parasite on the human body. Following homeopathic principles of 'like cures like' and applying his own version of homeopathic dilution and potentization (the more diluted the substance the more potent it becomes) he felt that tiny doses of the poisonous mistletoe plant could stimulate the body to rectify its so-called 'error' in producing malignant tumors. Mistletoe could coax the body back to a state of equilibrium and regulate the area where tumors had been allowed to develop.

"Today, it's estimated that the Germans alone spend more than $30 million annually on mistletoe preparations to fight cancer. A recent survey of 200 physicians in Germany revealed that nearly 80 percent were inclined to recommend unconventional cancer therapies to their patients, and mistletoe was a clear favorite. Nearly 45 percent reported prescribing this herb. The anthroposophically based Lukas Clinic in Arlesheim, Switzerland, is devoted almost exclusively to cancer treatment and has been using mistletoe for nearly 75 years.

"The U.S. Food and Drug Administration hasn't reviewed or approved the use of mistletoe in any form.

"For cancer support: In Europe, injections are given in the morning three to seven times a week, with doses adjusted over time based on the patient's general health, type of cancer, sex and age. The injection is given near the location of the tumor, and sometimes directly into a tumor on the liver, cervix and esophagus. Typically, treatment lasts several months to years.

"Cautions

"If you have cancer, see a doctor and discuss your desire to use mistletoe or any other herb. Mistletoe should only be considered as a complement to other cancer treatments, such as chemotherapy and radiation, that your doctor recommends.

"Because the mistletoe dosing schedule for cancer treatment is extremely complex, it should only be undertaken by a physician familiar with its use.

"It's particularly important to consult your doctor before taking mistletoe if you have heart condition, gastrointestinal disease or central nervous system problems.

"Never use the fruits (berries) of the mistletoe plant for any medicinal purpose; they are poisonous and can cause vomiting, abnormally low or high blood pressure, seizures, slow heart beat and even death.

"Because mistletoe has been shown to stimulate uterine activity in laboratory animals, pregnant or breast-feeding women should avoid the herb.

"Mistletoe cancer treatment with formulations available in Europe (not the homeopathic versions found domestically) can be quite expensive over time, costing as much as $160 (U.S. dollars) a day for nine to 21 days.

"Keep the mistletoe plant and all extracts and formulations made with it out of reach of children."

17. "Small (<2.0 cm) Breast Cancers: Mammographic and US Findings at US-guided Cryoablation—Initial Experience." (http://radiology.rsnajnls.org/cgi/content/full/233/3/857 (04/23/07 10:51:48)

"Small (<2.0 cm) Breast Cancers: Mammographic and US Findings at US-guided Cryoablation—Initial Experience1.

"Marilyn A. Roubidoux, M.D., Michael S. Sabel, M.D., Janet E. Bailey, M.D., Celina G. Kleer, M.D., Katherine A. Klein, M.D., and Mark A. Helvie, M.D.

"PURPOSE: To determine the mammographic and ultrasonographic (US) findings at cryoablation of small solitary invasive breast cancers and compare them with presence of residual malignancy after treatment.

"MATERIALS AND METHODS: Institutional review board approval and informed patient consent were obtained. Nine patients with small solitary invasive breast cancers diagnosed at core biopsy were treated with US-guided cryoablation and a 2.7-mm cryoprobe. Mean cancer size was 12 mm (range 8–18 mm); four were palpable. Tabletop argon gas–based cryoablation system with a double–freeze-thaw protocol was used to treat cancers in outpatient setting. Tumor sites were excised at lumpectomy 2–3 weeks after cryoablation. Findings at mammography and US before, during and after cryoablation were assessed to categorize densities and masses on mammograms and masses on US images with Breast Imaging Reporting and Data System (BI-RADS); maximum cancer size was measured. Imaging findings and clinical breast examination data were compared with histologic findings from lumpectomy specimens to determine presence of intraductal or invasive cancer.

"RESULTS: With US guidance, ice balls (maximal mean size, 4.4 cm) were formed around cancers. Before excision, eight patients underwent mammography; all had new focal densities (maximum size 2.5–5.0 cm) at cancer sites. Six patients underwent pre-excisional US; 100 percent of them had new hyperechogenicity in tissue surrounding cancer site. Seven (78 percent) of nine patients had no residual cancer; specimens contained fat necrosis. One patient had a small focus of invasive cancer; one had extensive multifocal ductal carcinoma in situ. Patients with BI-RADS category 1 or 2 densities on mammograms or nonpalpable tumors had no residual malignancy. No residual invasive cancer occurred in tumors 17 mm or smaller or in cancers without spiculated margins at US.

"CONCLUSION: After cryoablation, there was increased echogenicity at US and increased density at mammography; these findings were observed in areas that approximated location and size of the ice ball. Tumor size, mammographic density and US characteristics may be indicators of likelihood of complete cryoablation.

"Clinical Data

"All nine patients completed the cryoablation protocol according to the methods described. Maximum cancer size at US or mammography before core-needle biopsy was 8–18 mm (mean, 12 mm). No procedure was prematurely terminated because of patient discomfort or patient request, and no patient needed any conscious sedation or post-procedural narcotic pain medications. There were no major or minor complications, which included immediate or peri-procedural (within the time period up to extirpative surgery) complications.

"Prior to cryoablation, the mean distance from the most superficial margin (relative to the transducer and the skin) of the tumor or the biopsy site to the skin surface, as measured at US, was 9 mm (range, 5–12 mm); that is, the surface of some tumors was only 5 mm deep from the skin surface. The mean distance between the posterior margin of the tumor and the anterior side of the chest wall (ie, pectoralis muscle) was 8 mm (range, 0–18 mm); that is, at the time of US, some tumors appeared to be immediately adjacent to the pectoralis muscle. Despite the close margins of some tumors to either the skin or the chest wall, no complications occurred. There was no skin injury to suggest thermal injury, and there were no large hematomas or delayed occurrences of them.

The results are summarized in Tables 1 and 2, and they include precryoablation clinical patient data, maximum tumor size, core-needle biopsy data, mammographic and US findings and before and after cryoablation and histologic data. The patients are listed in chronologic order (i.e., patient 1 was the first one to undergo cryoablation and patient 9 was the last)."

18. "Cryoablation in China." http://www.bgwicc.org.cn/english/2281.html

"US Patent Application of Alexei V. Babkin, Peter J. Littrup and William J. Nydam for Method and System for Croyablation Treatment. The present invention pertains generally to systems and methods for performing a cryosurgical procedure. More particularly, the present invention pertains to systems and methods that use a probe having a cryotip for cooling biological tissues to cryogenic temperatures. The present invention is particularly but not exclusively, useful as a closed-loop system wherein a liquid refrigerant remains in a liquid state as it is cycles through the system between its source and the cryotip of a probe."

About the Authors

Laura Ross-Paul

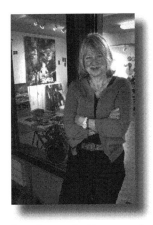

Laura attended Oregon State University in the late sixties. She was an anti-war activist, working as a political cartoonist for an underground anti-war newspaper. After graduating with her Masters of Fine Art from Portland State University in Portland, OR, she began her teaching career as an Adjunct Professor of Art specializing in painting and drawing the figure. She also began her continuing career as a gallery represented studio artist. That career blossomed and can be viewed at her website, LauraRoss-Paul.com and her gallery website, FroelickGallery.com.

Laura met her husband Alex while involved in the Vietnam War peace movement. They have three talented children, Sean, Louie and Emma who are college graduates and work independently in creative fields.

Laura had enough interest in science to receive an extra Bachelor of Science degree. Her curious mind

501

often pushes the envelope technically as she develops techniques for her paintings. She credits her ability to anticipate a successful outcome before having tried something new as a contributing factor in trusting Dr. Littrup's approach to using freezing to cure breast cancer.

Laura continues to keep a studio and exhibition practice going. She joins her husband in his many outdoor adventures, most recently adding stand-up paddling to her activity list. Laura and Alex spend the winters in Portland, OR and live in a small cedar cabin on the Oregon coast during the summer where Laura works in her yurt studio surrounded by huckleberries and firs. Her animated illustrations can be seen in her son's recent documentary, *2012, The End?* Her latest exhibit can be seen at FroelickGallery.com.

Dr. Peter J Littrup, M.D.

Professor of Radiology, Urology and Radiation Oncology Clinical Operations
Barbara Ann KARMANOS Cancer Institute

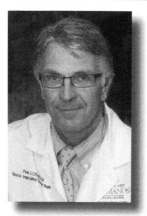

Dr. Peter Littrup's medical career has been dedicated to improved cancer diagnosis and image-guided treatments. His current areas of research include development of breast ultrasound tomography and its potential for non-invasive breast cancer treatments via drug delivery and focused ultrasound ablation. He's currently developing image-guided treatment programs focusing on cryotherapy, due to extensive experience with freezing treatments for nearly any anatomic location.

Beginning with prostate cancer, his cryotherapy work now extends to many organ sites and cancer types. One of the founders of American Cancer Society's National Prostate Cancer Detection Project, he is a leading authority on prostate cancer early detection using prostate specific allergan (PSA) and ultra-sound.

One of the early Radiology Society of North America Research Fellows, he was first to observe laser/microwave tissue ablation in the prostate by ultrasound and MRI. He translated this work with ablation imaging and cancer screening to come full circle with his current work in cryotherapy, breast ultrasound tomography and focused ultrasound. Littrup's CV includes over 60 publications, 4 patents and multiple research grants.

Littrup received his B.S. (1980) and MD (1985) from the University of Michigan and completed a Fellowship in Prostatic Ultrasound (1987) at St. Joseph Mercy Hospital, University of Michigan.

Alex Paul

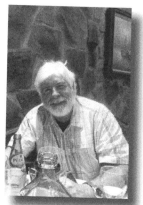

Alex received a Bachelor's and Master's Degree in Science from Oregon State University in Industrial Engineering. After graduating, Alex became a sales engineer for pollution control equipment, which led to Alex starting his own equipment sales business at an early age.

This was followed by a career as a real estate investor and developer, which culminated in the development of several retirement residences in Oregon. Alex and Laura still own and operate one facility, Beaverton Lodge Retirement Residence.

An early interest in poetry and writing blossomed into a writing career. His first novel, *Suicide Wall,* about Vietnam veterans and suicide, was published in 1996.

A middle-grade action-adventure novel series called *Arken Freeth and the Adventure of the Neanderthals* is now available on Amazon.com.

In addition, Alex acted as narrator, editor and ghostwriter for Dr. Littrup and co-author of this book, *They're Mine and I'm Keeping Them, or How Freezing my Breast Saved my Breast.*

Alex maintains websites for his writing work. SuicideWall.com provides a place for veterans and their families to record their experiences with veteran suicide while ArkenFreeth.com is about the Arken Freeth series.

Alex and Laura have been married since 1970 and have three children. Alex is an avid outdoorsman, fishing the ocean for salmon in the summer off the mouth of the Columbia River, surfing year round in Oregon and California, skiing the western states and Canada and hunting elk, deer and antelope in Oregon, New Mexico, Wyoming, Utah and Colorado.

Alex is also a musician, playing blues bass in the band, Skeleton Crew.